GUIDE TO PATIENT EVALUATION

History Taking,
Physical Examination,
and the Nursing Process

Fifth Edition

GUIDE TO PATIENT EVALUATION

History Taking, Physical Examination, and the Nursing Process

Jacques L. Sherman, Jr., M.D., F.A.C.P.
Consultant in Education, Veterans Administration Medical Center, Miami, Florida; Formerly, Professor of Medicine, Health Sciences Center School of Medicine, State University of New York at Stony Brook, Stony Brook, New York

Sylvia Kleiman Fields, R.N., Ed.D.
Formerly, Professor and Director, Baccalaureate Program and Projects, Nell Hodgson Woodruff School of Nursing, Emory University, Atlanta, Georgia; Formerly, Associate Professor of Nursing, Health Sciences Center School of Nursing, State University of New York at Stony Brook, Stony Brook, New York; Editorial Consultant, Medicine, Nursing, and Allied Health

Medical Examination Publishing Company

Medical Examination Publishing Company
A Division of Elsevier Science Publishing Co., Inc.
52 Vanderbilt Avenue, New York, New York 10017

© 1988 by Elsevier Science Publishing Co., Inc.

This book has been registered with the Copyright Clearance Center, Inc.
For further information, please contact the Copyright Clearance Center, Inc., Salem, Massachusetts.

Library of Congress Cataloging-in-Publication Data

Sherman, Jacques L.
    Guide to patient evaluation.

    Includes bibliographies and index.
    1. Physical diagnosis. 2. Medical history taking.
3. Nursing. I. Fields, Sylvia Kleiman. II. Title.
[DNLM: 1. Medical History Taking—nurses' instruction.
2. Medical Records—nurses' instruction. 3. Nursing
Assessment. 4. Physical Examination—nurses' instruction.
WY 150 S581g]
RT48.5.S53 1988   616.07'54   87-23978

ISBN 0-444-01158-7

Current printing (last digit):
10 9 8 7 6 5 4 3 2 1

Manufactured in the United States of America

To those we have learned from
and
To those who have learned from us

Contents

Foreword

In his foreword to the first edition of this book Dr. Edmund D. Pellegrino commented that, "Students in all health professions can easily share this knowledge [of assessment], which enhances the capacity of each to contribute to the assessment of the totality of the patient's needs." Very quickly the rationale for nurses to have sophisticated assessment skills and accurate data has changed from merely enabling a contribution to the patient's data base, to being necessary for clinical decision making: necessary for nursing diagnoses and interventions and necessary for the evaluation of a patient's progress in response to medical and nursing therapy for trauma and disease.

The shift in emphasis from data gathering as a new component of the nurse's role to decision making indicates the continuing evolution of the nurse's role in health care. As providers of health care, nurses use all the tools of scientific thought and application in their work. As we develop increasing skill and acumen in data gathering through history taking and physical examination, we appreciate the significance of nursing judgments in patient care. It has never been more true that nursing care improves the patient's chances of surviving a hospitalization and makes return to the home environment a positive option.

As complex as nursing care is, we must codify and document assessments, interventions, and rationales for interventions in a language that is commonly understood by collaborating nursing professionals. Communication of this nature documents the essentiality of nursing care.

I have observed the evolution of *Guide to Patient Evaluation* since its inception. When the book first was published it fulfilled the needs of many of our health science students here at Stony Brook; undoubtedly it will continue to meet the learning needs of nursing students and practitioners in the future because it has responded to the changes in health care delivery and the profession of nursing.

Lenora J. McClean, R.N., Ed.D.
Dean and Professor
Health Sciences Center
School of Nursing
State University of New York at Stony Brook
Stony Brook, New York

Foreword to the First Edition

Historians of twentieth-century medicine will easily be overwhelmed by the breakthrough and technological wonders wrought by the fruitful marriage in our era of medicine and experimental science. They may easily overlook some of our more human and equally difficult accomplishments in the organization and delivery of health care. One of these most surely is the emergence of the team concept and the sharing of clinical functions, formerly the sole province of the physician, by a variety of other health professionals.

To respond adequately to the social mandate to make health care available on an equitable basis for all, we must begin to make genuine progress toward the optimal use of all health manpower. In that endeavor, medicine and all the other health professions will undergo a redefinition of their roles and functions within new models of health care teams. The social utility of team care which will emerge may well come to rival our brightest technological triumphs.

If this is to happen, we must encourage the sharing of a common language among all who engage in clinical care of patients, enabling them to communicate with each other, as well as to exchange and share certain functions which the needs of patients may dictate. The ancient art and techniques of history taking and physical examination constitute the most basic common language. A first step in building an effective health team is fuller sharing of the responsibilities for collecting clinical data about the patient. Educators and practitioners now appreciate that future team members should be taught together if they are later to share some of their functions and to understand their own contributions more clearly. One of the most feasible and effective methods of interdisciplinary education is to teach the elements of pathophysiology and the detection of abnormal states by history and physical findings. Students in all the health professions can easily share this knowledge, which enhances the capacity of each to contribute to the assessment of the totality of the patient's needs.

Sherman and Fields' book is, therefore, a timely effort, consciously intended to introduce the essentials of history taking and physical examination to those who work most closely with the physician—physician's assistants and nurse practitioners. It is based on the authors' experiences in teaching this subject and in making use of its principles in an experimental model of team care in operation at the Northport Veterans Administration Hospital.

The book, as the authors point out, is not a replication of standard texts of physical diagnosis. The number of these abounds, and scarce justification can be found for producing yet another. Rather, the authors have aimed at a special category of new health professionals and their special requirements for these skills as members of a coordinated team. The same material will be valuable for the pharmacist, the dentist, and other health professionals as they too become less isolated from the mainstreams of medical and health care.

Sherman and Fields' manual will facilitate cooperation among health professionals by introducing nurses, physician's assistants, and others to the acquisition of a common set of terms, techniques, and criteria. The collection of clinical data about the patient by the time-tested method of history taking and physical examination will be improved thereby. This book meets an urgent present need and it will surely be followed by others.

Edmund D. Pellegrino, M.D., F.A.C.P.
Vice-President for Health Sciences
Director, Health Sciences Center, and
Professor of Medicine
Health Sciences Center
State University of New York at Stony Brook
Stony Brook, New York

September 20, 1973

Preface

Originally developed in 1974 for nurses and other mid-level health care practitioners focusing on primary care, this textbook was one of the first practical guides for teaching history and physical examination skills necessary for patient evaluation. Since that time the concept of health assessment as a signficant responsibility for all professional nurses has been adopted by practicing nurses and nursing education programs across this country and abroad. Therefore, each subsequent edition was revised and expanded in response to recommendations of clinicians and educators as new roles for professional nurses evolved and new learning needs were identified.

This text should assist beginning nurses as they prepare for the independent and interdependent professional functions of nursing, including health promotion, health counseling and health restoration for individuals of all ages, in hospitals, nursing homes, community health centers, and patients' homes. It will be of value to the many students preparing to participate collaboratively in health care delivery as nurse clinicians, nurse practitioners, midwives, and anesthetists, who have assumed responsibility for assessing and managing the health status of increasingly diverse populations in the United States and around the world.

During the intervening years since publication of the first edition of this text, major changes have taken place in our health care arena that affect nursing. New health problems have emerged, such as the devastating effects of the AIDS virus, the expanding and complex problems of homelessness, drug and alcohol abuse, and the explosion in teenage out-of-wedlock pregnancy. The new emphasis on wellness and focus on prevention, as well as development of new knowledge about risk factors, has reached the public, who have responded with alterations in life style. For example, a decrease in smoking among males, dietary restriction of cholesterol, and regular exercise regimens have led to decreases in death due to cardiovascular disease and perhaps cancer as well. New diagnostic technologies have been developed, such as echocardiography and magnetic resonance imaging. New therapeutics for cancer treatment; immunosuppressive drugs; and surgical interventions—including fetal surgery, coronary bypass, PTCA, heart and lung, liver, and soon brain transplantations—have prolonged the lives and quality of lives of our expanding and aging populations.

At the same time, major changes have taken place in our health care delivery system. (It has been said that more changes have taken place in the past 10 years than in the previous 50 years.) Some changes affecting professional nursing practice are economic in nature; others are humanistic. As new technologies have been developed, access to health care has been expanded, and wage and benefit packages negotiated by health personnel have been improved, the costs of health care have skyrocketed. In response, a variety of cost containment constraints, such as PSROs, DRGs, and utilization reviews, have been placed on traditionally independent medical practitioners and hospital administrators by third-party payers—the federal government and large insurance companies.

We must be aware that humanistic and ethical concerns have been raised by the new consumers of health care, who demand respectful treatment, education for health promotion and illness prevention, as well as the freedom to participate in therapeutic decision making. Therefore, quality assurance plays as urgent a role in health care facilities as cost consciousness; but what is most important is that all health care personnel, including nursing personnel, have to be accountable for the patient's continued care and/or hospital stay. *It becomes very clear that ongoing, systematic evaluations/assessments of the patient's needs and plan of care are necessary not only to clarify, verify, and justify the cost and quality of medical care, but to demonstrate the significance of professional nursing care as well.*

Although the goals for this fifth edition basically remain the same, there are some important changes from earlier versions. We continue to focus primarily on the skills necessary for the collection of data about the patient's health status (response to illness and therapy), but emphasize the application of this data to the development of nursing diagnoses and clinical decision making.

The text begins with a brief overview of both the nursing process (including the nursing diagnosis terminology developed since this text was last published) and the problem-oriented system. These serve as the framework for documentation and communication of the health assessment within the nursing care plan and/or patient progress record. We continue with discussions of the process of interviewing, methods of history taking, and general principles of the physical examination, which precede chapters describing specific examination techniques for each anatomic body system. We then provide information on nutritional assessment and laboratory procedures to complete the data base for the general screening examination.

To demonstrate adaptations of processes and techniques throughout the life cycle and during other stressful situations, we discuss assessment of the pregnant woman, the newborn, the infant and child, the adolescent, and the older adult. In addition, chapters on psychiatric/mental health assessment and the comatose patient are included.

Most of the chapters conclude with a sample write-up of normal findings as well as a list of potential nursing diagnoses. Many of these chapters also offer a patient problem situation with a brief model nursing care plan to demonstrate the clinical application of the assessment data. Complete write-ups of fictional patients are also provided in Appendixes III and IV; however, we do not want to imply that the actions included in the nursing care plans throughout the text or in the appendixes should be considered directions for practice.

We want to emphasize again that this is not a ''do-it-yourself'' textbook. It should be used in conjunction with a formal course taught by a clinical instructor or preceptor, audio visual and simulated models (when available), and laboratory practice. Students should first review standard textbooks of anatomy and physiology, since we offer only a few details immediately pertinent to the history and physical examination for reference. Although the major emphasis of the text is on history and physical examination skills and the description of normal findings, we also include a few descriptions and illustrations of abnormal findings to help the reader recognize deviations from normal. The student should be able to describe deviations so that a more experienced examiner can recognize them. It should be understood, however, that this is not information for simple memorization. Study and practice are needed. With clinical experience and further study of pathology the student will continually develop more skill in that regard and certainly make more confident judgments in assessment.

For this fifth edition we have continued following the suggestions of friends and colleagues who have assisted us over the years, and listened to the recommendations of new reviewers, students, practitioners, and educators. We appreciate all the interest, support, and encouragement we received; as a result, each chapter has been thoroughly reconsidered and often rewritten. Every effort has been made to include the most current topics of interest to clinicians in varied settings, such as the assessment of physical and sexual abuse of children and psychiatric and mental health assessment, including tools for assessment of anxiety and depression.

In earlier editions, we used the pronoun "he" to signify the patient and examiner, except in specific situations where examination was clearly only of the female patient. The use of the "he/she" pronoun form, or several others that were suggested, seemed much too awkward. Since this edition is primarily for nurses, most of whom are female, we considered changing the pronoun to "she." Sometimes, when it seemed natural we did; sometimes "he" seemed more appropriate. Most of the time we tried to eliminate any reference to gender by referring to the "examiner," "student," "reader," "practitioner," or "clinician."

The writing of this text represents a 15-year collaboration between two colleagues, with the assistance of many contributors from different disciplines. Now separated by geography and changes in professional interests, we needed the input of reviewers and associates more than ever. We want to thank all of our contributors (who we specifically acknowledge again later), especially Mildred Nagler, R.N., M.N., Field Representative, Joint Commission on Accreditation of Healthcare Organizations, and those contributors to earlier editions who we could not name because of space limitations. In addition, we want to give special thanks to Linda Weinerman, mother of Wendy in Chapter 25; Bernice Wissler and Mary Ellen D'Orazio in Philadelphia, professional associates and friends; and to Harriette Sherman and Frank Marzolf, our spouses, without whose support and encouragement on a day-to-day basis this writing would not have been possible.

Contributors

The authors are grateful to the many educators and clinicians representing several disciplines, whose advice and input have contributed to the development of *Guide to Patient Evaluation* from the introduction of the first edition in 1974 to this fifth edition. Although we would have liked to name each individual who participated in the "peer review" process for successive editions, we must limit this list to those who submitted significant contributions incorporated into the text for more than one edition or for this volume specifically.

Milton Agulnek, M.D., F.A.A.P.
Clinical Professor of Pediatrics
Health Sciences Center School of Medicine
State University of New York at Stony Brook
Stony Brook, New York

Carol T. Bush, R.N., Ph.D.
Professor of Nursing
Nell Hodgson Woodruff School of Nursing
Emory University
Atlanta, Georgia

Rose Cannon, R.N., M.N.
Assistant Professor of Nursing
Nell Hodgson Woodruff School of Nursing
Emory University
Atlanta, Georgia

Susan B. Dickey, R.N.C., M.S.N.
Assistant Professor
Temple University Department of Nursing
Doctoral Candidate, School of Nursing
University of Pennsylvania
Philadelphia, Pennsylvania

Janice B. Flynn, R.N., M.N.
Formerly, Assistant Professor of Nursing
Nell Hodgson Woodruff School of Nursing
Emory University
Atlanta, Georgia

Arthur H. Friedlander, D.D.S., F.A.C.O.M.S.
Associate Clinical Professor of Oral Surgery
Health Sciences Center School of Dental Medicine
State University of New York at Stony Brook
Stony Brook, New York

Steve L. Goldman, M.D., F.A.C.P.
Associate Professor of Clinical Medicine
Health Sciences Center School of Medicine
State University of New York at Stony Brook
Stony Brook, New York

Edward M. Gotlieb, M.D., F.A.A.P.
Director, Institute for Adolescent Studies
Stone Mountain, Georgia

Sandra Jaffe-Johnson, R.N., Ph.D.
Assistant Professor of Psychiatry-Mental Health
Health Sciences Center School of Nursing
State University of New York at Stony Brook
Stony Brook, New York

Elizabeth Mabry, R.N., Ed.D., C.G.N.P.
Professor of Nursing
Nell Hodgson Woodruff School of Nursing
Emory University
Atlanta, Georgia

Patricia Martinell, R.N., M.N., C.F.N.P.
Formerly, Assistant Professor of Nursing
Nell Hodgson Woodruff School of Nursing
Emory University
Atlanta, Georgia

Judith Metcalf, R.N., M.N.
Formerly, Clinical Specialist, Neurology and Neurosurgery
Thomas Jefferson University Hosptial
Philadelphia, Pennsylvania

Mildred Nagler, R.N., M.N.
Field Representative
Joint Commission on Accreditation of Healthcare Organizations
Chicago, Illinois

Rose Richmond, R.N., M.A.
Formerly, Assistant Professor
Health Sciences Center School of Nursing
State University of New York at Stony Brook
Stony Brook, New York

Rita Wieczorek, R.N., P.N.P., Ed.D.
Professor and Dean
College of Nursing
Health Science Center
State University of New York at Brooklyn
Brooklyn, New York

GUIDE TO PATIENT EVALUATION

History Taking,
Physical Examination,
and the Nursing Process

Part One

FRAMEWORK FOR DOCUMENTATION AND COMMUNICATION

chapter 1

The Nursing Process

Patients and Clients

Levels of Health Care

Phases of the Nursing Process

The Nursing Care Plan

Interrelationship between the Nursing Process and the Problem-Oriented System

This book is about health assessment within the role of professional nursing. While it does not include everything you need to know about nursing, it does provide most of what you will need to know about nursing assessment as the first phase of the nursing process.

Although we focus primarily upon the specific assessment skills necessary for patient evaluation — interviewing, observation, physical examination, and selected laboratory methods — it is important to understand the context in which they are used within the nursing process and the written records. To provide a patient information data base common with other health professionals, a medical model for history taking and physical examination is defined throughout the text. The nurse, however, has the opportunity to selectively adapt or enlarge upon this design to encompass the information necessary for development of a nursing care plan specific to each patient.

In this initial chapter we examine the nursing process and describe briefly the principles necessary for developing the nursing care plan, the problem solving recording method specifically developed for nursing. However, since nurses in many settings must also be adept at recording the results of their assessments on patient care records developed with the problem-oriented system, Chapter 2 focuses on that system. Succeeding chapters of this text are devoted specifically to learning the principles and methods of health assessment we are talking about: history taking and physical examination for all age groups and special populations.

At the ends of many chapters there are examples of how to "write-up" the data collected in the framework of both a nursing care plan and a problem-oriented record. Nurses in diverse clinical settings will find many recording methods incorporating modifications to the frameworks we present; however, we believe that while the structures may vary, the principles are for the most part consistent. It is also important to understand that there are many similarities between the nursing care plan and the problem-oriented system. Many of the concepts presented, therefore, will be alike.

PATIENTS AND CLIENTS

As nursing roles have expanded and practice extended from the hospital to the community and home, the relationship between the professional nurse and the consumer of nursing (individual, family, and/or community) has become more like a contractual agreement. As a result, especially in primary care, the term "client" has entered the health care professional's vocabulary to replace the more dependent sounding term "patient." Taber's Medical Dictionary defines "client" as the "patient" of the health care professional. However, we believe the term "patient" is more universally used by professionals and consumers alike. To avoid the use of the double term "patient/client" throughout this book, we have chosen to retain the term "patient" in most chapters.

LEVELS OF HEALTH CARE

Whether as generalists or specialists, nurses are involved in all levels of health care, and patient evaluation

skills are required in varying degrees for all levels. Levels
of health care[1] include:

Primary Care — (in clinics or community settings) providing
   independent nursing interventions such as preventative
   care, health counseling, and management of selected
   common health problems, often within medical protocols.

Secondary Care — (in homes, hospitals, and long-term care
   institutions such as hospices and nursing centers) providing
   general and specific independent and interdependent
   (medically delegated or prescribed) intervention.

Tertiary Care — (in hospitals and rehabilitation centers) providing all of the above and requiring sophisticated technology or highly specialized skills.

PHASES OF THE NURSING PROCESS

   In every situation, the nursing process incorporates four
main phases — *Assessment, Planning, Implementation,* and
Evaluation — beginning and ending with the collection of information about the patient's health status. These phases
are fluid and overlapping, providing a feedback loop demonstrated in Figure 1.1. The determination of what information
or data to collect and what diagnostic judgments to make is
based upon the level of care and the clinician's goals and responsibilities during each unique nursing situation. A concep-
tual framework (or theoretical approach) for the nursing
process will provide a structure as well. This generalized
way of looking at the world should be within the accepted
procedures and guidelines of the educational institution or
employing agency.

Assessment

   The first phase of the nursing process focuses on assessment, the collection and analysis of information (data) to

[1]Levels of care patients require, not levels of prevention,
   which refer to the Intervention Model.

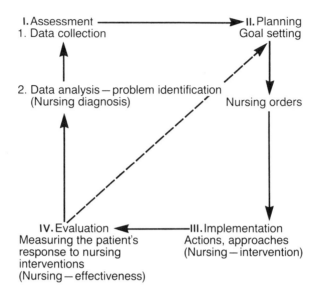

Figure 1.1 The nursing process.

identify problems and make a diagnosis. It is important, however, to distinguish between *health assessment* and *nursing
assessment.* They may or may not fulfill the same goals, although nurses may be involved in both processes. Health assessment and nursing assessment are orderly and systematic
processes for the collection and analysis of data describing
an individual's physical, psychologic, spiritual, and social functioning. Data for health assessment may be contributed by
a *nurse, physician, social worker, student,* or other *member
of the health care team,* while data for nursing assessment
are collected for the most part by *nurses.* Data for health
assessment are usually collected to determine a *medical diagnosis* while data for nursing assessment are collected to make
a *nursing diagnosis.* For example, a nurse practitioner in a
primary care setting while conducting a health assessment for
a patient seeking a pre-employment physical may take a
health history and perform a complete physical examination
to determine his health status. She will probably record findings using the medical model on the appropriate employment
form indicating that the patient is well enough to perform the

necessary job functions. Meanwhile, a nurse admitting a patient to a medical unit in the hospital may conduct only a partial physical examination herself, but may utilize information gathered by the emergency room physician or nurse to determine the nursing care plan.

Health Assessment

The *initial health assessment* including health history (subjective data), physical examination, and basic laboratory data (objective data) may be conducted by a house officer, medical or nursing student, professional nurse, or attending physician, depending upon the presenting events and the organization of the specific health care system (e.g., emergency, preventive care, chronic illness follow-up).

Continuing health assessment, including observation and recording of events and patient responses, may be the responsibility of one or more members of the health care team, e.g., nurse, physician, etc. Recording of these data may be in the form of problem-oriented records (discussed in Chapter 2) or in other similar styles and formats.

The guidelines for collecting health assessment data according to the medical model are described in much detail later in this text. In most situations the health history includes information gathered through interview with the patient and/or the family, or through review of past records related to the following areas.

Health History. (This information is considered *subjective data.*)

Chief complaint (CC) (or reason for contact)

History of present illness (HPI) or patient's perception of
    current health status if there is no illness present

Past health history (PH)

Family health history (FH)

Personal/sociocultural history (PSH)

Review of systems (ROS)

Patient profile, including self-concept, role relationships,
    coping patterns, lifestyle, and summary of risk factors
    identified (e.g., genetic diseases, alcohol or drug abuse,
    cigarette smoking, divorce, loss of mate)

The physical examination includes information collected through observation, specific inspection, palpation, percussion, auscultation, and measurement. All of these techniques may be considered during a general screening examination, but body systems will be selectively examined based upon (1) the nature of the presenting complaints, (2) the acuteness of the event, (3) known risk factors, (4) the patient's general health status, and (5) the goals of the examiner.

Physical Examination. (This information is considered *objective data.*)

General survey — mental status — vital signs

Skin, hair, and nails

Head, face, and neck

Eyes, ears, nose, and throat

Chest (heart, lungs, and breast)

Abdomen

Back and extremities

Neurologic

Male and female genitals

Selected Laboratory Studies. (Also considered *objective data* and may include one or more of the following.)

Complete blood count (CBC)

Urinalysis

Chest x-ray

Electrocardiograph (ECG)

and many others, depending upon presenting signs and symptoms, risk factors identified from history and physical exam, and diagnostic questions.

Nursing Assessment

Nursing assessment does not use the biomedical systems model described above as a framework for data collection, but may use one of several nursing frameworks developed in

Table 1.1 Functional Health Patterns[a]

Health-Perception/Health-Management
Nutrition-Metabolic
Elimination
Activity-Exercise
Cognitive-Perceptual
Sleep-Rest
Cognitive-Perceptual
Self-Perception/Self-Concept
Role-Relationship
Sexuality-Reproductive
Coping-Stress-Tolerance
Value-Belief

[a]This integrated approach to health patterns developed by M. Gordon and colleagues presents areas of assessment nurses are familiar with and which are applicable to all patients.

recent years. One model that has gained many followers is the *functional health patterns model* described in Table 1.1. Much of the data is consistent with health assessment information listed previously; however, as mentioned earlier, the nurse is primarily interested in developing nursing diagnosis, and not medical diagnosis. The nurse focuses on the patient in relation to the personal, interpersonal, and social impact of illness, disability, and hospitalization, as well as the physical effects (see Table 2.1). An example of a nursing assessment recording form is also provided in Appendix III.

The *nursing history* emphasizes the patient and his responses to illness, not the dysfunction or disease process itself. It includes psychosocial information related to the patient's understanding of his illness, coping methods, family support systems, self-awareness, etc., and patterns of living such as sleeping, eating, exercise and activities, elimination,

alcohol and drug use, smoking, hobbies, sensory/communication, risk factors, or potential problems.
Physical examination by nurses upon initial contact may or may not be as complete as in a traditional health assessment. It may be limited to a general survey, vital signs, and selected body systems related to the functional health patterns in Table 1.1. There are many factors influencing the extent of nursing assessment including the setting, the level of care described earlier (primary, secondary, or tertiary), and the specific goals for care. As a result, each nursing assessment situation is unique and the development of each nursing care plan individualized.

Nursing Diagnosis [2]

The American Nurses Association defines *nursing* as the "diagnosis and treatment of human responses to actual and potential health problems" and this definition has been incorporated into the ANA's *Standards of Nursing Practice*. Specifically, nursing diagnosis is a concise statement of a patient problem or potential problem that can be helped by nursing intervention. Nursing diagnosis expands upon the concept of problem identification to view the patient's problems from the patient's perspective. The diagnostic statement is not a symptom of disease or a pathological syndrome, but an acknowledgment of the patient's response to his condition or situation that is actually or potentially unhealthful. It is a change, dysfunction, impairment, deficit, or disturbance in the patient behavior or health status. Some examples of nursing diagnosis include:

noncompliance with drug therapy

sleep pattern disturbance

self-care deficit

fluid volume deficit, potential

The nursing diagnosis has two parts: first, a statement of the patient's unhealthful response (the problem), e.g., alteration in comfort (pain), and then the probable cause of the problem, e.g., due to distention. (It is important to remember that the nurse should not make assumptions regarding the probable

[2]NANDA 7th Conference incorporated the use of defining characteristics, e.g., risk factors, related factors, and major and minor indicators.

cause of the unhealthful response. There are legal ramifications related to the recording of a medical diagnosis as the cause of a problem.) Other examples include *alterations in sleep-rest patterns due to cough* and *alterations in self-concept due to unemployment.* Based upon previously learned scientific knowledge, nursing theory, past experience, judgment, and consultation, the nurse interprets the information collected to identify problems and formulate a nursing diagnosis. This is a dynamic analysis subject to review and revision. Continuing communication with the patient and family, as well as continuing observation and assessment, will be necessary to determine and validate actual or potential problems and to establish priorities as patient goals are formulated and nursing actions designed.

The reader is referred to several excellent references at the end of this text for a more detailed description of how to formulate the nursing diagnosis, and we have included the current (1987) listing of diagnoses accepted by the National Conference Group on the classification of nursing diagnoses in Appendix II.

Planning

Once the data are collected and analyzed, problems identified, and the nursing diagnosis stated, the plan for nursing and/or health care management is developed. Before the plan can be outlined, however, the nurse must determine goals and objectives for the plan. Practical goals must be clearly identified (in behavioral terms), and actions by nursing to assist the patient to meet those goals designed. Together with the patient and his family, realistic expectations should be established. These give impetus to the patient and his family to work with the nursing team toward the goals set. Nursing actions should be outlined for all health care team members so there is consistency in approach to the patient and the patient's movement toward these objectives promoted by all who communicate with him. These are *nursing orders,* and they represent the nurse's unique role in patient care. Nursing orders refer to *independent* nursing actions, such as health counseling and teaching for self care, to physical care to meet daily living needs the patient cannot do for himself, and to *interdependent* nursing actions (physician prescribed actions such as dressings and administration of medications). What is most important to remember is that all nursing orders must be individually determined to meet the specific needs of each patient as a unique person.

Implementation

The implementation phase incorporates the actual carrying out of the nursing orders designed to help alleviate a patient's problem or to prevent a potential problem that has been identified. For example, if the nursing diagnosis is *fluid volume deficit . . . due to elevated temperature and diaphoresis,* the nursing order could be *Encourage clear fluids as preferred to 200 ml every two hours. Assess and document intake and output.* These orders should be written in the nursing care plan of the patient's record and on the Kardex (or other nursing service format), and all team members alerted to the need to fulfill this order. The patient and his family, who are of course involved as well in the planning for actions, must first be advised of the need to carry out this order to alleviate the problem. Their participation, or at least cooperation, may make the difference between successful or unsuccessful accomplishment of goals.

Evaluation

Throughout the nurse-patient interaction, the nurse is concerned with the patient's response to his condition or situation as well as his response to therapy initiated, so continuous monitoring and assessment is an inherent responsibility. As new data are collected and analyzed, new problems may emerge, strategies designed may be considered unsuccessful, and new problem solving plans deemed necessary. The *evaluation phase* therefore overlaps the *implementation phase* quite clearly. However it is inversely related to the *planning phase*, since it focuses on the goals established for the patient in conjunction with the actual or potential problems identified. Evaluation is a way of assessing the patient's progress toward the goals, and the way of measuring the effectiveness of the nursing interventions, although not directly.

Evaluation therefore focuses on the patient's progress toward goals, specifically physical, emotional, or attitudinal responses, as well as his capacity for self-care.

THE NURSING CARE PLAN

Development of a nursing care plan based upon the scientific problem solving method described above is the nurse's responsibility for every patient care situation, regardless of the setting (see Figure 1.2). In fact, the Joint Commission on Accreditation of Hospitals requires a written nursing plan for each patient. Third party reimbursement is dependent upon documentation of nursing care plans, actions, and evaluation of a patient's response to treatment. In any event, this "blueprint" for nursing care should be based upon nursing process derived through systematic assessment of the patient's actual or potential health problems and it should always be written.
All nursing care plans should include the following:

1. Assessment of subjective data (health history) and objective data (physical findings and laboratory reports)
2. Nursing diagnosis (actual or potential problems, needs, and limitations)
3. Statement of patient goals (objectives in relation to each problem)
4. Nursing orders (actions or interventions), such as continuing assessments needed, teaching, physical care, and interdependent functions consistent with the medical regime (medical therapy) designed to assist the patient to reach stated goals. Documentation of the reason or the scientific rationale for decision making may be necessary.
5. Evaluation in the form of ongoing records of patient responses to nursing intervention and medical therapy.

The care plan must be flexible, reviewed regularly, and updated and modified as necessary if it is to be practical and useful. All members of the health team, including the patient (when feasible) and/or the family, should participate in developing and carrying out the plan.

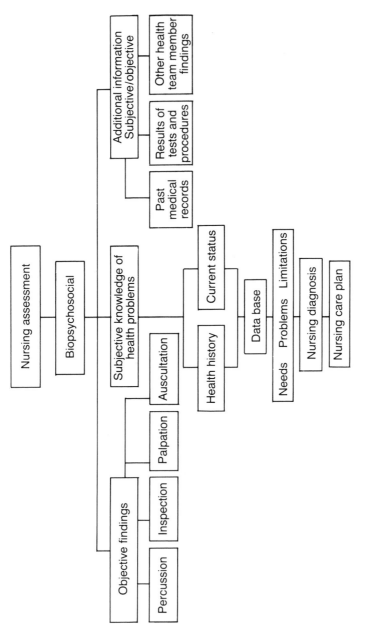

Figure 1.2 Development of the nursing care plan. From *Nursing Management* 13(4):20, reproduced by permission.

INTERRELATIONSHIP BETWEEN THE NURSING PROCESS AND THE PROBLEM-ORIENTED SYSTEM

In this chapter we have reviewed the nursing process and its written record, the nursing care plan, to indicate to the reader the importance of patient evaluation skills in the nursing process. In Chapter 2 we present background material on the problem-oriented system, since many nurses will find themselves using this system or some modification of it within their practice. In many settings the recording method used is an integration of both of these systems. You can see the similarities readily in Table 2.1. What is very clear is that in both systems the practitioner needs skills of assessment or patient evaluation to establish a data base for problem identification and/or diagnosis, planning, implementation, and evaluation.

chapter 2

Problem Orientation

The Problem-Oriented System

The Method

The concept and method for implementation of problem-oriented medical records (POMR)[1] were developed several years ago by Dr. Lawrence Weed to bring a logical system into the recording of information, opinions, and plans related to a patient's problems. The organization of the POMR is based upon the scientific method and is designed for problem solving and for preserving the logic used in arriving at solutions. Its primary purpose is to provide a method for communication among all professionals responsible for providing health care. The recording method serves to establish the initial history and physical and to maintain the integrity of initial plans. It provides a method for evaluation of patient care management and of educational programs as well.

THE PROBLEM-ORIENTED SYSTEM

This brief outline of the POS serves as only an introduction to the concept. Nonetheless, students may gain an idea of the way in which such a system may help to organize their

---

[1]Often referred to as problem-oriented record (POR) or problem-oriented system (POS).

thinking in the process of patient evaluation. The system has undergone modification since Weed first introduced the concept, and various agencies and institutions have adapted the system to their individualized needs. Major advantages of the POS are its flexibility and adaptability.

The problem-oriented system is a tool to aid in the management of the patient's problems — not nursing or medical problems — and it organizes these problems for assessment, management, and evaluation. All of this also leads to another advantage of the system — it is ideal for teaching. Schools of medicine, nursing, and allied health professions have readily identified these additional benefits and encourage implementation of this system in locations where students are having clinical learning experiences together.

The concept of the POS is simple, data must be presented in a form that makes sense for problem solving. The POS identifies the patient's important problems and provides a uniform system of recording so that anyone who deals with the patient can use the record. It should reflect the plans for management of the whole patient and his/her problems: holistic patient care.

No diagnostic or therapeutic regimen is sufficient unless it is complete and properly executed. No method of communication is of value if the information is inaccurate, incomplete, or illegible. A problem-oriented record openly displays thoroughness or sloppiness in record keeping or in patient care. It can help in management of a single problem or of the whole patient, but it cannot perform this management.

THE METHOD

The system includes four basic components for a POMR.

1. Data base: The record of the patient's physical and psychosocial history, physical examination, and laboratory reports.
2. Problem list: Delineation of the assessment of the patient's identified and potential problems which require a separate plan for management.
3. Plans: Written goals (measurable, behavioral) for each major identified problem (including preventive goals

relative to potential problems), further studies or observation, interventions, treatments, and patient education
for self-care.
4. Action phase: The records of implementation of plans
and of the patient's progress toward the planned goals.
These include orders (diagnostic and therapeutic), consultations, records of additional information from history,
or further physical examination, and records of the
monitoring of the patient's responses to treatment and
interventions.

All of these actions generate new data which modify
the database and lead to continued reevaluation of the problem list.

These components are represented in the flow diagram
that reflects the "closed loop" nature of the system (Figure
2.1).

The Data Base

This information is collected and recorded in standard
format for the health history, the physical examination, and
laboratory results. (See Appendix II). The data base also
contains important data from previous medical records.

In this system the data base is well defined so that
every practitioner, whether nurse or physician, will gather
the same basic information. A complete data base should
contain the same information required for health assessment
in Chapter 1:

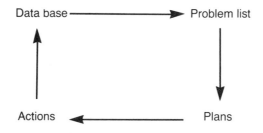

Figure 2.1

1. The chief complaint or reason for contact
2. History of present illness(es) or patient's perception of current health status if there is no illness present
3. Past health history
4. Family health history
5. Personal/sociocultural history
6. A logically arranged review of systems, including functional health patterns
7. Patient profile, including self-concept, role relationship, coping patterns, lifestyle, and summary of risk factors
8. Complete physical examination
9. Results of initial laboratory tests

Each of these elements of the data base will be described in the chapters to follow.

The initial collection of the data base should be as thorough as the patient's comfort and physical condition will allow. Uniformity and thoroughness of the data base will enable easier assessment of the patient's problems and need for education as well as individualization of the plan of care.

The Problem List

No better description can be given to the problem list than Dr. Weed's: it is a "table of contents" and an "index" to the patient's problems. The precision and skill with which the patient will be managed may often depend upon the precision and skill with which the patient's problems are defined.

A problem is defined as any *significant* deviation that has influenced, is now influencing, or may influence the patient's state of health or ability to function normally. It may be of medical, psychiatric, or social significance. This definition is not very precise, and titles will not always be the same in the hands of different clinicians, but that minor deficiency is not comparable to the benefits to be derived from such an index.

Note that problems are not necessarily diagnoses. In fact, the initial entry on a problem list is quite often a sign, a symptom, or a syndrome, but is *not* a diagnostic possibility or "rule out." The problem entered is the most specific possible at the time — one defines the problem in terms of exactly what one knows about it — *no more and no less.* The following list illustrates various classes of problems.

1. A proven diagnosis, e.g., pulmonary emphysema
2. A physiologic entity, e.g., congestive heart failure
3. A syndrome, e.g., hyperventilation (rapid breathing)
4. A sign, e.g., hepatomegaly (enlarged liver)
5. A symptom, e.g., chest pain
6. An abnormal lab value, e.g., elevated alkaline phosphatase
7. An allergy, including drug sensitivities (this should *always* be an active problem), e.g., anaphylaxis to penicillin
8. An operation, e.g., subtotal gastrectomy
9. A risk factor, e.g., two-packs-per-day smoker
10. A psychologic problem, e.g., depression
11. A social problem, e.g., unemployment
12. Functional health pattern problem, e.g., insomnia (due to anxiety)

The problem list will contain two types of problems: active and inactive (or, resolved). An *active* problem is any major or significant problem that is *presently* affecting the patient, e.g., diabetes, schizophrenia, blindness, unemployment, rectal bleeding. An *inactive* (or resolved) problem is any past problem of major significance that is *not* presently affecting the patient, e.g., an appendectomy, history of pneumonia, a fracture that healed without sequelae. The words *major* and *significant* are critical, for if every hangnail, childhood disease, and upper respiratory infection are recorded, the problem list could become pages long and thereby lose its effectiveness.

The physician or nurse enters problems at his level of understanding. For example, patient Z gives a history of myocardial infarction in 1986 and angina since 1987. Practitioner A may list two separate problems: (1) myocardial infarction, 1986; (2) angina pectoris, 1987. Practitioner B may list one problem: (1) arteriosclerotic heart disease, 1986. Both are correct; the latter merely indicates an understanding that the infarction and the angina are part of the same disease entity. However simple or complex, the problem list must contain only factual data, not speculations.

Since both the patient and his health status are subject to change, the problem list must also be dynamic and expected to change as well. As more information is gathered, some of the problems listed initially may turn out to be parts of a single problem, and the problem list will reflect this modification. Changes indicate that thinking is going on, not necessarily that the clinician has made errors. For example, when several problems turn out to be separate manifestations of a single problem, the problem list is modified. If problems such as arthritis or pericarditis are later recognized as being due to lupus, then the two entries are eliminated as separate problems, and a new problem, lupus is entered on the problem list.

When nurses use the POMR, nursing diagnoses would be entered on the problem list, e.g., "alterations in mobility due to hip joint pain." In this situation, the nursing problems do not change with the diagnosis, except to activate new problems relative to the patient's response to lupus as a diagnosis or disease entity.

As problems are clarified, altered, or further delineated, the original problem list is modified accordingly. This modification is not accomplished by erasure, but by insertion of the new statement. In the example that follows, this is illustrated in entries 1, 2, and 3, each of which has been changed from the original entry.

Although the techniques used for modifying the problem list vary from place to place, one principle is constant: keep the problem list up to date.

Minor episodes may arise in the course of a patient's illness that the practitioner may hesitate to define immediately as a significant problem on the problem list. This should be recorded in a *progress note* and entitled Temporary Problem. If it is subsequently decided that the problem is significant, it is then entered on the *problem list*. If not, a note on the progress sheet should indicate that it is a transient episode of little significance. An example might be a brief episode of "constipation probably due to inability to use the bedpan."

A hypothetical problem list that might appear on the face sheet of a hospital record will demonstrate its value as an index to the record (Table 2.1). Note that this interprofessional record is maintained for both physicians and nurses.

At a glance it can be seen that on 28 June the practitioner dealt with the initial health problems of cough, fever, hyperglycemia, and the psychosocial problem of retirement. Three days after admission, problems 1 and 2 were judged to be the single problem of pneumonia, which was then considered resolved eight days after admission. Problem 3 presented as the laboratory finding of hyperglycemia, and on the sixteenth hospital day was refined to the problem of diabetes mellitus.

Table 2.1 Problem List: Sample of Hospital Record Face Sheet

Problem	Approx. date of onset	Date problem recorded	Active problems	Inactive/ resolved problems	Date resolved
1	6/24/88	6/28/88 7/1/88	Cough Pneumonia		7/6/88
2	6/24/88	6/28/88 7/1/88	Fever Pneumonia		7/6/88
3	Unknown	6/28/88 7/14/88	Hyperglycemia Diabetes mellitus		
4		6/28/88		Subtotal gastrectomy	8/1963
5	Unknown	6/28/88	Alteration in self concept due to retirement		
6		6/28/88		Appendectomy	1938

Doe, John M
SS# 123-45-6789
D.O.B. 1/12/1920
Admitted 6/28/1988

University Hospital, HSC, Stony Brook, N.Y.

From this "table of contents" a reviewer cannot tell on what basis problems 1 and 2 were made into the single problem of pneumonia, or why it took three days to make that judgment, but she knows that a progress note entitled *Pneumonia* should have been written on 1 July that should explain the situation. That progress note should have all of the pertinent data, the practitioner's reasoning, and a plan for therapy and patient education on the problem of pneumonia. The reviewer should not need to look through the laboratory slips, x-ray slips, or nurses' notes to find the story. Similarly, the reviewer might want to know why the problem of hyperglycemia took over two weeks to resolve. She also would be interested in the impact of retirement or the subtotal gastrectomy on the patient's current status.

As mentioned in Chapter 1, variations in recording systems are commonly found. In some settings using the POMR, nurses may record nursing diagnoses on the problem list in the following way.

1. Alterations in oxygen exchange due to cough
2. Alterations in sleep-rest patterns due to fever
3. Alterations in nutritional patterns due to hyperglycemia
4. Alterations in health management pattern due to knowledge deficit regarding newly diagnosed diabetes mellitus

In the last situation, the nursing process may activate potential problems relative to a *standard of care* for a patient newly diagnosed for diabetes.

The Initial Plan

In a problem-oriented record, significant problems will be discussed in terms of a plan designed to resolve that problem. Before determination of the plan, a summary of pertinent data is noted and an assessment of the situation established, which should reflect the practitioner's thinking about the problem. The format that is used later for progress notes includes the number and problem title and follows the "SOAP" outline.

S. Subjective: Pertinent complaints, observations, and past history elicited from the patient, his family, or his previous records related to a specific problem.

O. Objective: Current physical findings and laboratory data
    collected by the practitioner.
A. Assessment: Analysis and synthesis of the data, interpre-
    tation and evaluation of the problem, the data, possible
    implications, and the prognosis. This is the place for
    opinions, guesses, and "rule-outs."
P. Plan: The Plan may be organized into three sections —
    diagnostic, therapeutic, patient education — *discharge
    planning* — in which the clinician will outline a program
    of further management.

JCAH standards require both nursing and medical staff
to write treatment goals. The plan may be further organized
according to the priorities of the problems. Under patient
education, a statement is made as to what the patient has
been told about the illness, possible course, and what should
be known and understood about necessary medications, therapy,
and self-care for benefit in the future. It may indicate collaboration with other health personnel or the patient's family.

It is important to note here that a plan is generally
formulated for each active problem on the problem list, with
the corresponding number of the problem on the list. If no
actions are considered necessary, this should be specified.

After an initial plan has been written, subsequent modifications of the plan are incorporated into the progress notes.

Action Phase

As stated earlier, these are records of the actions taken
for resolution of the patient's problems. In acute and chronic
care settings, clinical practitioners other than the MD/DO staff
may function under protocols. (If this . . . , do this . . .)
and follow the medical regimen. This includes interdependent
and independent actions.

Orders should be organized and titled. The first set of
orders should be entitled General and include such items as
medication for pain, position (e.g., ambulatory), and vital
signs. All other orders should appear under separate headings
corresponding to a problem on the problem list. This organization helps the practitioner to group orders related to one problem and assists other health personnel in their understanding
of the program for the patient.

The Progress Notes

Progress notes are always dated and include the number and problem title for each note, as well as information about the specific problem. The information then follows the SOAP outline. In every care setting, a nursing staff assessment should be performed regularly to review the whole patient and to identify progress towards the initial goals.

Properly titled and organized progress notes will enable any practitioner to read all data regarding a single problem by locating those numbered and titled entries, without having to search through information pertaining to other problems. Communications are thus simplified and are more clearly defined than the traditional entries in which several problems may be cited in a single paragraph.

All data, however, do not have to be recorded in narrative form. As part of the progress record, data essential to the patient's problems that require frequent monitoring may be recorded on a *flow sheet*. Flow sheets similar to the graphic chart used to record vital signs can be designed for individual situations, e.g., diabetes, postpartum, renal dialysis, and hypertension. Flow sheets have often been used to record routine daily activities, such as hygiene, activity, and diet. The flow sheet may include space for a variety of entries, such as medications administered, significant laboratory test results, vital signs, intake and output, all correlated and coordinated for the evaluation of treatment regimens for individual patients and their problems. If flow sheets are used for complicated problems, an entry under "objective" in the progress note may simply state, "see flow sheet." (See Chapter 29.)

There is a place in the progress note for general information, e.g., "constipation has been relieved" or "patient's morale is greatly improved" — items that may not relate to a major problem. Such entries are perfectly acceptable and should appear under the heading "General."

Individual institutions may elect to maintain separate consultation sheets; however, these notes should preferably be in the same format as for progress notes (SOAP).

Evaluation

The POS has been in use for several years in a variety of institutions. Many schools, clinics, offices, and hospitals have adapted the system to meet their own special interests or needs. Although it has proved to be an excellent teaching device, allowing for better auditing of the patient's record, tending to emphasize data rather than memory, and serving as a tool for communication among members of a health care delivery team, it has sometimes seemed unwieldly and cumbersome. Many institutions, therefore, use a combination of methods with nursing care plans and progress recording maintained separately on patients' records. The similarities in the methods, however, are clearly shown in Table 2.2. Sample problem-oriented progress notes are included to illustrate the method at the end of some chapters. Note that only items considered pertinent to the problem under discussion are included. This selection of data is a matter of judgment, subject to review, discussion, and differences of opinion, all of which are of use to the patient and to the teaching process.

Table 2.2 Interrelationship between Nursing Process and Problem–Oriented System

Nursing Process	Problem–Oriented System

I. Nursing Assessment
   1. Collecting the data
      Patient's history
      (subjective data)
      Physical examination
      (objective data)
      Laboratory results
      (objective data)
 	
   2. Nursing Diagnosis
      (analyzing the data)
      Statement of the patient's response
      to his condition or situation that
      is actually or potentially unhealth-
      ful, a deficit, dysfunction, impair-
      ment or disturbance in behavior or
      health status, amenable to change
      through nursing action
	I. Database
	      Patient's history
	      (subjective data)
	      Physical examination
	      (objective data)
	      Laboratory reports
	      (objective data)
	
	II. Problem List
	   A. List of the patient's identified problems
	      which require a separate plan for
	      management
	      1. A proven diagnosis
	      2. A physiologic entity; e.g., congestive
	         heart disease
	      3. A syndrome
	      4. A sign
	      5. A symptom
	      6. Abnormal lab value
	      7. Allergy
	      8. Operation
	      9. Risk factor
	     10. Psychologic problem
	     11. Social problem

II. Planning (patient/client goal setting)
Goals or objectives to be attained for each problem (mutually understood and accepted desirable outcome of nursing intervention.)
Design of orders, approaches, activities and actions based on diagnosis; i.e., teaching, physical care, and delegated medical therapy

III. Nursing Implementation
Planned nursing actions actually carried out

IV. Evaluation
Measurement of client's progress toward stated goals, physical condition, psychological state and knowledge of self-care, as well as nursing effectiveness (indirectly)

III. Plans
A written plan for each major problem identified, including the writer's own assessment of the factors involved and processes occurring, with goals established and recommended further studies, treatment and patient education
    Dx
    Rx
    Pt. Ed

IV. Actions
The records of implementation of plans and of the patient's progress; these include, orders (diagnostic and therapeutic) consultations, records of additional information from history, or further physical examination, and records of the monitoring of the patient's response to treatment

V. Evaluation
All of these actions generate new data which modify the data base and lead to continued reevaluation of the problem list, etc.

Part **Two**

ESTABLISHING THE DATA BASE: INTERVIEWING AND HISTORY TAKING

chapter 3

The Process of Interviewing

Dynamic Interviewing

Cultural Diversity and Interviewing

General Techniques

Aphorisms

The development of an accurate data base is essential for conducting a successful health assessment of an individual. It is from this base that one begins to identify specific problems, as well as the appropriate treatment plan. Much of the desired completeness and accuracy of the first portion of the data base — the health history — is dependent upon the examiner's ability to set up effective communication with the patient. The interview is the first step in this process.

Successful interviewing requires that several objectives be kept firmly in mind and that these objectives be reached as rapidly as possible. These are:

1. To establish a working relationship between the patient and the practitioner
2. To obtain accurate and precise information about the patient's physical and emotional state of health
3. To give the patient an understanding of his state of health with information for maintaining health and identifying deviation from normal through the period of treatment and follow-up

The patient interview comes first in evaluation because it is the most important tool in establishing the patient's problems and diagnoses. A careful health history can provide 70% or more of the data necessary to diagnose most commonly encountered health problems. A skillful interviewer will be able to obtain data that are both *accurate* (unaffected by bias or interpretation), and *precise* (sufficiently detailed to draw a clear, medically useful picture of the illness). The first step in this process is to understand that interviewing is dynamic and that all the information obtained must be filtered through the practitioner-patient interaction itself, as well as through the patient's underlying beliefs and expectations.

DYNAMIC INTERVIEWING

When people are faced with health problems, they experience a wide range of reactions. In addition to the impact of the diagnosis itself, these reactions are determined in part by age, sex, personality, and cultural, social, and economic circumstances. These facets of the patient's life need to be considered when conducting a health assessment, for understanding them provides the key to an accurate interpretation of both the verbal and nonverbal communications of the patient.

The patient who seeks professional health care frequently experiences fear and anxiety, because the impact of the health problem on his present and future is uncertain. Even if these fears or emotional responses are not founded in reality, it is still necessary for the examiner to know to what extent they exist in the mind of the patient. Even though it may differ from that of the clinician, the patient's perception of reality must always be respected.

It is essential that the clinician be attuned to the feelings of the patient from the earliest moments of contact, so that he may encourage the expression of these feelings and follow up with appropriate support throughout the period of health care. The health professional must have a strong grasp of the principles of human behavior and an appreciation of the psychosocial forces that affect the patient's life.

First and foremost, the practitioner must develop a sense of caring. Mary Donahue stated so beautifully, "Caring is the essence of nursing—caring for, caring with, and caring about."[1] Francis Peabody,[2] in his well known essay entitled *The Care of the Patient,* concludes: "One of the essential qualities of the clinician is interest in humanity, for the secret of the care of the patient is in caring for the patient."

The practitioner should demonstrate two basic qualities during the interview: respect for the patient and empathy. Respect is manifest in such actions as: (1) introducing oneself clearly, (2) not using the patient's first name during an initial interview, (3) arranging for the patient's comfort, (4) sitting at the patient's level where one can be easily seen and heard, and (5) encouraging the patient to ask questions.

Empathy means getting on the patient's own "wavelength." It means demonstrating that you have listened to and understand the entire content of his communication, both the words and the meaning. Empathy requires listening without bias, listening to the total communication and responding in a way that neither minimizes or exaggerates the person's expressed beliefs or feelings.

Through teachers and experience, the practitioner will develop certain verbal skills and techniques. In addition, however, the ability to respond to an individual with warmth, concern, and support must be cultivated. Occasionally, a patient is embarrassed or has difficulty in expressing certain thoughts or ideas. Quick recognition of this problem may enable the interviewer to assist the patient. Simple *verbal* acknowledgment of the patient's difficulty is frequently supportive and may develop or strengthen rapport.

CULTURAL DIVERSITY AND INTERVIEWING

To communicate effectively, the practitioner must learn as much as possible about the health beliefs and practices of diverse cultural groups. The patient must be seen as an individual within the framework of a cultural background that may have influenced attitudes toward sickness

[1]Donahue MP: *Nursing: The Finest Art.* St. Louis, CV Mosby, 1985, p 468.

[2]Peabody F: The care of the patient. *JAMA* 1927;88:877.

and health. Denigration of the patient or of his previous
treatment must be scrupulously avoided, for the patient will
be sensitive to bias and an important opportunity for good
communication may be lost. The essence of professionalism
is maintaining a nonjudgmental attitude when learning of
health care practices and beliefs that seem unusual and are
unfamiliar.

Folk medicine, often based on a holistic view of the
interaction of the mind, the spirit, and the body, may com-
bine religious or mystical beliefs and behaviors with the
use of herbs and plants as well as other techniques, such as
massage or special dietary additions. Within Latin communities in this country, for example, there may be found the
"yerbero," a specialist in herbs and spices, "curanderos" who
heal by rituals, herbs, massage, and ventriloquism, and
"espiritualists" who analyze dreams.

The inclusion of religion and philosophy in the health
practices of Asian culture is common. First generation
Asians may rely heavily on the use of herbs, foods, massage,
acupuncture, and special prayers, but more assimilated or
established residents generally accept the Western health
system.

The health care practices of American blacks, as in all
cultures, vary according to socioeconomic status, educational
level, and housing location, with middle- and upper-income
groups using the modern American fee for service health
care system more often than lower-income groups.

The African heritage focused on medicine men who
served as priest-physicians, using herbs and special rituals,
while family and community played important roles in the
healing process. The slaves brought to this country learned
to treat themselves when sick or relied on fellow slaves,
especially the elders who had learned survival medicinal
practices. Sometimes they included treatments observed
in white households or experienced in hospital wards as well
as methods shared with American Indians. Since modern
health care is often expensive or inaccessible for poor rural
and urban blacks, reliance on traditional folk medicine has
often been sustained. Survival takes priority over preventive
health care and, as a result, poor blacks often seek care at
a later than optimum time.

It follows, then, that specific interviewing techniques
must be adapted to conform to the patient's cultural pattern.

Remembering that questions about bowel habits or sexual activity may be offensive to those from Eastern cultures or that Latin women may be reluctant to share personal information with male examiners will add sensitivity to the clinician's interviewing skills.

Even when the patient appears to speak and understand English, language barriers may interfere with clear communication and understanding. It is sometimes helpful to have a family member or a co-worker familiar with the language and/or culture assist during the interview process.

One should not only expect people whose culture is different from one's own to have specific health beliefs that influence the transmittal of information or compliance with recommendations; everyone, in fact, has such beliefs that derive from their family experiences, what they have read, the opinions of their friends, and so forth. Many of these beliefs are fragmentary and contradictory: a person may be a strong believer in the "naturalness" of taking vitamins, while at the same time being a cigarette smoker, a very "unnatural" assault on the body. Particularly in cases of chronic illness, or illness that seems to be getting worse despite adequate medical therapy, it is important to inquire explicitly what the patient believes about the illness, what he thinks caused it, and what he thinks is required for it to get better.

A vast commonality of human needs runs through all cultures and it is a wise interviewer who remembers that people are more alike than different.

When interviewing older patients, special attention should be given to possible sensory impairments, levels of fatigue, and anxiety that may arise from cultural, generational, or personal concerns. Older adults are generally creditable historians when patience and understanding are provided during the interview.

GENERAL TECHNIQUES

Although each professional functions in accordance with his/her own unique characteristics and patterns of behavior, effective communication channels can be best established with the patient when certain principles and techniques are understood. These general guidelines must always be modified to suit the specific situation, but they do apply in most practitioner-patient relationships.

Privacy

The place selected for the initial interview and subsequent contacts should always assure the maximum possible privacy for the patient. Unnecessary interruptions or noise should be avoided and every effort expended to focus on the patient with his concerns.

Identification

The position of the interviewer in the health care delivery team should be made clear to the patient at the outset. The patient has initiated the interview by seeking help, and he is entitled to know with whom he is dealing. If the interviewer is a student, it is often useful to have him introduced by name to the patient by a more senior member of the team; but, in all cases, it is important to present the interviewer to the patient for what he is — student, nurse, physician's assistant, or physician.

Listening to the Patient

This sounds simple, obvious, and unnecessary to say, but is, in fact, none of these. Imagine for a moment the following exchange:

Interviewer: Now, Mr. Smith, tell me just what happens when you walk for several blocks during the cold weather. Do you get chest pains in that situation?
Patient: Yes.
Interviewer: Now, tell me about the type of chest pain that develops. Is it a sharp pain, or is it heavy, with some shortness of breath?
Patient: Er — would you repeat that, please?

Although the patient has 100% of the desired information, it is the interviewer who has been talking for 90% of

the time. This method of interviewing — direct questioning —
which requires a *yes* or *no* answer — is more useful *after* the
general story has been told by the patient.
An example of a more open-ended exchange might go
something like this:

Interviewer: Mr. Smith, you said that you've had some chest
pain. Please tell me all about it.
Patient: Well, I don't know just what to say. It hurts only
some of the time. (Pauses)
Interviewer: Some of the time?
Patient: Yes. After meals mostly, but I've noticed recently
that walking makes it feel bad, especially on cold days.
(Pauses)
Interviewer: It?
Patient: Oh, the pain. Well, it starts here (pointing to
substernal area) and it feels as if someone's sitting on
my chest. Doesn't last too long — perhaps only a minute
or two — but it hurts. Oh, yes. Last week when I was
having the pain, it also seemed to hurt here in the shoulder. Did I tell you that I've had this pain only for the
past few months? Never had it before. Is it serious?
Interviewer: I can't say yet. But are there any other things
you can tell me about the pain? Tell me more. Are
there any other symptoms you notice when you get the
pain?
Patient: Well sometimes my hand seems to tingle . . . .

(Continues)

Listening Without Bias

It is extremely important to listen to all of the patient's
history before coming to a judgment. Premature conclusions,
or "snap diagnoses," triggered by some aspect of the story,
may turn off the clinician's thoughtful perceptions of what
the patient is saying, or cause the examiner to cut off the
patient's flow of information. Dangerous *prejudgment* must
be forcefully and deliberately resisted.
Here is an example of a clinician who decided, too
quickly, that a 67-year-old woman complaining of shortness
of breath had congestive heart failure:

Patient: When I go to do anything I have trouble catching my
    breath and I have this . . .
Interviewer: (interrupting) How about at night. How many
    pillows do you sleep on?
Patient: I've always slept on two pillows.
Interviewer: Do you get short of breath through the night?
Patient: Well, not exactly short of breath . . .

This distressing series of closed-end questions to support the
clinician's diagnosis of congestive heart failure never uncovered the critical information that the patient had a productive cough and a 30 pack-year smoking history. She turned
out to have chronic obstructive pulmonary disease.

Listening to Everything

Listen to what the patient is saying, even though it does
not come in the order in which you want the information or
in which you will record it. The next chapters will outline
the preferred form for reporting a history. Make very brief
notes as the patient is talking, but make no attempt to fit
the patient's story into your format. Later, when you wish
to verify a point or a time relationship, clarification will be
given freely by the patient who is pleased that you have
listened. There are few things so frustrating and annoying
to the patient as having an examiner ask a question that
shows that he was not listening when the patient explained
that particular point.

Patient: . . . when my father died of cancer. Actually, that
    was around the same time this pain started.
Interviewer: (later in the interview) And are your parents
    still alive?

The interviewer who does not listen appears disinterested.
As much as possible, it is the interviewer's task to get
the patient talking and, as long as he is providing pertinent
information, to keep him talking. Listen carefully, for these
are the most important physical sounds you will ever hear—
the sound of the patient trying as best he can to tell you just
what is wrong with him. It is the patient's job to tell his story
and it is the clinician's job to listen.

Using open-ended dialogue allows the patient — not the clinician — to do most of the talking. The examiner's role is to keep the story going, to keep it from wandering too far afield, and to obtain necessary details. One can assist in keeping the story moving by short periods of silence or by use of cues or *facilitators* such as "Yes?" or "Tell me more," or repeating the patient's last words. Before turning off the patient's story in order to get in some of your own words, remember that you have *no* information and the patient has *all* the information regarding his problems, so listen carefully before deciding that no further useful information is forthcoming.

Consensual Validation

Each person uses familiar language to convey needs, describe complaints, and identify problems. As patients tell their stories to interviewers, mutual understanding of what is being said is very important. Under stressful circumstances, the interviewer may sometimes accept what is being said by · the patient but attribute meaning to an expression that the patient did not intend.

For example, if a patient says he is bothered by "diarrhea," the interviewer should make sure that what the patient means by diarrhea is what the interviewer thinks it means. An appropriate question might be "What do you mean by diarrhea?" While you might think that most people define diarrhea (as you do) as frequent watery bowel movements, the patient may reply, "Well, it's after breakfast only, I get this real strong urge to go to the bathroom and it's kind of loose."

As another example, if a patient says he is bothered by "arthritis," the interviewer should not record that the patient is bothered by arthritis until he knows precisely what the patient means by the word "arthritis." He may attribute the aching in his legs (actually from peripheral vascular disease) to arthritis, he may have been given a diagnosis of arthritis by someone else, or he may actually have stiffness and pain in certain joints.

So that the interviewer reports what the patient says and *only* what the patient says, it is helpful to summarize what the patient has said periodically during the interview and ask for the patient's agreement. For example: "Now as I understand it, you said you have had stiff and swollen joints in your legs and feet for eight days. Is that correct?" Then the patient has the opportunity to validate these data as being correct or in error.

Nonverbal Communication

The student must continually remind himself of the great importance of nonverbal forms of communication in the establishment of rapport and in transmitting information. Nonverbal cues are a part of our normal communication and will be used naturally by both the examiner and the patient; these cues are often unconscious and not subject to the same "censorship" as our words are. Discipline over the use of certain words and phrases is often readily learned by the interviewer, but failure to learn control over nonverbal situations or actions can effectively prevent the establishment of rapport or obtaining information. For example, dirty fingernails may "turn off" a patient within moments of the introduction, as may an inappropriate smile when the patient expresses fear of cancer over an insignificant skin blemish.

Proper understanding of nonverbal signs can be used positively to encourage the patient to continue a story, to assure him of your interest, to shift to another subject, to comfort him, and to relieve some of his anxieties. Watching the patient's use of nonverbal signs may assist in obtaining information, both at this point and later on during the physical examination. You are observing but you are also being observed.

The "Third Ear"

There is another aspect of receiving communications that is commonly referred to as listening with the third ear. This means that the interviewer pays close attention not only to the words per se, but also to the way in which they are expressed. Changes in the quality of the voice, such as its tone and loudness, may be clues to the importance of

[3]Reik T: *Listening with the Third Ear.* New York, Farrar, Strauss and Co, Inc, 1948.

what is being said. Facial expressions, body movements, hand positions, and nervous mannerisms are nonverbal signs that modify the words being spoken. In addition, the third ear listens to what is *not* said. Important omissions, vagueness, evasiveness, and sudden changes in the subject are all methods for avoiding expression of thoughts that are sensitive or disturbing to the patient.

For example, the patient who delays answering a usually straightforward question may be using the delay to censor material:

Interviewer: Have you ever been pregnant?
Patient: . . . No . . .

(Censored material: Patient had a first trimester therapeutic abortion.)

APHORISMS

There are a few other guidelines that are important in the health assessment interview process. These may be briefly stated.

1. *Never* express surprise or judgment at the patient's statements. You are a data collector and a health professional, not a judge.
2. Always express interest and concern for the patient's problems. The patient's problems are the basis for your profession.
3. Remember that there is no adequate way to measure pain other than the taking of a careful history that elicits specific descriptions from the patient.
4. Try to respect your patient for who he is. He will recognize your sincerity and become a more willing partner. Diagnosis and treatment will be made easier and more effective.
5. Do not believe everything you hear. Patients forget; they may deliberately suppress information (often because of fear), they may unconsciously repress information, and they may falsify because of embarrassment or perhaps for purposes of compensation or insurance payments.

6. Try to avoid too many "why" questions, for they are often challenges to the patient's competence. The question "Why did you stop taking medication?" can lead to confrontation and hostility, whereas more neutral and open-ended expressions such as "Tell me about your reasons for not using the medication" may maintain rapport and obtain information.
7. Do not express judgment about the previous course of treatment given the patient by other practitioners. It is a safe assumption that neither you nor the patient has adequate information to make such judgments hastily.
8. Be *certain* that words used by you and the patient mean the same things. *You* know that all tumors are not cancers — does the patient? Use medical jargon carefully to avoid misunderstanding and be sure that the patient understands your words and questions clearly, or his answers may be inaccurate.
9. Try to get the patient to be as quantitative as possible. "Once upon a time . . ." is a pleasant way to start a fairy tale but is inadequate for a medical history. "At 2:00 p.m. yesterday, about one-half hour after eating a large meal, Mr. X arose from the table and vomited about 2 qt of partly digested food mixed with bright red blood . . ." may not be a pleasant way to start a story, but is quantitative and informative. However, do not badger the patient into a quantitative history where none really exists. Some illnesses have a rather vague onset that does not lend itself to such a precise description.
10. Keep in mind the patient's reason for seeking professional help. If he came for treatment for a cold, do not forget this complaint as you get involved in the important but incidental finding of high blood pressure.
11. During the health assessment interview you also should be completing the first portion of the physical examination on the patient; observing general state of alertness, body build, skin tone, eye lesions, hair problems, muscle tics or tremors, and voice quality. This will be discussed further in Chapter 7.

Remember that you are the health professional, and therefore, the guide in this relationship between you and the patient. Together you can achieve the goals desired of the health assessment interview — the establishment of a good working relationship and accurate information regarding the patient's physical and emotional health.

There are several fine texts on interviewing, a few of which are suggested at the end of the book. Needless to say, it is impossible to learn interviewing skills by reading. It is most advantageous to practice, under observation, with fellow students. The video camera is an excellent tool for recording the interview and then for reviewing the effectiveness of the examiner's skills. Whenever possible, an experienced interviewer should be available to critique performance and offer advice.

chapter 4

The Health History: Part I

Chief Complaint

Present Illness

Past History

Types of Questions and Responses

A health history is the first element of the data base because it is the single most important element in establishing the patient's problems. A comprehensive history should give the examiner a picture of the person's current and past health problems and information about the individual as a whole in his environment.

The basic content of the health history should not vary if it is to be complete and comprehensive, but the format for recording the history differs somewhat from author to author. The format presented in this text is a medical model for a complete history to be ascertained during an initial patient contact to establish a data base; however, it can be used by all health professionals for all levels of care. During subsequent visits the examiner selectively elicits information related to current events and new problems.

Nurses in secondary and tertiary care may find it appropriate to determine only a "nursing history" if the initial examination has been conducted upon admission to the emergency room or unit by a house officer or attending physician. This health history will vary from setting to setting, but, as described in Chapter 1, usually focuses on the patient's perception of his health status, response to his illness, coping strategies, and ability to carry on activities of daily living. All of these elements will be explored in the comprehensive health history described here.

The health history consists of the following elements: chief complaint, present illness, past history, family history, personal/sociocultural history, review of systems, and patient profile. Each of these elements has a specific goal, or set of goals, that must be clear to the practitioner, so that when he has achieved his purpose with one element, he will know that it is time to shift and explore the next. Briefly stated, the objectives of each element are as follows:

Chief complaint (CC): to establish the major specific reason for the individual's seeking professional health attention *now*

Present illness (PI)): to obtain all details related to the chief complaint from the time the patient first became ill to the present

Past history (PH): to give the examiner a picture of the patient's previous illnesses and injuries

Family history (FH): to identify the presence of genetic traits or disease that have familial tendencies; to learn if the patient has had prolonged contact with a communicable disease in a family member; and to assess the patient's ability to cope with stress related to the disease or death in his family

Personal/sociocultural history (PSH): to develop an understanding of the patient as an individual, as a member of a family, and of a community

Review of systems (ROS): to bring to light any additional health problems or symptoms related to the PI or the PH that were not mentioned earlier

Patient profile (PP): to summarize in the examiner's mind the totality of the individual within the context of his medical, psychologic, spiritual, and socioeconomic background, with consideration for risk factors, self-care knowledge, and abilities for discharge planning

In actually taking a history, the practitioner should let the patient report any information in any order, as long as it seems pertinent to the complete history. Do not force the patient to conform strictly to this outline, but rather, keep him talking. However, the practitioner can, and should, *report* the history using the above format by rearranging the elements given to him by the patient.

While the interviewer may guide the patient to present the details of his history in a certain order, a fact pertinent to the present illness may turn up in the past history or review of systems. Facts should be rearranged later when writing up according to this or another outline.

CHIEF COMPLAINT

The chief complaint represents the specific reason for the patient's visit to the office or admission to the hospital. Since the CC may be thought of as the title, and the PI as the story of the patient's major problem, the two are often intermixed as the history is being evolved. It is important to determine, as much as is possible, the major problem facing the patient at the moment, and its duration. Often, there may be no problem or complaint. The individual may want a routine annual check-up or may require a preemployment examination. This is simply listed as the reason for contact. Sometimes the stated chief complaint is not the actual reason for the patient's visit. In these cases, a physical symptom might serve as a "ticket of admission," but the patient's real problems lie elsewhere and may be difficult for the patient to discuss. It is important for the practitioner to be sensitive to this phenomenon and "recheck" the chief complaint before the end of the visit. Later in the interview, after some rapport develops, the patient may be able to express his actual chief complaint.

The CC should be briefly recorded, using the patient's own words (in quotation marks) where possible. An attempt should be made to have the patient identify the major problem, even if there seem to be several closely related complaints. These other problems will be recorded elsewhere. It may not be possible for the patient or the examiner to isolate one chief complaint, in which case the CC may contain several entries.

The examiner should begin the history taking with an *open-ended,* neutral question or statement, as free as possible of confrontation, judgment, or misinterpretation. "How may I help you?"; "Tell me about what is bothering you"; "What problem led you to seek help?"; and "What is your trouble?" are relatively good ways to start. The question, "What is your sickness?" implies that the patient is, in fact, sick. "What brought you to the hospital?" may readily be answered by "The ambulance!" or "My wife!" and the interview could begin with an unnecessary humorous note or with some hostility, which may adversely affect the patient-practitioner relationship. There is no single question that is guaranteed to get the interview started without a possible negative reaction on the part of an already hostile patient, but the neutral questions suggested above are frequently successful.

The following are samples of desirable recordings because they are brief, specific, to the point, and serve as titles for the story (PI) to follow:

CC: "terrible chest pain," 2- to 3-hour duration

CC: "I think I've got a fungus," 2-days duration

CC: cough, fever, insomnia of 4-days duration

CC: coma, unknown duration

Reason for contact: routine annual examination

Be sure not to confuse *description* with *interpretation*. Medical shorthand can be useful, even essential, for clear communication once a diagnosis is established. However, at the level of initial patient evaluation, if the examiner interprets the finding, he or she introduces a bias that will reduce the accuracy of the data. If the chief complaint was of passing black stools, it should be recorded as such, not as gastrointestinal bleeding. Chest pain should be described with accuracy and precision; it should not be referred to as angina pectoris, atypical chest pain, heart attack, or any other such term until the diagnosis is established.

A chief complaint with multiple entries often confuses the examiner, the reviewer, and the consultant, as well as the patient. Thus CC: "high blood pressure, chest pain, numbness of fingers, palpitation, nausea, cough, and vomiting of several-days duration," presents a series of problems that may or may not be related. The examiner may be unable to focus in on just what bothered the patient most or what made

him concerned enough to seek help now. Were all these problems "of several-days duration," including the high blood
pressure?

Remember that the chief complaint refers to why the
patient sought help *now*. Patients may have suffered for a
long time from a variety of symptoms caused by two or more
chronic diseases. The patient may seek help for chronic
symptoms at a given point in time because the symptom itself has become more severe; because something else has
happened to make the patient more worried about the symptom (e.g., his sister died of cancer and she had abdominal
pain); or something entirely different is bothering the patient, but he is using the chronic symptom as a ticket of
admission.

PRESENT ILLNESS (PI)

A clear history of the present illness will be a narrative,
beginning with the earliest onset of the complaint and
describing its progression to the present. It is important to
obtain information about the reason for the patient's seeking
help *now*. In a history of arthritis, for example, it might
well be found that the acute attacks that began five years
ago recurred once four years ago, then twice in the next
year, and have become almost monthly in frequency in this
current year. Such a story, presented to the appropriate
consultant, would suggest the characteristic progression of
gouty arthritis.

How does a student learn which questions to ask without knowing, for example, that acute attacks of gouty arthritis generally become progressively more severe and occur
with increasing frequency? This comes by dissecting the
story into its critical parts:

The details of *onset*

The complete *interval history*

The *current status*

The reason for seeking advice *now*

An expert would achieve the results more quickly but he
must obtain the *same* critical bits of information as the

novice: onset, interval history, current condition, and reason for being in the office today.

Thus, a CC: "cough and fever 3-days duration" should prompt the examiner to find out why the patient came today, not 2 days ago or yesterday. Did the cough become worse? Did the fever become worse? Did the cough change? A CC of "arthritis of 5-years duration" must be explained, in the PI, in terms of how it began 5 years ago, what went on over the 5-year period, and what it is like now. The story should end with a statement of the reason for the patient's visit to see the examiner *today*. Many valuable diagnostic clues will be uncovered by obtaining the history of a complaint from its onset, through the interval period, and up to the present moment. Additionally, a fair amount of insight into the patient's personality and motivation may be uncovered by digging into details of the story. In the example cited of "CC: cough and fever 3-days duration," the clinician might uncover, as a reason for coming *today*, the fact that the patient's cough was no worse, but that he became afraid that he had tuberculosis or cancer.

It must be remembered that patients seek help because of changes in their *clinical* status; because of *behavioral* changes (increase in anxiety, loss of tolerance to pain); and because of *social* pressures (increased stress at home or at work). Any one or all of these may play a part in the patient's decision to seek help today.

There are some basic bits of information about various problems that are important to obtain and the student must develop a pattern of history taking that will elicit these vital facts. No one could, or should, memorize a series of routine questions but the student should learn what basic information must be obtained.

Knowledge of pathophysiology will enable the student to develop a background of knowledge of syndromes or clustering of symptoms characteristic of specific problems. For example, when the patient's chief complaint is "difficulty in urinating," it becomes important to branch from that complaint to the commonly found associated symptoms of blood in the urine, dribbling, burning, and incontinence

If there is no problem or chief complaint, as for the person who comes for a routine examination, Present Illness (PI) may be retitled Current Health Status, and will record the patient's perception of his state of health.

Recording Pain

One useful way of characterizing symptoms is to use a series of "Wh" questions that specify with precision the story of the symptoms or illness.

Where: Where exactly is it on your body?

What: What does the symptom feel like?

When: When does it occur? Is it episodic? Does it fluctuate? What is the frequency?

How: How is it altered by life circumstances? By sleep, by food, by exertion?

Why: Why does it occur? What provokes it? Why do you think you have it?

Who: Who is affected by it? Does it affect only you or does it interfere with your relationships with others?

An excellent example of a pattern to be followed is in dissecting the story of pain, an extremely common complaint. One convenient outline for the critical features of pain is:

1. Type
2. Location
3. Severity
4. Duration
5. Influencing factors
6. Associated symptoms

A report that incorporates each of these characteristics will be complete and informative. For example, here is such a history recorded in highly condensed form:

Crushing, heavy (type), substernal pain radiating to left shoulder and arm (location), which causes a patient to stop all activity (severity), occurring for past 3 months at about 7- to 10-day intervals, each attack being only 1-2 minutes in duration (duration). This often occurs about an hour after meals, especially while walking; brought on by severe job tension, cold weather, large meal, climbing two flights of steps; relieved by stopping activity (influencing

*factors); associated with sweating of few-minutes
duration and fear of impending death; does not recall if he is short of breath during attacks (associated
symptoms).*

This, of course, is the typical pain of angina pectoris
due to coronary heart disease.

Note that there are entries for each of the critical
features of pain. The type of information desired for each
of these features of pain will not vary no matter what pain
syndrome is being investigated. A few details regarding
each of these features may assist in obtaining all the necessary diagnostic information.

Type

The character of pain is of great importance and it is
useful to have the patient's description. Let him choose the
words as long as you understand just what the pain is like.
"Like a headache," is not adequate, since there are many
types of pain associated with headache; but "like being stab-
bed with an ice pick" is highly specific. In the PI recorded
above, the patient used the term heavy to describe his pain,
and this is clear enough for the clinician to distinguish the
type of pain from sharp, knifelike, throbbing, or sticking.
One caveat: certain pains are very difficult for patients to
describe; then it is best to ask the patient to describe it in
familiar terms such as "like a menstrual cramp, only worse."

Sometimes the patient is unable to describe the type
of pain in his or her own words. It is useful in these cases to
provide a *menu* or *laundry list* of options: "Would you
describe the pain as sharp, burning, dull, or constricting?"
When doing this, however, it is important *not* to ask the
question in a leading way so that the patient feels that you
expect a certain answer. An example of such a leading
question is, "The pain is sharp like a knife, rather than dull,
right?"

Location

Try to ascertain just where the pain is perceived. The
patient may need to be helped to locate pain by indicating
to him the importance of such localization. "Head pain" is
an inadequate description of pain located deep behind both

eyes, or in other locations such as over the left occiput, over the left eyebrow, at the top of the head, at the right mastoid process, at the angle of the jaw, or across both temples. Each of these is, indeed, head pain, but each is possibly due to a different disease process in a different structure. Often the patient may add nonverbal means of description by pointing with a fingertip, as with the epigastric pain of peptic ulcer disease, or by spreading an outstretched hand over an area. A clenched fist pressed against the midsternum may be used to describe both location and type of pain, as with angina pectoris.

Location should also be defined in terms of the patient's perception of whether the pain is superficial or deep, whether it is diffuse or localized, and whether or not it radiates to some other anatomic site. For example, radiation to the left shoulder and arm, or into the neck, is often associated with pain of coronary heart disease; radiation from the low back down the posterior thigh and calf frequently is found with sciatic nerve pain; radiation to the tip of the right scapula from the abdomen may help in identifying gallbladder disease.

Severity

This feature is generally best described by having the patient tell you how the pain affects his normal *activity.* Adjectives are used too frequently and too loosely. Thus, an attack of "terrible" pain during which the patient goes on with playing cards, walking, or other usual activities may not be regarded by the clinician as being truly severe, despite the patient's words. Pain, on the other hand, which causes the patient to stop in midstride, or halfway up a flight of stairs, to fall to the ground, to double up, or to lose consciousness, is clearly understood by the examiner. It is always preferable to record the effect of the pain on the patient's activities of daily living, than to quote adjectives. Any apparent discrepancy between how the patient describes his pain and its effect on his activities is very useful in understanding the patient's perception of his problem and coping style.

Duration

This feature should include the duration and timing of a single attack as well as the frequency of attacks, since the onset of the problem.

Influencing Factors

These include a wide range of factors that seem to the patient to *precipitate* the pain or to make it worse, or that partially or totally *relieve* the pain. Factors such as exercise, excitement, meals, medication, smoking, standing, bending over, cold or hot environment, fatigue, time of day, or season of the year, may all be pertinent in tracking down the possible cause of pain or its relief.

Associated Symptoms

This category will include symptoms in body regions not directly involved by the primary pain. Thus, in the example of angina pectoris given above, sweating and fear of impending death were considered to be *associated* with the chest pain. If the patient had noted nausea as an accompaniment of the angina, it would properly be included here.

The student must memorize these six critical features of pain. With these guideposts and experience an accurate history can be obtained that will often enable a reviewer to make a diagnosis, suspect a particular disorder, or, at the least, to focus attention on a specific organ system. This outline, designed for eliciting a history of pain, sometimes cannot be followed exactly for other symptoms, but should give the examiner a general pattern of questioning to follow. Complaints such as blurring of vision, chronic cough, constipation, palpitations, nausea, or fever will require somewhat different guideposts, but questions about *type* (or character) of the symptoms, *severity, duration, influencing factors,* and *associated symptoms* are all as pertinent for these symptoms as they are for pain.

PAST HISTORY (PH)

Having obtained enough information about the CC and the PI, the examiner then directs the interview toward other medical and surgical problems. This is ordinarily an easy shift to make. A convenient organization of this element of the history is *medical, surgical, injuries, allergies, immunizations,* and *current medications.* As before, in obtaining a CC and PI, the patient is encouraged to "tell me about all other illnesses and operations you have had." This is an open-ended invitation for the patient to detail what *he* thinks important. If later in the interview other important facts turn up, the examiner may have obtained information about the patient's memory, or perhaps about his reluctance or fears in revealing information earlier. If such a delay occurs, the examiner should use this situation to reinforce the rapport and confidence developing between practitioner and patient, but must never confront or chastise the patient over such a lapse, no matter what the reason.

Entries here are previously established *diagnoses* with dates of occurrence, severity, and complications, if any. Try to establish the fact that the diagnosis reported by the patient was provided by a nurse or physician and not simply assumed to be a diagnosis by the patient. Thus, with a report of "a heart attack in 1972," the examiner should inquire as to how the diagnosis was established, the length of hospital-ization and convalescence, and the name of the primary care provider of record. A reply such as, "Oh, I had some chest pain and I thought that it might have been a heart attack," is improperly classified as indicating a true coronary occlu-sion. Such a story should be entered in the review of systems where *symptoms* are recorded.

By such evaluations the examiner makes the PH a list-ing of *known* and *established* medical facts. Relationships between these facts and the PI may or may not exist, but until they are clearly recorded, it is impossible to evaluate such relationships adequately. Since the entries are estab-lished diagnoses, questioning can be brief, and need not go into much detail beyond confirming the fact that the patient is reporting the diagnosis accurately. Use quotation marks to indicate that you are recording a diagnosis as reported by the patient, but not confirmed, for example, by review of old records.

Translation into brief medical terminology is desirable here, so that if the patient describes pain in the right lower quadrant, vomiting, and removal of an inflamed appendix three years ago, the entry may simply be: "appendectomy — 1984."

Medical

Included here are *diagnosed* and medically *important* illnesses. Remember that symptoms and complaints that are undiagnosed belong in the section on review of systems. Historical data relevant to the current problem should be recorded as part of the history of the present illness. If the patient was hospitalized for heart failure ten years ago, and has continued to have episodic cardiac decompensation since then, this information is actually part of the story of the current illness.

Entries should be as brief as possible, e.g., "pneumonia, right — 1986"; "cholecystitis — 1987, no attacks since, no stones." Some illnesses may require more details to give an adequate picture, e.g., "hypertension discovered in 1979 on routine checkup; BP said to be moderate requiring no treatment; more severe by 1981 when medication (type unknown) was begun; patient discontinued Rx in 1982 and has taken none since."

Listing of usual infectious childhood diseases such as measles, mumps, or chicken pox may be of importance in the evaluation of an adolescent patient or pregnant woman (has she had rubella?), but is unlikely to shed much light on the overall medical status of an 80-year-old widower suffering from depression. Whether or not to inquire about and record such information remains a matter of judgment.

To assist the patient in recalling significant diseases, it is often useful to ask about any illnesses that confined the patient to bed for several weeks or that required hospitalization.

Surgical

This is primarily a listing of operations; examples are:

Appendectomy — 1960, Mountainside Hospital, NY

Partial hysterectomy — 1982, for prolonged bleeding due to fibroids; no malignancy reported; Westview Hospital, NJ

In more complicated situations, include as much information as is necessary to indicate exactly what the disorder was and the results, for example, "kidney stone passed 1979; second stone 1980 removed by surgery; third stone removed surgically late 1980 led to workup for parathyroid disease and parathyroidectomy in 1981; no stones since."

Injuries

The history of old or recent accidents may shed as much light on the patient's balance and stability as on the possible consequences of the injury. In obtaining the history of a fall, it is important to ascertain *why* the patient fell as well as learning what injuries occurred. Learning the reason for a fall may reveal the first clues to such diverse disorders as night blindness, epilepsy, stroke, vertigo, or syncope.

Obviously, a history of repeated falls or accidents must be carefully reviewed with the patient to find a reason, if possible, for his being accident-prone. Damage to the brain, heart, lungs, liver, spleen, kidneys, bladder, and other organs may follow blunt injury whether or not there were fractures, so the interviewer must not discard the story of such trauma simply because the patient is sure that "no bones were broken."

Allergies

The patient should be asked about commonly known allergic disorders such as hay fever or asthma and also about any unusual reactions to food, drugs, or contact agents such as fabrics. It is important to clarify what your patient means by the term "allergy" or "allergic." People may confuse the known side effects of a drug with an allergic response to it. Thus, a patient might say he is allergic to aspirin, but further inquiry reveals that he develops nausea because of GI intolerance to the drug. True drug allergy must be carefully recorded in this section of the history and also brought forward to the summary of abnormalities and the active problem list, if the POMR is used. Sometimes patients will also say they are allergic to a treatment when they mean that they perceive the treatment was unsuccessful. For example, a patient may say she is allergic to flu shots because she attributes her subsequent bouts of bronchitis to an ineffective influenza vaccine.

Immunizations

This is of particular importance in the examination of infants and children for whom a record should be made of immunizations to diphtheria, pertussis, tetanus, poliomyelitis, measles, and vaccination against smallpox. Information on tetanus boosters is usually adequate for adult patients; older patients should be asked whether they have had recent influenza and pneumococcal vaccines.

Current Medications

A complete list of the medications being taken by the patient may be invaluable to an understanding of his past or present illnesses. This list should include vitamins as well as nonprescription medications, such as antacids and laxatives. Although some of this information may have been recorded in the PI, all medications should be listed here including *name, dose, schedule, duration,* and *reason* for the treatment. If circumstances are appropriate, ask the patient to bring in, on his next visit, all such medications for your review, particularly if there seem to be many. It is not unheard of to have the patient return with a large bag containing a dozen or more vials and bottles, including two or three sedatives, several stimulants, and several other similar medications prescribed by different physicians. The current medications being taken will often provide useful information about the patient's physical and emotional health. Additionally, since many of the modern potent drugs are capable of producing illnesses themselves the list may offer significant diagnostic clues.

TYPES OF QUESTIONS AND RESPONSES

There is no one type of question appropriate for the entire clinical interview. The practitioner will be unable to obtain an accurate and precise medical history by using only open-ended questions because the patient may not know what details are important for specification and clarification. On the other hand, a too directive interview consisting only of closed-ended questions will not allow the patient to explain what is really bothering him and will inhibit the development of patient-practitioner rapport. Moving from general to specific is ordinarily best in the interview: from open-ended questions to help sketch the nature of the problems to more directive questions that request important details.

There is a place for yes/no questions, which are the most closed-ended of all. They should be used as screening questions in taking the review of systems (see Chapter 5) or in inquiring about habits. "Do you smoke?" They ordinarily should not be used except to check specific details already stated in the history of the present illness.

Summarizing is a useful technique to verify the information the patient has provided on a given topic, to demonstrate that the patient is understood, and to provide a transition from one topic to another. The practitioner simply repeats or paraphrases in a few sentences what he or she understands the patient has said: "Okay, I understand that you've had the severe watery diarrhea 10 or 12 times a day for the last week, and that sometimes you've noticed a little blood in the diarrhea. Now I want to ask you about nausea and vomiting." When parts of the story appear to be contradictory, it is important to request clarification: "You said the diarrhea first started last week but then you just mentioned you've been off work two weeks now because of illness. Did I misunderstand you?"

chapter 5

The Health History: Part II

Family History

Personal/Sociocultural History

Review of Systems

Activities of Daily Living

Patient Profile

    In obtaining the chief complaint (CC), present illness (PI), and past history (PH), it is desirable to use open-ended questions and/or prompting to assist the patient in telling you his health story. The remaining sections of the complete health history will require more direct guidance on the part of the examiner. It also may be more difficult to obtain prompt cooperation from this point on, since the lines of questioning may seem to be leading further away from the patient's CC, which is *his* main concern. Therefore, a brief explanation is in order to assure the patient that you have not forgotten the prime reason for his having come to the office or hospital. Both the practitioner and the patient need to be aware of the reasons for obtaining further history. that is, the details of the medical, social, familial, and economic *background* on which the current problems are based. Accurate evaluation is usually not the product of inspiration, but more often depends upon carefully putting together all of the information about the person himself, not just his disease.

FAMILY HISTORY (FH)

As stated earlier, the family history can shed light on the potential existence of hereditary diseases in the patient, on the patient's reactions to illness and death in the family, and the possible exposure to communicable disease. Ask first: "Are there any illnesses that seem to run in your family?" Then: "Is there anyone in your family who's had symptoms like yours?"

In most situations, brief questioning about first-order relatives (parents, siblings, children) is adequate. Questions should be asked about disorders that tend to run in families, such as heart disease, hypertension, diabetes, cancer, bleeding disorders, sickle cell anemia, allergies, and mental disorders.

Unless there are other family members with disorders similar to those of the patient, further exploration usually is not necessary. If a full history is deemed necessary, it may well be deferred to a subsequent visit, since this may require as much as an hour and the construction of a genogram or a table (Figure 5.1).

PERSONAL/SOCIOCULTURAL HISTORY (P/SH)

Information on the "patient as a whole" in his socioeconomic environment is needed in the process of evaluation. Sir William Osler's dictum — that it is as important to know what kind of patient has a disease as to know what kind of disease the patient has — is as pertinent as ever in our complex, stressful world.

Questioning the patient at this point in the interview is generally easier, since good rapport may have been developed. The patient may not construe this questioning as "prying" if he has confidence in the practitioner's interest in him and his problems. However, rapport is not automatic and if the clinician is aware of some hostility on the part of the patient, the questioning about personal and private matters must be done carefully, sensitively, and minimally. Back off as necessary if the patient does not wish to discuss certain topics. You may return to these areas later if more trust develops.

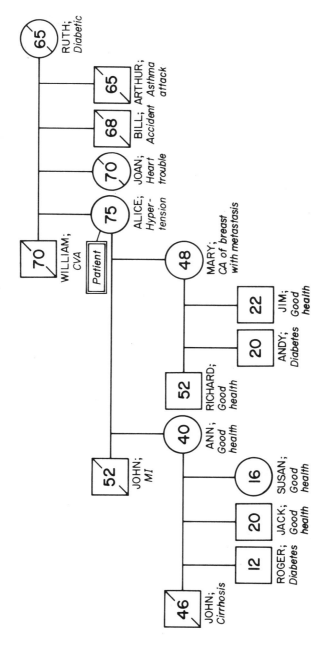

Figure 5.1 Example of a genogram.

As with other elements of the history, the amount of
detail sought by the clinician must depend on clues and leads
that develop during the patient-practitioner contact. Thus,
if the examiner senses that the patient is someone who seems
to be psychologically sound and whose problem appears to be
a straightforward organic one, the personal and social history
can be brief. On the other hand, patients who seem tense or
anxious and who present with obvious psychic or psychoso-
matic disorders deserve more detailed interviewing about
personal and social aspects of their life (see Chapter 28).
Skill in differentiating signs of emotional illness from psycho-
pathology develop with experience.

Geographic Exposure

Important items regarding geographic exposure are
birthplace and travel or residence in tropical or subtropical
areas that have a high incidence of certain diseases. Inquiry
into professional service in this context is necessary; even
people who have "lived their entire life" on the Eastern Sea-
board may neglect to mention a tour of military service in
Korea, Africa, the Middle East, or Vietnam.

REVIEW OF SYSTEMS (ROS)

This portion of the history reviews all *current* and pertinent *past* symptoms to be sure that no important clues have
been overlooked by either the patient or practitioner. The
history of the PI should include a complete review of the
system related to the CC, so additional questioning on that
system is often unnecessary. For example, if the CC was
"cough of 6-weeks duration," the examiner should have obtained at least as much information in the PI as is suggested
for the review of the respiratory system in the listing that
follows. Do not make the patient repeat his story here, but
add only any information on those systems not obtained in
the PI.
The listing of items of data to be obtained in the ROS
is, to some degree, arbitrary. There is no practical limit to
the number of questions that might be asked, but those suggested were selected as ones relating to the more common

problems found in adult practice.   The suggested order is also arbitrary and is roughly in anatomical order, starting with
the head and working down (which is also less intimate to
more intimate), so that the reviewer can proceed with questioning in some sort of systematic way.   Questioning will, of
course, vary with circumstances.   The items pertinent only
to adults will not be asked of the parent of the infant or
child.

Although medical terminology is listed here, the questioning must be in words commonly used and *clearly* understood by the patient.   Failure of the patient to understand
will lead to responses that are inaccurate and misleading.
Each of the items is briefly asked about and, if denied, may
be so recorded.   If positive responses are elicited, additional
information is obtained according to the guidelines provided
in Chapter 4 for "pain."   Thus, for example, a "yes" answer
to the question, "Have you ever been told that you had high
blood pressure?" should be pursued with either an open-ended
statement such as, "Tell me more about it," or with a series
of more direct questions.   The examiner should know, regardless of which interview technique is used, additional details
such as when hypertension was first found, how it was discovered, how high pressures were, how or if it was investigated, how persistent or transient it was, what treatment
was suggested or taken, whether it was followed regularly,
what the most recent pressures were, etc.

In reporting the ROS, remember that this is a part of
the history, so that the patient's *responses,* and *not physical
findings,* are recorded.   Physical findings will come later.
A useful technique for this review is to start with general
questions for a system, e.g., "Have you ever had any problems with your lungs or your breathing?"   Specific questions
can be asked later to cover items not mentioned by the
patient.

General: overall state of health, fatigue, unexplained weight
changes, exercise tolerance, fevers, night sweats, frequent infections, ability to carry out activities of daily
living

Integument: eruptions, rashes, pruritus, pigmentation, unusual hair growth or loss, disorders or deformities of nails

Head: headache, trauma

Eyes: visual problems, pain, lid edema, use of glasses, date of last examination, tests for glaucoma, scotomata, excessive tearing

Nose: smell, nasal obstruction, epistaxis, sinusitis

Mouth, teeth, and gums: dental problems, fit of dentures (if present), last visit to dentist, soreness of tongue, bleeding or swelling of gums

Throat and neck: frequent sore throat, hoarseness, tonsilitis, neck stiffness or pain

Breast: discharge, bleeding, lumps, soreness

Respiratory: wheezing, cough, hemoptysis, sputum production, shortness of breath at rest or on exertion, orthopnea, paroxysmal nocturnal dyspnea, last chest x-ray

Cardiovascular: chest pain, palpitations, heart murmur, peripheral edema, hypertension, claudication, varicose veins, thrombophlebitis

Gastrointestinal: dysphagia, appetite, food intolerance, jaundice, abdominal pain, indigestion, bleeding, flatus, nausea or vomiting, bowel habits, laxatives, blood or mucus in stools, tarry stools, clay-colored stools, use of antacids

Genitourinary: dysuria, frequency, urgency, hesitance, incontinence, nocturia, force of stream, odor and color of urine, bleeding, stones, venereal disease, discharge, hernia, prostatitis, sexual activity[1]

Gynecologic: menarche, character, frequency, duration of menstrual flow, date of last menstrual period, type of contraception (if used), dyspareunia, postcoital bleeding, vaginal discharge, pruritus, infertility, date and result of last Pap smear, sexual activity (see footnote 1)

Obstetric: pregnancies, full-term deliveries, abortions, living children, complications of pregnancies

Musculoskeletal: weakness, neck, back or joint stiffness, pain or swelling, radicular pain, muscle cramps, deformity

---

[1]This may be a natural time to introduce discussion of sexual concerns.

Neuropsychiatric

1. General: syncope, seizures, vertigo, dizziness, insomnia, nightmares, consciousness
2. Motor: tremor, paralysis/paresis, tic, spasm
3. Sensory: paresthesia, hyperesthesia, hypesthesia
4. Affect: anxiety, nervousness, depression
5. Cognitive ability, orientation, memory

Lymphatic and hematologic: lymph node swellings, excessive bleeding or bruising, anemia, blood transfusions

Endocrine: intolerance to weather changes, thyroid disorder, sugar in blood or urine, polydipsia, polyphagia, polyuria, excessive sweating, change in voice

ACTIVITIES OF DAILY LIVING

A convenient way to begin this segment of history is to say, "Tell me about the way you spend an average day." You will want to hear specific details about the patient's occupation and education, recreational activities, sleep, diet, use of tobacco, alcohol, or drugs of any type. If sufficient detail is not given, prompting or direct questioning will help in obtaining specific information.

Occupation and Education

Record present occupation, level of education, certification, and general history of work or school patterns. An individual who, for example, has held 15 to 20 jobs in as many years, or a student who has dropped in and out of school, never completing a program, may be giving you useful information about a person who is chronically ill or chronically dissatisfied. The type of job may provide clues about environmental hazards, such as coal dust for a miner, asbestos fibers for a construction worker, or toxic fumes for a factory worker. Find out exactly what the patient *does.* A patient who works in a mill may be anything from a secretary to a heavy equipment operator.

Knowledge of the patient's occupation also will be useful in the clinician's judgment about the patient's ability to continue working or the convalescent time that might be required upon discharge, if the patient is hospitalized.

If the patient is unemployed or retired, he will generally discuss his financial problems and may readily go on to express hostility or resentment toward society or individuals, if these feelings are present.

Recreation

Leisure time activities will often provide clues to a person's social environment, personality traits, and, occasionally, toxic exposure, as in the case of any office worker whose hobby is repairing and cleaning old guns using carbon tetrachloride as a solvent.

Diet

The examiner should obtain an estimate of the patient's average food and fluid intake. Several useful and simple techniques for obtaining this information are contained in Chapter 21, Nutritional Assessment. A typical 24-hour food intake pattern is recorded in the sample history in Appendix IV.

Habits

The pattern of use of over-the-counter drugs, tobacco, alcohol, and coffee or other high-caffeine beverages should be explored in quantitative terms. Cigarette smoking at present or in the past should be estimated in packs per day and "pack-years." Since the terms "social drinker" or "a few drinks" are nonspecific, the time of last drink and actual weekly intake of beer (number of bottles, cans, or glasses) should be ascertained. Similarly for hard liquor and for wine, some estimate of specific amounts is needed in terms of drinks per day, fifths of liquor per week, or other measurement of intake.

The regular use of over-the-counter drugs or vitamins provides an important clue to symptoms that may not have been uncovered earlier, and again, the clinician's task is to try to identify the types and amounts of the use of such drugs.

Vinegar, molasses, certain teas, herbs, or spices may be a patient's equivalent to over-the-counter drugs, and it is important to ascertain the health reasons for using such items regularly. Obviously, a patient's admission that he is using narcotics, "uppers," "downers," or other dangerous substances will provide the examiner with a significant lead, requiring investigation into the patient's reasons for starting or continuing use of these agents and the nature of the addiction. It is important to reemphasize the point, made earlier, that the examiner's personal bias or prejudice about drugs must not be expressed, nor should it interfere with the conduct of the interview.

Sleep

Information about the average number of hours of sleep, the frequency of waking during sleep, position during sleep, and recent alterations in sleep patterns will help to clarify the patient's physical and mental status. This may be included as part of the review of systems.

Marital and Sexual History

Sexual health is closely related to both physical and emotional health, so that failure to gather information about sexual functioning may lead to omission of important data vital to patient welfare. Depression, anxiety, and alcoholism may follow conflicts over sexuality, while these same problems resulting from other stresses may lead to reduced sex drive and unsatisfactory sexual functioning. Drug ingestion has been identified as one of the leading causes of desire and performance problems. Many couples experience vague somatic symptoms such as headache and back pain as a result of sexual incompatibility, while for others medical conditions may interfere with sexual satisfaction. Male impotence may result from diabetes, or certain antihypertensive drugs, while the female may experience painful intercourse as a result of postoperative or postpartal adhesions. Uncovering and correcting such problems may be of tremendous help to the patient, providing relief of much tension.

Despite the openness and frankness on sexual matters of our society, many people are still reluctant to discuss their own problems. New stresses have been created due to social pressures and expectations. Professional interest and the ability of the professional to talk with ease about sex may help to overcome reluctance to discuss sexual concerns. Sexual history should be attempted during the initial full health history so the patient is aware of the practitioner's concern for the importance of sexual health and willingness to offer help. Although discussion may be prompted early during the review of systems with open-ended questions such as, "What concerns do you have about your sexual life?", more time may be needed with the clinician before the patient feels comfortable expressing sexual concerns. The discussion may be better facilitated when topics are introduced in a nonjudgmental way with the assumption that most people have experienced the phenomenon or problem. Statements such as, "Many people experience problems—what has been your own experience?" may be helpful. The denial of problems during the initial interview, however, should not lead the practitioner to believe that problems do not exist. Perhaps, during a follow-up visit when greater trust has been established, additional communication may take place if the subject is reapproached.

The practitioner needs to be aware of his beliefs and values related to sexual practices so he does not overtly or covertly project judgmental attitudes. Patients who are at high risk for exposure to the AIDS virus need special sensitivity here.

Interpersonal Relationships

While it is important to identify sources of hostility and/or conflict in the patient as well as strengths and supports, detailed questioning about all contacts is not desirable or necessary. The clinicians should have picked up clues from earlier portions of the history that may be pursued, or he may simply ask the patient about any difficulty in "getting along" with family members, friends, or co-workers. Ask, "Are there any problems at home or work that cause you much concern?

Interpersonal Evaluation

The patient may be asked to give a brief view of himself, his life-style, his way of coping with stressful situations,
his own strengths, and weaknesses, his usual mood, and his
current concerns. Coming at the end of the interview an
open-ended request for such information is often well received and may produce a picture of the patient's self-image.

PATIENT PROFILE (PP)

This is *your* evaluation of the patient as a whole. All
the data will have been collected and recorded before this
evaluation, so the PP will not provide additional information
from the patient. A summary of risk factors will be noted here.
Review, briefly, the patient's socioeconomic status,
his current family structure (with whom does the patient
live?), his income in terms of meeting basic needs for food,
shelter, and clothing, his support systems, and his potential
for self-care. Give your opinion of his adjustment to his
situation (e.g., "This 45-year-old ex-Marine is employed
full time and lives at home with his wife and three children,
ages 9, 11, and 14. His wife works to help support the family.
He seems well-adjusted but is afraid of spending too much
time in the hospital because of concern about losing his job.").
Ignoring this evaluation may occasionally lead to missing the
real problem.
An illustrative actual case is the story of an elderly
man who had repeated admissions to a hospital for "intractable congestive heart failure." Properly managed on each
admission, he was placed on a low-salt diet, appropriate
medications, and adequate rest with good results, and then
was discharged. A *careful* history, finally taken on about
his fourth admission, revealed the facts that he lived alone
in a fourth-floor walk-up apartment and that his income
was inadequate to purchase the more expensive low-sodium
foods prescribed for him. When the PP was properly written
about this poor, quiet, shy old man who had to walk four
flights of steps daily to buy his food, the "medical" problem
of intractable heart failure was supplemented by a socioeconomic problem of poverty, loneliness, and overexertion

that required referral to the proper agencies. Knowledge about both types of problems allowed for adequate total treatment of the patient.

The student should review the purposes of each of the elements of the complete health history in relation to potential nursing diagnoses (see Chapter 4), and should then examine the models of a history (Appendix IV A and B).

Part Three

ESTABLISHING THE DATA BASE: THE SCREENING EXAMINATION

The Physical Examination

The basic premise in performing a physical examination is that the examiner, by use of all of his senses, can detect variations from the normal state that will become the second part of the data base on a particular patient. It is apparent from this premise that the examiner must know the range of normal findings for each of the modalities of the physical examination. This knowledge is based upon a sound foundation in anatomy and physiology and is developed with practice under the guidance of experienced instructors. There are, of course, some abnormalities that are obvious to even the untrained individual, but most abnormalities that will be of importance in the establishment of a good data base are not obvious without learning, training, experience, and practice — and more practice.

The student must learn how to inspect and observe —
not just to see; to feel accurately and sensitively; and to
use techniques of percussion and auscultation that are outside
the realm of everyday experience. The chapters that follow
will assist the student in developing the needed skills and in
establishing a systematic pattern of examination so that important findings will not be missed or forgotten.

The examination described is a sound, basic routine
evaluation that will identify almost all significant abnormalities. It must be recognized, however, that it does not represent a complete examination. There are hundreds of observations, signs, and tests that are not described in this text. For
example, in *Dorland's Medical Dictionary,* under the term
"sign," there are 695 entries, almost all of which relate to
the physical examination! Every specialist can add tests and
evidence of abnormalities that would expand the material
presented here. Thus, in the real world, there is no such
thing as a "complete physical examination" for every patient.

At the same time, every nursing interaction does not
call for a "complete examination" as described in this text.
The nursing students will learn early that the basic skills of
observation and general inspection for each body section as
determined by the faculty in relation to curriculum goals.
The special skills of palpation, percussion, auscultation, and
measurement will be incorporated into the teaching-learning
plan appropriately according to program objectives and then
selectively applied during each patient assignment.

With each new experience the student will expand these
special skills of physical assessment and will soon feel comfortable with most of the procedures described in this text.
The nurse who can perform the described examination well
and thoroughly need have no concern regarding the effectiveness of evaluation, for this is an excellent screening examination that will identify the presence of almost all important
findings.

As in the history taking, when one finds an abnormality,
further and more detailed examination is indicated. For example, it is not ordinarily necessary to listen over each square
centimeter of the lung during routine auscultation. But if
rales are heard in a particular area, it then becomes mandatory to cover that entire area — centimeter by centimeter —
to determine the exact extent of the abnormality. The
history provides the practitioner with clues relating to certain

areas deserving special attention. During the physical examination, the clinician will frequently find things not mentioned by the patient during the history taking. Significant skin lesions, scars, deformities, rales, muscle weakness, heart murmurs, etc., may require a continuation of questioning. As mentioned earlier, history taking is a *continuous* process extending throughout the physical examination, at the discussion after the examination, and at each subsequent visit.

Interviewing and teaching are continued during the examination to obtain additional information and often also serve to place the patient at ease. The examiner should explain what is being done and what the patient may expect. Surprises must be avoided. Where patient cooperation is required, clarity and patience will most often be rewarded by a better examination and the development of confidence. Maintenance of eye contact with the patient will assist greatly in development of good rapport and may often provide clues to assist in evaluation of the degree of pain induced by any movement or pressure during the examination. However, individuals of certain ethnic groups do not care for direct eye contact, so the examiner must not feel that the lack of it is indicative of aloofness. Of utmost importance is the professional demeanor of the examiner. Careless behavior, lack of preparation, inappropriate jokes, impatience, lack of proper draping, and other evidence of lack of consideration for the patient may all inhibit a proper relationship and a thorough examination.

The clinician must always guard, very carefully, verbal and nonverbal behavior when something unexpected is found. Inappropriate reactions will often frighten the patient or may "turn him off" as a partner in the necessary interchange between patient and clinician.

At the completion of the physical examination, after the patient is dressed and the examiner and patient are together for a summing up, it is useful for the clinician to ask the patient, "Is there anything else that you'd like to discuss with me?" By this time the patient should have more confidence in the examiner and may give additional, and often important, information he withheld earlier.

ORGANIZATION

As much as is practical, the physical examination will be described in this text by general body regions such as the head and neck, the thorax and its contents, the abdomen, etc. Thus, the examination of the peripheral vascular system, for instance, will not be described in any single chapter, but rather will be incorporated into the examination of the neck, the abdomen, and the extremities. While there are some exceptions to this format (e.g., skin, neurologic system), the teaching of examination by body region will more nearly match the technique of the actual physical examination.

TECHNIQUES

The four classical techniques of the physical examination are *inspection, palpation, percussion, auscultation.* These will be described separately and should, in general, be performed one at a time in sequence.
With certain major exceptions, the right and left sides of the body are nearly symmetrical. The heart extends into the left hemithorax more than into the right. The liver lies in the right upper portion of the abdomen, the stomach and spleen in the left upper, and on both sides these organs are covered by the thoracic cage. Thus, the examiner will find normal asymmetry during examination of both the thorax and upper abdomen. In the remainder of the body, symmetry is to be expected, and abnormalities may be identified by comparing one side of the patient with the other. There are slight deviations from side to side which fall within the normal range, so the observer must not expect perfect symmetry but must learn by experience when deviation is to be considered abnormal, and therefore notable.
An important part of the physical examination is the evaluation of function of the part or organ as well as examination for anatomic change. For instance, in the examination of the head and neck, the facial muscles are tested for strength and symmetry of motion, the eyes for motion and vision, the ears for hearing, the jaw for motion, the tongue for motion, the pharynx for swallowing, etc.

SOUND PRODUCTION

Since interpretation of sounds is extremely important in the examination, a few basic points should be reviewed at this time.

All sound is produced by vibration of an object or substance. Strings in vibration produce the sounds at the guitar or violin, reeds vibrate in the clarinet, the player's lips vibrate in the trumpet, the head of a drum vibrates, and an air column vibrates in a pipe organ. Physiologically, we hear vibrations of the larynx in voice production, vibrations of the air passages during breathing, vibrations of the thorax and abdomen as we percuss them, vibrations from the passage of air and fluid through the intestines, and vibrations produced by closure of the heart valves.

While it is not necessary to describe pitch in absolute numbers, it may be of interest to know that middle C on the piano is tuned to 262 cycles per second (cps), the tuning fork recommended for the diagnostic kit has a pure tone of 128 cps, and the normal human voice ranges from about 80-2000 cps. Heart sounds are of relatively low pitch, 30-70 cps, while some murmurs reach 600 cps. In the abdomen, normal peristaltic sounds are generally below 1000 cps, while peaks of over 2000 cps may be produced in intestinal obstruction.

The important qualities of sound for the clinician are pitch and loudness. Pitch is related to the number of vibrations (frequency) per unit of time. The fewer vibrations per second, the lower the pitch of the sound will be. Striking a firm, hollow object (such as a drum) will produce a low-pitched, booming sound that will have a long duration since the drumhead vibrates freely. On the other hand, a soft, solid object (such as the thigh), which does not vibrate freely, produces a very short, high-pitched sound. Loudness of sound (intensity) is related to the force that produces the sound, and the ability of the object to vibrate. Thus, in the example above, striking the thigh gently will not produce a very loud sound. Striking it more forcefully will produce a louder sound, but the pitch will not change.

SOUND TRANSMISSION

To hear a sound, the vibrations produced at the source must be transmitted through various media to the air and thence to the eardrum. Thus, closure of the heart valves will vibrate those valves, this vibration will be transmitted to the chest wall, to the stethoscope, through the air column in the stethoscope to the eardrum.

Factors that influence the transmission of sound are of great importance in understanding physiologic and pathologic phenomena. In general, sound vibrations are best transmitted through firm *solids* (e.g., metal, wood), less well through *fluid*, and poorest through *air*. For example, when one applies a stethoscope to a patient's chest and asks the patient to speak, the vibrations are transmitted from the larynx, through the trachea, the bronchi, the air-filled lung, the chest wall, and thence through the stethoscope to the examiner's ear. However, if there should be a consolidation of the underlying lung (as with advanced pneumonia), the voice sound will be transmitted *much better* than normally. This finding (see Chapter 12, bronchophony) will indicate to the observer that the underlying lung is more solid than normal — a definite pathologic finding. These principles must be kept in mind during the examination by percussion and auscultation to interpret the findings by these techniques.

SEQUENCE OF EXAMINATION

There is no single, perfect, "right" way to do a physical examination and various patterns are used by different practitioners. (See Chapter 20 for a recommended sequence.) No matter what the exact sequence may be, however, no general physical examination is adequate that neglects to consider examination of each area and region by all the necessary techniques. It is an absolute rule, however, that *inspection* of the part to be examined should always come first.

PHYSICAL EXAMINATION

Inspection

Most of what we have learned in life has come through our sense of sight and a great deal of the data on which a diagnosis will be based will come from inspection. It is a psychologic truth, however, that we perceive more of what we look *for* than what we look *at.* Skill in inspection will come in learning what to look for and how to observe carefully.

The master detective, Sherlock Holmes, used to astound Dr. Watson with his deductions based on observation. In one story Holmes asked Watson how many steps there were on the stairway leading to their flat. When the doctor admitted that he did not know, Holmes pointed out that while Watson had *seen* those steps for years, he had never *observed* them. We all see all there is to see, but the trained eye observes, and that is the essence of inspection in physical examination.

Adequate lighting and proper exposure of the area being observed are essential. Instruments such as a penlight, otoscope, ophthalmoscope, nasal speculum, and vaginal speculum are aids in the inspection process.

Palpation

Because the sense of touch is highly developed, with training and experience it can become an important diagnostic tool. The hand can distinguish many variations between hard and soft (e.g., a nodule within a thyroid gland), rough and smooth (e.g., a fine papular skin rash from a macular rash), stillness and vibration (e.g., absent fremitus from diminished fremitus), and heat and cold (e.g., increased temperature surrounding an early inflammation from normally warm skin). In general, the fingertips are most sensitive to touch, the palm and ulnar surfaces of the hand to vibrations (fremitus), and the ulnar and dorsal surfaces of the hand to temperature. Sensitivity to touch can be dulled by heavy pressure on the fingertips and by continued pressure. Thus, as a rule, light palpation is preferred for most examinations. It is often necessary to increase pressure to make certain distinctions, and better discrimination will result from pushing down several times rather than holding the fingertips in place for a long period.

Deep palpation is necessary to accomplish a thorough examination of the abdominal contents. A preferred technique for deep palpation is to place the fingers of one hand over the area to be palpated, and then to place the fingers of the other hand immediately in front of the first set of fingers and to push deeply with both hands (Figure 6.1). Bimanual techniques also include using both hands to entrap an organ or mass between the fingertips or to fix an organ in place with one hand while palpating with the other.

Another useful technique of palpation is *ballottement.* The term comes from the French verb meaning to toss or bounce a ball. This consists of a bouncing or tapping motion of the fingertips. Performed very lightly, ballottement of the eyeball through the closed lid may sometimes give a better sense of eyeball tension than will simple gentle pressure. Light ballottement is also useful in the initial palpation of the abdomen where the fingertips are rapidly bounced along the abdominal wall from the lower to upper portion. A sense of resistance which may be missed by firmer palpation can often be appreciated in this way.

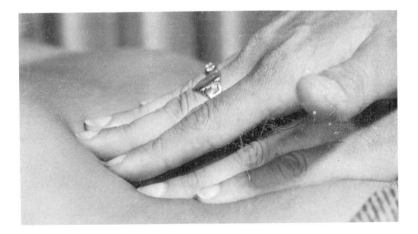

Figure 6.1 Position of fingertips for deep palpation. Note the overlapping.

Percussion

Percussion is the act of striking a portion of the body to evaluate the condition of underlying structures. Blunt percussion will produce tenderness in an underlying inflamed tissue or organ. Thus, striking a blow over the kidney may produce pain if there is renal infection (see Figure 16.3) and tapping over an infected sinus will often induce pain. A special form of blunt percussion over a tendon is used to stretch the muscle and produce a reflex used in the neurologic examination.

Another purpose of percussion is to identify and demarcate underlying structures by vibrating an area of the body surface. This is ordinarily performed by placing the middle finger of the left hand (for right-handed examiners) flat and holding it firmly against the area to be percussed. This is called the *pleximeter* finger. The percussion blow is struck by the *tip* of the middle finger of the right hand (Figure 6.2). Obviously, the fingernail must be trimmed short; otherwise the examiner will use the pad of his finger, producing a poorer sound. The target for the percussing fingertip is the area immediately distal to the last joint of the pleximeter finger.

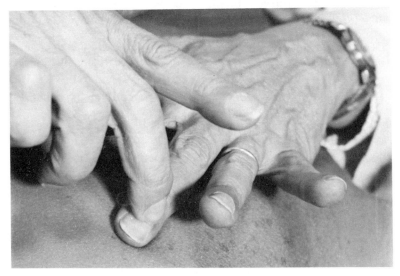

Figure 6.2 Percussion. Only the pleximeter finger is flat on the chest wall. The distal phalanx is struck by the tip of the third finger of the other hand.

Those who have played percussion instruments will know without further instruction that in order to produce a sharp, crisp note, the flow of the percussing finger must be brisk and short; otherwise the vibrations produced will be damped and muffled. The wrist should be used to produce the striking force and the blow should be controlled so that the percussing finger bounces off the pleximeter, rather than poking it.

In addition to listening to the sound produced by percussion, the examiner should concentrate on the vibrations *felt* by the pleximeter's finger. Both the sense of touch and the sense of hearing will assist the examiner in detecting changes as the pleximeter finger is moved from one area to another. This technique cannot be learned by reading the above description alone. After obtaining assistance from an instructor, the student should practice this technique until it is easily performed. One can produce the important percussion notes by practicing on one's own body, if no other cooperative one is at hand.

The vibrations produced by percussion depend upon the nature of the tissue underneath the pleximeter. Verbal descriptions of the various notes are nearly useless, so definitions are best given in terms of example. *Normal* percussion notes over the thorax and abdomen are resonance, dullness, and tympany:

Resonance: the low-pitched sound produced by percussion over normal lung (e.g., right anterior thorax above the level of the breast)

Dullness: a higher-pitched sound produced over more solid tissue (e.g., over the heart or liver). Dullness is a normal note over the heart or liver, but is *abnormal* when heard over normally resonant areas

Tympany: an even lower-pitched sound produced by percussion over an air-filled organ (e.g., most of the abdomen)

Two abnormal percussion sounds are flatness and hyperresonance:

Flatness:[1] an extreme degree of dullness sometimes referred to as "absolute dullness." This is higher pitched than dullness and may be simulated by percussion of a totally non-aerated tissue, such as the thigh

Hyperresonance: an even lower-pitched sound than resonance, produced over an abnormally air-filled lung, such as in a severe emphysema or pneumothorax

It is not necessary to produce a loud percussion sound. On the contrary, the best diagnostic information is obtained by quiet percussion since, by striking lightly, the examiner vibrates only a small area and can pick up smaller lesions or variations from the normal.

One final point is that percussion will not produce vibrations of deep structures. Therefore, any organ or mass more than 4 or 5 cm deep will not be detectable by this technique, and structures smaller than 4 or 5 cm cannot ordinarily be detected.

Auscultation

The most important factor in being able to do diagnostic auscultation is an adequate stethoscope that fits. This is the one piece of equipment that must be *fitted for you* and that you must own, carry, and use. When you come to the examination of the ear and use the otoscope, you will appreciate the fact that there is great variation in the diameter and angle of individual external auditory canals. There may be variation also between one's own left and right canals. It then will be obvious to you that no one stethoscope can possibly fit all ears.

---

[1]Some authors describe the normal percussion sound over the mid-portion of the heart or liver as "flat." It is our preference to reserve this term for an abnormal note such as that produced over a large pleural effusion.

The earplugs must be of the right size; the metal earpieces must be properly angled for each of your canals; the tension spring must hold the earpieces tightly enough to block out most extraneous noises but not so tightly that your ears are uncomfortable; the tubing should be of 1/8 in. internal diameter, of fairly thick outer diameter, and about 12–15 in. long; there must be no leaks anywhere in the tubing or connections; the instrument should have both bell and diaphragm chestpieces. Anything less than this may be adequate for taking blood pressure, but nothing less than this will do for clinical auscultation. The time spent with a box of extra earplugs, a pair of pliers, an otoscope, and an instructor will be one of the most important investments you will make in learning auscultation.

The *diaphragm* of the chestpiece amplifies sounds and transmits *higher-pitched* sounds better than lower frequency sounds. When using the diaphragm, press it firmly against the chest wall to get maximum benefit from its ability to amplify sounds. The *bell* filters out high-pitched sounds and is therefore useful in listening for *low-pitched* sounds. The bell should be placed lightly on the skin, just enough to make good contact. If pressed tightly, the bell will stretch skin across its orifice and, in effect, will become a diaphragm chestpiece. Both diaphragm and bell are used in the routine examination of the heart, whereas the diaphragm is generally adequate for examination of lungs, since most of the chest sounds are of higher pitch. There are areas in thin persons and children where the diaphragm will not lie flat, such as at the lung apices above the clavicles or between ribs where the bell may be needed.

EQUIPMENT

As has been suggested, a properly designed, carefully adjusted stethoscope is the one piece of equipment the examiner must own. All other instruments can be borrowed or are usually available at diagnostic stations.

Additional equipment necessary includes:

Penlight

Reflex hammer

C-128 tuning fork (128 cps)

Tape measure (180-200 cm)

Transparent ruler (15 cm)

Blood pressure set (with adult and pediatric cuff)

Otoscope-ophthalmoscope set

(Carrying bag for the above items)

VITAL SIGNS AND MEASUREMENTS

It should be obvious to all that no physical examination is complete without certain vital signs and measurements. Yet, all too often these elements are absent or taken casually. Routine blood pressures — even in only one arm — may not be recorded in certain offices and clinics, particularly in some of the specialty areas. Many patients will depart from a hospital stay without a single body weight ever having been recorded.

The practitioner must incorporate these simple but vital examinations into his practice. The measurements, made routinely, should include, *at a minimum,* height, weight, pulse, temperature, respiration, and several blood pressures. While there are, of course, circumstances in which height and weight cannot be measured immediately, these must not be forgotten and must be recorded at the first opportunity. All of these measurements serve as a part of an adequate data base and may give important clues during the follow-up period.

Blood pressure should be taken in both arms and in at least two positions. A useful routine is to take pressures after the patient has been supine for a few minutes. Record pressure in one arm, move the cuff to the other, record pressure, then with cuff still on the arm, ask patient to sit up and repeat pressure. Pressures should not normally vary from one arm to the other by more than 10 mmHg and on sitting up (or standing), there should be no more than a 10 mm lowering of either systolic or diastolic pressure. Variations in either situation of more than 10 mm warrant rechecking at some time before completion of the full physical examination. Conditions such as orthostatic hypotension, paroxysmal hypertension, and coarctation of the aorta, among others, may be first suspected by careful measurement of blood pressure and repeated recordings at each visit.

As an aid in patient evaluation, other measurements can assist in determining variation from normal standards and in evaluating change. The student and practitioner are encouraged to use the metric system. A 15-cm transparent pocket ruler and a 180- to 200-cm tape measure are essential ingredients of the diagnostic kit and should be used often. In addition to recording height, weight, and blood pressures in the infant, head circumference and crown-rump height are also routinely measured. To these, one should add measurement of significant asymmetry of any part of the body, the size of masses, the size of organs (such as the liver), the degree of swelling of an extremity with thrombophlebitis, etc. The simple act of carrying a ruler and tape measure at all times will assist in making such measurements a matter of routine practice.

RECORDING

The development of skill in reporting is important to provide a record of the findings at a particular time. Communication of these findings is necessary for others who may examine the patient and to the examiner himself when he repeats parts of the examination at a later hour or date. Remember that the focus is on what the examiner sees, feels, hears, or measures, not subjective information he has read in the patient's chart or learned from the history.

Examples will be given in each chapter to assist in learning this skill. In general the term "normal" is used sparingly. Rather, the report should describe what has been done and found. For instance, a report "pharynx normal," communicates no information as to what was examined, and is therefore an inadequate report. A report: *"pharynx* — mucus pink, no lesions, tonsils absent, uvula rises in midline on phonation, gag reflex present bilaterally," is specific, useful for communication, and serves as a basis for comparison at a repeated examination.

Vital signs and measurements are best recorded in traditional tabular form:

Ht: 163 cm (5'4")

Wt: 61.4 kg (135 lb)

Temp: 37°C (98.6°F) oral

Pulse: 80 reg.

Resp: 16 reg.

BP: RA 135/80

   LA 130/80 supine

   LA 130/80 upright

chapter 7

General Survey

The Patient as a Whole

Mental Status

Body Development

Nutritional State

Sex and Race

Stated Age Versus Apparent Age

Presenting Appearance

In the very few moments while the patient walks into the health center office or is wheeled by stretcher from the emergency room to the hospital nursing station, physical examination, starting with inspection, will be unobtrusively underway. The astute observing nurse will have collected dozens of bits of information as she greets the patient and assists him to the chair or bed. She will be aware of the patient's sex, race, apparent age, personal hygiene, nutritional status, and gait. She will know whether the patient's skin is dry or sweaty and will have observed the presence or absence of skin lesions, pallor, flushing, cyanosis, jaundice, or facial scars. Respiratory difficulty, cough, facial tics, jerky uncoordinated limb motion, obesity, hearing deficits, speech impediments or foreign accent, and many other characteristics will have been noted.

Not all of these findings — positive or negative — will be recorded as part of the general survey, but all will find

their way into the patient's record, and all will have given
the clinician some leads into the history taking and the physical examination.

THE PATIENT AS A WHOLE

"Mrs. A is an alert, cooperative, ambulatory, well-
developed, small, moderately obese, well-groomed 47-year-
old white woman appearing of about stated age who is in
mild respiratory distress. No speech defects." We recommend such a general introductory statement to the physical
examination report.[1] There can be no rigid rules for such
a statement, its purpose is to present a reviewer with an
immediate general image of the patient so that the details
that follow can be put into a general context.

Most of these observations are not related to a single
body system, but reflect constitutional factors which give a
picture of an individual's general state. The recommended
elements of this introduction are *mental status, body development, ambulation, nutritional state, sex and race, chrono-
logical versus apparent age, presenting appearance, posture,
and speech.* Remember that these introductory statements
are intended only to sum up the gross total appearance of the
patient and do not need to be detailed descriptions. For instance, Mrs. A's "mild respiratory distress," noted in the
sample introduction, will be described fully in the report of
the physical examination of the thorax and lungs.

MENTAL STATUS

This is a brief general statement of how an individual
behaves, feels, and thinks. It should describe the patient as
alert, and responsive, or dull, lethargic, and drowsy; oriented
or confused; anxious and fearful or confident and assured.
It should make a statement about appropriateness of personal
grooming and dress. Any indication of a change in behavior

[1]Individual institutions may establish guidelines for the nurse,
incorporating more or fewer of the characteristics described
in this chapter.

or mentality is specifically significant. This component will be expanded upon in the examination with specific reference to orientation, memory, general level of education, intelligence, reasoning ability, learning potential and distortions of thought, perception, or sensation (see Chapters 19 and 28).

BODY DEVELOPMENT

The nurses judgment, related to description of body development, is influenced by experience with diverse individuals of varying ethnic and racial backgrounds. Any patient whose height and body build fall within the wide range of acceptable normal for age and sex may be simply characterized as well-developed. (The 5 ft. 2 in., one hundred twenty pound male of Asian descent may or may not be considered underdeveloped when compared to other members of his family.)

There are some pathologic variations the nurse should recognize readily, such as gigantism, usually due to hypersecretion of growth hormone prior to maturation, in which the height and weight are well beyond the normal range. This condition is also usually associated with retarded sexual development. Where the anterior pituitary hypersecretion occurs after full body growth has been completed, the condition is called acromegaly. Here, there is enlargement of the nose, jaw, hands, and feet, producing the characteristic appearance seen in Figure 7.1. The opposite of gigantism is dwarfism. The ateliotic dwarf or midget is simply an abnormally small adult with normal body proportions. Another type of dwarf is the achondroplastic dwarf, in whom the head and body are frequently normal size but the extremities are very small and short.

There are other congenital and metabolic disorders that produce abnormalities of body size, shape, and proportion. Any such abnormalities should be reported here.

NUTRITIONAL STATE

Nutritional state may be reported in terms of malnourishment, the normal state, and obesity. A record will be made

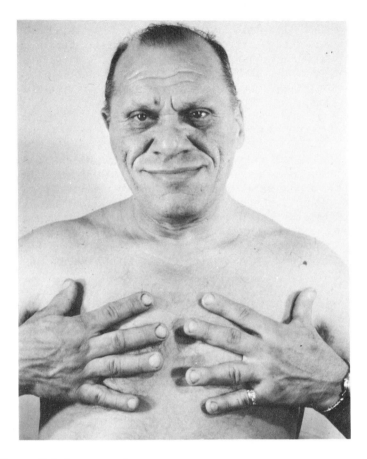

Figure 7.1 Acromegaly.

of actual height and weight so that the evaluation of over-
weight or underweight will not depend totally upon the examiner's concepts of the ideal. Height and weight charts
should be available to the examiner for subsequent discussion
with the patient who falls outside the normal range (see
Table 21.1). In infants and children such data should be recorded on standardized growth charts. In Chapter 21 we
discuss nutritional assessment in more detail.

SEX AND RACE

The patient's sex, of course, will usually be obvious to
a reviewer, but it is useful to state it here for the record to
assist in presenting a picture of the patient as a whole to
any reviewers or consultants. Occasional errors have occurred.
Since there are disease entities which are predominant-
ly found in persons of a particular racial origin, this factor
must also be recorded. Sometimes racial origin may not be
as obvious as we think. Consulting the patient, if you are not
certain, requires much sensitivity. In most cases, this question is raised by admission clerks in a very matter-of-fact
manner, so race appears on the identification stamp or band
worn by the hospital patient. However, you may have to
validate the information presented with the patient to be
certain you are correctly identifying racial origin.

STATED AGE VERSUS APPARENT AGE

There is often a difference, to the examiner's eye, between these ages. While this is admittedly a matter of subjective judgment, it is important to record such an apparent
significant difference. Frequently, the person harboring a
chronic disorder may appear definitely older than his actual
age, and the notation of such a clue may assist in uncovering
such a disease, if it exists. Sensitivity in interviewing is critical here. Challenges should not be made to the patient.
Pathologic extremes such as *progeria* or *precocious puberty*
are rarely seen.

PRESENTING APPEARANCE

This is reporting of a specific observation such as, "in
acute respiratory distress" or "writhing in pain." More general
subjective observations such as "appearing chronically ill,"
"in no acute distress," or "seeming to be in excellent health"
also assist in providing the desired overall survey of the
patient.
There are general abnormalities that may well fit into
this introductory report, such as obvious amputation and blindness. One of these general abnormalities is the patient's

position, often referred to as station. The examiner's interest here is not in simple poor posture due to habitual stooping or slumping, nor in skeletal deformities, which will be examined carefully later on. Rather, the abnormalities of station are those related to physiologic disturbances such as the position taken by the patient in severe respiratory distress. Here, he will lean forward, bracing his arms so that he can use the accessory muscles of respiration (see Figure 12.7). In left-sided congestive heart failure with severe pulmonary edema, the patient will sit or stand nearly upright and will not lie supine comfortably. He may lean to one side to splint a fractured rib or have his knees drawn up to relieve abdominal pain. Station refers to *any* feature of the patient's position; where pertinent, station should be specified if it helps to give a picture of the whole patient.

Abnormalities of *speech* should be recorded here initially and then described in detail in the neurologic examination. Speech is a highly complex act that involves mental processes, the cerebellum, several cranial nerves, the mouth, palate, tongue, larynx, and the respiratory system. As with many other problems, the exact mechanism for speech defects may not be known at the completion of the history and physical examination, but a careful, complete description of the defect will have important diagnostic value.

As stated earlier, many observations will be made at the very outset of the interview. In general, however, it is a useful procedure to describe abnormal findings in the system or region in which they are located, and to reserve this general survey for a brief, orienting, introductory picture of the patient as a whole.

chapter 8

The Integument, Masses and Lymphatics

Topographical Anatomy

Physiology

Technique of Examination

Examination of the Skin

Examination of Masses

The Lymphatic System

Recording

Potential Nursing Diagnoses

Patient Problem

Since the skin is the individual's showplace to the world, it becomes a medium through which the personality is frequently expressed. Tattooing, use of makeup, wigs and hairpieces, and other cosmetic aids are also considered when the practitioner is making a psychological assessment, since their use may reflect the individual's self-image, as well as his cultural identity.

Examination of the skin, hair, and nails begins with general inspection during the interview, early in the process of health evaluation, and continues throughout the physical examination of each body organ or body system. The condition will ordinarily be described along with other elements of a particular reigon. Thus, absence of genital hair will appear as a part of the inspection of the genitalia, and a skin rash limited to the abdomen will be described in the report on that region. However, if there is a condition that involves all or nearly all of the body, it is useful to describe it in this general section. Examples of widespread abnormalities that belong here are total absence of hair, absence of skin pigment (albinism), jaundice, or generalized rash.

TOPOGRAPHICAL ANATOMY

Figure 8.1 is of value in identifying the different layers of the skin and its appendages, but its inclusion here is primarily to help the examiner establish a framework for further study.

PHYSIOLOGY

The skin is an organ that serves many functions in addition to protection of underlying vital organs, such as controlling temperature, maintaining fluid balance, carrying sensory nerve endings, and forming a barrier against penetration of harmful agents, including microorganisms of infection. The normal skin and appendages, the hair and nails, vary according to sex, age, race, endocrine influence, and genetic messages. They are also especially affected by factors of climate and nutrition, and reflect the internal as well as external environment of the body. Many disease processes alter their function and appearance. The general color and a number of pigmentary alterations are examples of inherited characteristics.

It is important to remember, however, that a variety of alterations in character and consistence may be quite normal in certain individuals. The child's skin is normally thick, elastic, and well-lubricated; but as the years advance, changes occur that result in thinning, decreased elasticity, drying, and wrinkling. Also, the skin long exposed to sunlight is coarser, dryer, and rougher.

The amount of hair growing over the skin varies from individual to individual and is also a genetic endocrine-determined trait. Thus, males develop hair on the face and

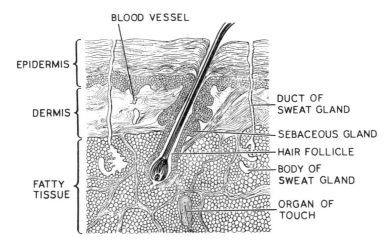

Figure 8.1 Cross-section of skin.

chest in addition to the axillae and pubis at puberty. The rapid rate of hair loss from the male head after age 25 is certainly a well-accepted fact of normal development.

Figure 8.1 shows that the sweat glands lie within the deeper layers, but they are of epidermal origin. Sweat glands are distributed generally over the skin, particularly on the palms, soles, and forehead. Sebaceous glands arise from hair follicles and are a frequent source of infection and cyst formation, especially over the scalp, neck, back, and genital area.

TECHNIQUE OF EXAMINATION

For the most part, the methods used in examination of the skin and its appendages require few special instruments, only the technique of inspection and palpation, good light, and a transparent flexible pocket ruler for measurement of any lesions found. The examiner must remain constantly aware of the fact that many skin changes and skin lesions are manifestations of underlying systemic disease. This fact makes it even more important to notice and carefully describe skin changes.

EXAMINATION OF THE SKIN

General Phenomena

Color

There are no practical methods of measurement of skin color. This remains a matter of individual judgment and skill. Although daylight is the best source of lighting, it is often unavailable, so one must make do. Worst of all sources is the flashlight. The examiner should note the general skin color and identify deviations such as pallor, flushing, cyanosis, and jaundice. Each of these may involve one or more small areas (e.g., cyanosis of lips and nail beds) or may be present over the entire body.

Skin color change is more difficult to detect and evaluate in brown-skinned individuals, and is most difficult to determine in those with deep black skin. One must search those areas where *melanin* (which reflects brown and black color), *melanoid* (yellowish), and *carotene* (yellow orange) are least concentrated. Some of these areas are the sclerae, palpebral conjunctivae, nail beds, lips, palms, soles, and mucous membranes of the mouth.

Pallor decreases the underlying reddish tones of skin leading to a near absence of skin color in whites, a yellowish brown in brow-skinned persons, and an ashen gray in blacks. Flushing is very difficult to detect in blacks and may be missed. Cyanosis must also be searched for more diligently in dark-skinned persons than in whites. When present, it is seen best in lips, conjunctivae, facial skin (ear lobes, cheeks, around the mouth), tongue, and nail beds. Jaundice is generally best seen in the sclerae and mucous membrane of the hard palate in light- and dark-skinned individuals. However, occasionally in the latter, there is a tendency for fatty deposits in the sclerae to take on a yellowish hue, which can be confused with jaundice. These deposits are often more prominent near the inner and outer canthi of the eyes, which assists sometimes in the differentiation from the generalized yellowing seen in jaundice.

When the practitioner notices any areas of increased or decreased pigmentation, further history from the patient should be elicited regarding their duration. There are some changes in pigmentation that are temporary or of no real significance. Chloasma gravidarum, for example, consists of brown patches on the forehead and cheeks of the pregnant women, known as the mask of pregnancy. This increase of pigmentation usually disappears spontaneously after childbirth. Table 8.1 identifies some of the color and pigmentation alterations that may be observed and require recording.

Texture

The texture or turgor of the skin should be assessed by grasping a small section between the examiner's fingers (see Table 8.2). It may feel thin, inelastic, and dry, due to lack of moisture within the skin itself, or thick and mushy if the skin is overhydrated. When the water content of the skin is excessive, edema is present and is characterized by pitting upon pressure (see Fig. 16.1).

A special type of thickening called *myxedema,* often seen over the tibia, may be present in hypothyroidism; it has the sensation of mushiness, but does not pit. More extensive hardness of the skin is seen in systemic sclerosis where the changes tend to be symmetrical, involving the face, extremities, and anterior chest. Thickening and hardening of thin and fragile skin may be due to disease and should always be described as accurately as possible.

Temperature

In general, increased warmth of the skin is due to increased blood flow as a result of the body's response to inflammation and attempt to lower the body temperature. Increased coolness is frequently due to reduction of blood flow to the integument in an attempt to preserve body heat or to supply vital organs, as in shock. Local coolness usually exists in extremities as a result of decreased blood flow, peripheral vascular disease, vascular spasm, or combinations thereof.

Local Phenomena

Skin

Skin Lesions. The skin is subject to so many types of lesions that the principal task of the examiner is to describe lesions accurately. They should be described according to

Table 8.1 Color Changes of Skin

Color Change	Basis	Examples
Erythema, reddish tint	Increased amounts of blood flow or RBC	Fever, sunburn, polycythemia vera
Cyanosis, bluish tint	Increased amounts of deoxygenated blood	Pneumonia, congenital heart disease with right-to-left shunt
Pallor, whitish tint to ash gray	Decrease in hemoglobin content	Anemia, shock
Greenish yellow	Increased bilirubin in skin or sclera	Jaundice due to blood pigments in hemolysis or biliary tract obstruction
Orange yellow	Increased amounts of carotenoid in skin but not sclera	Ingestion of excess amounts of food with carotene, occasionally in pregnancy
Gray	Deposition of metallic salts such as silver, gold, and bismuth	Prolonged ingestion of such salts
Increased or decreased pigmentation	Absence or excess of melanin	Exposure to sunlight, Addison's disease, albinism, vitiligo
Localized pigmentation superficially	Injection of carbon-containing particles	Tattoo

Table 8.2 Changes in Skin Texture

Texture and Turgor	Basis	Examples
Excessive moisture	Autonomic nervous system stimulation	Perspiration
Dryness	Endocrine imbalance, dehydration	Hypothyroidism, postmenopausal fluid loss
Wrinkling	Loss of skin elasticity	Rapid weight loss, aging
Velvety smoothness	Endocrine imbalance	Hyperthyroidism
Puffiness and indentation on pressure	Fluid and electrolyte imbalance, venous or cardiac insufficiency	Edema
Thickening without dryness	Endocrine imbalance	Myxedema

distribution and location, size, contour, and consistency. The data in Tables 8.3 and 8.4 have been prepared to assist in the recognition and recording of lesions. It is important to understand that eruptions consist of one or more primary lesions, which result directly from disease (Table 8.3) that can be either discrete or confluent, and with or without secondary lesions (Table 8.4). Certain lesions localize preferentially on exposed areas (e.g., poison ivy, sunburn), while others prefer typical locations such as the trunk and neck in pityriasis rosea, or the root of a nerve in herpes zoster (Figures 8.2 and 8.3).

An important test of the practitioner's examination ability requires that he differentiate among lesions that are commonly found, those that are premalignant, and malignant neoplasms which require immediate attention. Pigmented nevi or moles are usually raised dark brown or black lesions varying in a diameter from the size of a nodule to a tumor

Table 8.3   Primary Skin Lesions[a]

Types	Description	Size	Examples
Macule	A flat circumscribed area of color change without elevation of its surface	1 mm to several cm	Freckles, flat pigmented moles, vitiligo, cafe-au-lait spots
Papule	Circumscribed solid elevation of the skin	Less than 1 cm	Acne, lichen planus
Nodule	Solid mass extending deeper into dermis than does a papule	1-2 cm	Erythema nodosum, pigmented nevi
Tumor	Solid mass, larger than nodule	Over 2 cm	Epithelioma, dermatofibroma
Cyst	Encapsulated fluid-filled mass in dermis or subcutaneous layer	Over 1 cm	Epidermoid cyst
Wheal	A relatively flat localized collection of edema fluid	1 mm to several cm	Mosquito bites, urticaria (hives)
Vesicle	Circumscribed elevations containing serous fluids or blood	Less than 1 cm	Herpes simplex, herpes zoster, chickenpox, smallpox
Bulla	Larger fluid-filled vesicle	Over 1 cm	Pemphigus, second-degree burn

Table 8.3 *(continued)*

Types	Description	Size	Examples
Pustule	A vesicle or bulla filled with pus (larger collections of pus are called furuncles, abscesses, or carbuncles)	1 mm– 1 cm	Acne vulgaris, impetigo

*a*Some dermatologists include *plaques* as primary lesions, while some do not. In any event, a plaque may be defined as a flat, elevated lesion, more than 1 cm in size. Some plaques appear to be made up of clusters of papules which have co-alesced into a single lesion.

and may or may not contain hairs. Although commonly found and usually benign, they may occasionally develop into malignant melanomas (Figure 8.4). It is important to ascertain historical data relative to the duration of their existence and change in characteristics. If there is evidence of rapid enlargement, change in color, consistency, crusting, or bleeding, it may signify malignant degeneration, and warrant excision.

Vascular Lesions. The examiner should note the presence of unduly dilated superficial veins, telangiectasia, or spider angiomas. Some of these are caused by interference with normal blood flow and are usually significant in determining diagnosis, depending on location. Some are more related to severe pathology than others. *Telangiectasia* are localized, fine red lines due to dilated blood vessels that may be venules, capillaries, or arterioles. They frequently appear on the alae nasae of almost every adult but may occur at any age, in both sexes, and anywhere on the skin or mucous membranes. Their presence is rarely of diagnostic value. *Spider angiomas (vascular spiders)* are cutaneous lesions frequently found in areas drained by the superior vena cava. They have a central red pulsating arteriole representing the body from which small fine vessels radiate like the legs of a spider over

Table 8.4 Secondary Skin Lesions

Type	Description	Examples
Crust	The dried exudate of serous oozing, blood, or pus	Eczema, vesicular or pustular eruptions, impetigo
Scale	Flakes of skin	Psoriasis, pityriasis rosea
Excoriation	Scratch marks	Pruritus, needle marks
Fissure	A crack in the skin, usually through the epidermis	Eczema, chapping
Ulcer	A circumscribed loss of epidermis which may extend deeply into the corium and subcutaneous tissue	Chancre, malignant growth, stasis ulcer as with severe varicose veins
Scar	Replacement of destroyed tissue by fibrous tissue or excess collagen	Postoperative scar, keloid
Striae	Long, slightly depressed lines, appearing like scars but without disruption of the skin, often shiny and colorless when due to stretching of subcutaneous tissue, or reddish purple when due to excess adrenal steroids	Pregnancy, marked obesity, Lupus erythematosus, Cushing disease

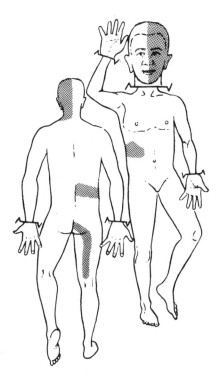

Figure 8.2 Herpes Zoster dermatomal distribution. From Lazarus G, Goldsmith L: *Diagnosis of Skin Disease,* Philadelphia, FA Davis, 1980, p 267, by permission.

a reddened area 1-10 mm in diameter (Figure 8.5). When the central arteriole is compressed, the branches become blanched, and upon release, fill again from the center. Although they may occur in normal individuals, and during pregnancy, they are most frequently found in association with chronic liver disease.

Bleeding Lesions. The term purpura, strictly used, means a disorder characterized by hemorrhage into the skin. There are two purpuric lesions that are important to differentiate because of their different causes.

The presence of individual tiny red or red brown capillary hemorrhages known as *petechiae,* no more than 0.5 mm in diameter, located within the skin papillae, may be indicative of capillary fragility due to vitamin deficiency, blood

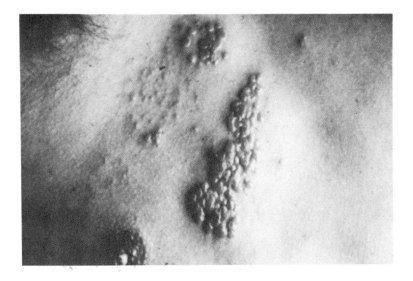

Figure 8.3 Erythematous papules develop to vesicles. From Lazarus G, Goldsmith L: *Diagnosis of Skin Disease,* Philadelphia, FA Davis, 1980, p 267, by permission.

dyscrasias, or severe infections (Figure 8.6). Larger hemorrhages under the skin, referred to as *ecchymoses,* or bruises, varying in size from several millimeters to several centimeters, may be due to trauma or blood dyscrasias.

Hair

There are many normal variations in hair distribution but only a few abnormalities are of importance. These are unexpected general or local hair loss (Figure 8.9), distinct change in the character of the hair, and excessive hair growth in women. Any of these findings should be the subject of a careful history to be sure that a change has occurred. Baldness is certainly not unusual in middle-aged or elderly men, but is worthy of questioning and reporting in a man under 25 years of age or in a middle-aged woman. Disappearance of body hair from a region where it is ordinarily present (see Figure 16.9) should be reported.

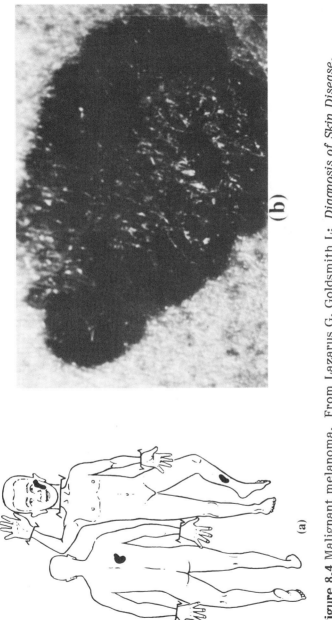
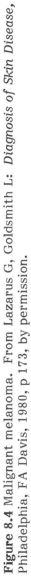

Figure 8.4 Malignant melanoma. From Lazarus G, Goldsmith L: *Diagnosis of Skin Disease*, Philadelphia, FA Davis, 1980, p 173, by permission.

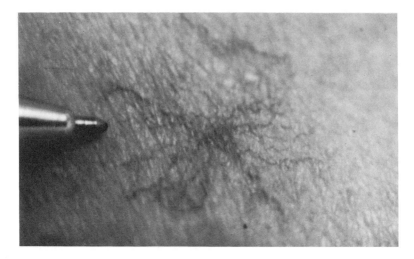

Figure 8.5 Spider angioma.

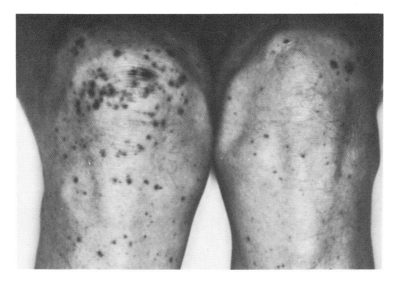

Figure 8.6 Petechia. From Lazarus G, Goldsmith L: *Diagnosis of Skin Disease,* Philadelphia, FA Davis, 1980, p 348, by permission.

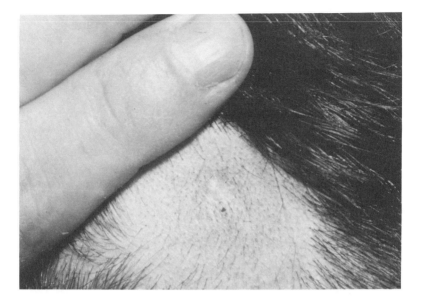

Figure 8.7 Alopecia areata. Note the normal area of loss of hair without scaling of the scalp and with normal hair elsewhere.

A change from normal hair texture to rapidly thinning, fine, silky hair is often associated with hyperthyroidism; in hypothyroidism the hair becomes dry and brittle and may begin to disappear from the lateral portions of the eyebrows.

In women who have excessive hair, the areas that should be carefully examined are the face and chest. The presence of coarse hair forming a beard or an excess in hair across the anterior chest are suggestive signs of hirsutism due to an endocrine tumor, while excessive hair on the arms, upper lip, or abdomen is more often an abnormality without known cause. Since this disorder may be a serious one from either an endocrine or cosmetic point of view, the presence of excess hair on a woman should always be a matter of report.

Nails

The nail bed can be seen through the transparent nail and it may be one of the first places that cyanosis will be seen. The appearance of badly mutilated, bitten nails may alert the examiner to consider the presence of an emotional or personality disorder. Nails grow outward at a regular rate that is ordinarily interrupted only by disorders such as a major operation or serious infection. As the nail continues to grow, a deep horizontal line across each nail will become visible. These are called *De Beau* lines, and the time of occurrence of the illness that caused them can be roughly calculated by remembering that outward growth is at the rate of about 1 mm every 10 days.

A most important lesion to identify is clubbing. This is an abnormality involving both the nail and the terminal phalanx, but is evident earliest in the nail. The normal nail meets the skin fold (called the eponychium) where the cuticle develops, at an angle (Figure 8.8). As clubbing develops, the proximal portion of the nail is elevated, eliminating this angle. Light palpation of the base of the nail will identify a softening of the nail bed. As clubbing becomes more severe, it also becomes much more obvious. The nail becomes curved (watch-glass deformity) and the terminal phalanx becomes widened and rounded (drumstick deformity). Clubbing is frequently a sign of chronic oxygen lack often seen with certain congenital heart diseases, chronic pulmonary disease, and arteriovenous shunts. It may also be a normal, familial trait, or be secondary to nonthoracic disorders such as sprue, certain kidney diseases, or leukemias.

The nail should be inspected for chronic infection and for "splinter" hemorrhages which are thin, brownish, flame-shaped lines in the nail bed. These most often are a result of tiny emboli associated with subacute bacterial endocarditis, which occur throughout the body but are not visible under the skin.

EXAMINATION OF MASSES

Any swelling or tumor larger than 2 cm in diameter is generally referred to as a mass. Its significance, of course, depends upon the nature of the mass. While the observer may

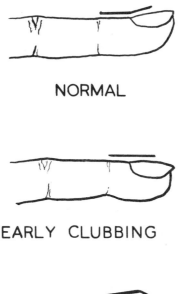

NORMAL

EARLY CLUBBING

SEVERE CLUBBING

Figure 8.8 Clubbing of nail. Note the normal angle between the eponychium and the nail. This is true even with curved nails. The loss of angle seen in early clubbing is replaced by a reversed angle as the proximal nail bed elevates.

not be able to identify its nature, every mass must be examined critically and described so accurately that a skilled reviewer may be able to identify it from the description alone. There are several fundamental attributes of all masses that must always be described: *location, shape and size, consistency, mobility,* and *tenderness.* Additional features that should be described, if present, are pulsations, temperature, and changed color of overlying skin.

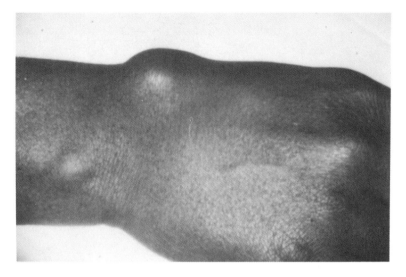

Figure 8.9 Ganglion. From Lazarus G, Goldsmith L: *Diagnosis of Skin Disease,* Philadelphia, FA Davis, 1980, p 230, by permission.

Location

Describe both the general anatomic region and the specific location as exactly as possible (e.g., left forearm just above wrist) (Figure 8.9).

Shape and Size

Describe the shape of the mass (e.g., spherical, oval, irregular, nodular) and draw a simple sketch to show the outline of its surface. Measure the greatest length and width and record these in centimeters. Measure depth, if possible, or give an approximate measurement.

Consistency

Use the most descriptive terms possible. Adjectives such as stony hard, hard, firm, rubbery, plastic, soft, mushy, and fluctuant are often used (Figure 8.10).

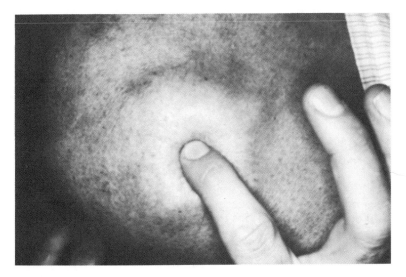

Figure 8.10 Lipoma. From Lazarus G, Goldsmith L: *Diagnosis of Skin Disease,* Philadelphia, FA Davis, 1980, p 222, by permission.

Mobility

The movement or fixity of a mass is related to the structures to which the mass is attached and is of considerable diagnostic importance. Note carefully the mobility of any mass in relation to both deeper and overlying tissues.

Pain and Tenderness

Pain refers to a spontaneous uncomfortable sensation, while tenderness means the induction of pain by pressure on or movement of a part. These characteristics should be noted in any description of a mass.

Other Features

If pulsation is present, it is important to determine the reason for this motion. Taking the mass between the fingers may assist in making this distinction. An aneurysm of an artery will pulsate in all directions, while a mass being moved

by an underlying artery will pulsate only upward. The temperature and color of the skin may be changed by the mass and,
if so, should be noted. Occasionally, the actual color of the
mass may be identified through the skin.
While the characteristics listed above are used for the
description of masses, they are useful also in the description
of enlarged organs such as the thyroid, liver, spleen, and
testes.

THE LYMPHATIC SYSTEM

The lymphatic system is an extensive system consisting
of a capillary network, larger collecting vessels, lymph nodes,
and organs. Its functions include production of lymphocytes,
return of tissue fluid to the major circulatory system, filtra-
tion and destruction of bacteria, removal of some foreign
particles, and transportation of digested fat from the intestine.
Under normal circumstances, only the tonsils and a few
patches of lymphoid tissue will be found in the pharynx on
physical examination. Inflammation of larger lymphatic vessels (lymphangitis) may be seen as reddish streaks near the
skin surface leading from an area of infection or, sometimes,
from the site of a malignancy.

Lymph Nodes

A special type of mass is the enlarged lymph node.
Under normal circumstances lymph nodes are not palpable,
as they are small (1-5 mm in diameter), soft, mobile, and
underneath the skin. While there are many lymph nodes
throughout the body, there are only three regions where enlargement is frequently found: the *neck,* the *axillae,* and
the *inguinal* area (see Figure 9.14).
Palpable nodes often occur in clusters, although solitary
nodes are occasionally seen. The most common cause of enlargement is infection somewhere in the body region from
which lymphatic channels drain toward the nodes (Table 8.5).
Metastases from neoplasms are often trapped in the nodes,
leading to enlargement, and there are systemic disorders that
sometimes lead to generalized lymphadenopathy, including
infectious mononucleosis, rubella, and rubeola, as well as

Table 8.5 Lymph Node Enlargement

Sites	Body Region Drained	Examples
Submaxillary	Mouth, pharynx	Abscessed teeth, carcinoma of mouth, tongue, etc.
Anterior cervical	Mouth, pharynx	Tonsilitis, pharyngitis
Posterior cervical	Scalp	Severe dandruff, lice
Supraclavicular:		
Right side	Right lung	Tuberculosis, sarcoidosis
Left side	Left lung, upper abdomen	Sarcoidosis, carcinoma of stomach
Axillae	Breast, chest wall	Mastitis, carcinoma of breast
Inguinal-femoral	Lower extremities, pelvic area, genitalia	Syphilis, skin infections, lymphogranuloma venereum
All or many	—	Hodgkin's disease, lymphoma

neoplastic lesions of the lymphoid tissue itself, such as Hodgkin's disease, lymphomas, and leukemias.

There is a general tendency for nodes that are draining infections to be of moderate size, firm, separate, and tender. Nodes involved by metastatic disease are often stony hard and are, as a rule, not tender. With involvement of the nodes by lymphatic neoplasm, the nodes are firm or rubbery and have a distinct tendency to be matted together as though bound by fibrous tissue. These are not absolute rules, by any means, since there can be a great variation in characteristics.

Palpation for nodes in each of the common locations will be described in the examination of each region later in the text. It should be noted, however, that sites other than these common ones may show lymph node enlargement. These include the areas immediately anterior to and posterior to the ear lobes, the epitrochlear area just above the median condyle of the humerus, and the popliteal space. Whenever and wherever lymph nodes are visible or palpable, all of the characteristics described for masses in the previous section must be included in the examination and report. In addition, since lymph nodes tend to appear in clusters, it is important to determine if they feel like separate masses (like grapes on a stem) or if they seem to be matted and bound together in lumps.

It is preferable to report lymph node enlargement (lymphadenopathy) in the specific locations where it is detected. Even for generalized lymphadenopathy, description region-by-region provides more accurate information.

RECORDING

Skin: pink in color, good turgor, warm to touch, no excoriations or lesions

Hair: normal distribution and consistency

Nails: no deformities, nail beds pink, no clubbing

POTENTIAL NURSING DIAGNOSES

Skin integrity, impairment of: actual

Skin integrity, impairment of: potential

Potential infection

PATIENT PROBLEM

Mr. T. J. R. is a 17-year-old white adolescent with a chief complaint of "skin lumps" of 2-years duration.

Problem: Skin Masses (Figure 8.11)

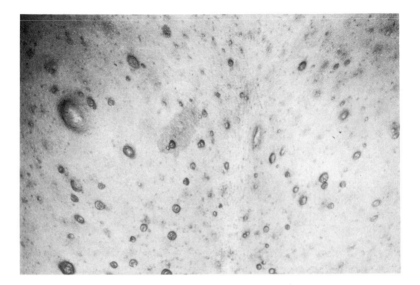

Figure 8.11 Neurofibromas of the back. Note the multiple nodules of varying sizes. A café au lait spot can be seen just left of the center of the photograph.

Subjective (S): History of development of nontender lumps on the back over the past 2 yr, most of them within the past 6 months; no family history; pt. is concerned that this may be veneral disease.

Objective (O): Skin: Pink color, freckled, good turgor, warm; there are about 10-12 light brown macules over the back averaging 2.5 cm in diameter without inflammation or excoriation. Masses: There are hundreds of scattered lesions of the skin varying in size from papules to tumors over 4 cm in diameter. These are distributed principally over the back, neck, and posterior surface of the arms, with a few on the thorax and abdomen; none on face or genitalia. They lie in the skin but protrude above the surrounding surface. They are not fixed to subcutaneous tissues and are firm and generally nontender.

ASSESSMENT: Coming on after puberty, associated
               with freckles and large brown macules
               (café au lait spots), these fit the descrip-
               tion of neurofibromas; not a venereal
               type of lesion.
               Nursing Diagnosis: Skin integrity;
               actual impairment of.
               Potential alteration in body image and
               self concept due to skin lesions.
               Knowledge deficit of sex and venereal
               disease.

PLAN: Goals: To determine cause of skin
               lesions and facilitate improvement.
               To verbalize the importance of accurate
               facts about sex and venereal disease.
               To verbalize the importance of keeping
               an appointment with the dermatologist.
               Nursing Orders:
               Diagnostic: Refer to dermatologist.
               Therapeutic: None.
               Patient Education: Facilitate open
               discussion about feelings relative to
               body image and to provide peer help
               group information.

IMPLEMENTATION: Patient told that these are probably not
                venereal, malignant, or contagious, but
                that examination by a specialist is
                mandatory.
                Discussion of patient's sexual activity
                cleared up several misconceptions.

EVALUATION: Patient visited dermatologist.
               Patient participated in a self-help group.

chapter 9

The Head,
Face and Neck

Topographical Anatomy

Physiology

Examination

Recording

Potential Nursing Diagnoses

Patient Problem

This chapter describes the examination of the head, including the face and the neck, leaving for other chapters the examination of the eyes, ears, nose, and mouth. Evaluation of the head and neck is principally accomplished by inspection and palpation, supplemented by percussion and auscultation to a limited degree. Nursing assessment of the functional abilities of the patient includes observing for appropriateness of facial expressions.

TOPOGRAPHICAL ANATOMY

As seen from front or back, the head, face, and neck are nearly perfectly symmetrical on the right and left sides. Slight normal differences should be readily discernible to the observer. Viewed from the side, the short cervical portion of the spine is seen to have an anterior concavity (Figure 9.1).

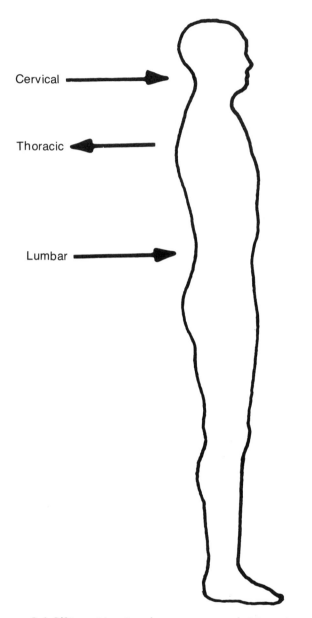

Figure 9.1 Silhouette showing proper upright posture and normal curves of the cervical, thoracic, and lumbar spines.

The sternomastoid muscles, which extend from the sternum (and the medial portion of the clavicles) to the mastoid processes, divide the neck into anterior and posterior cervical triangles (Figure 9.2). The carotid artery (Figure 9.3) courses upward from the thorax, passes under the sternomastoid muscle, and extends to a point just anterior to the angle of the jaw.

The upper portion of the thyroid cartilage (the Adam's apple) is found in the midline of the neck, and the thyroid gland is attached to its lower portion and to the trachea (Figure 9.4). Below the thyroid cartilage, the trachea extends

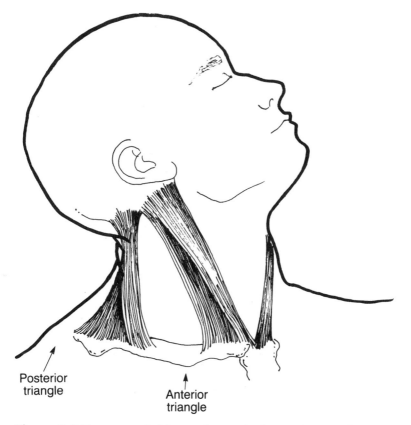

Posterior
triangle

Anterior
triangle

Figure 9.2 Sternomastoid muscle: anterior and posterior cervical triangles.

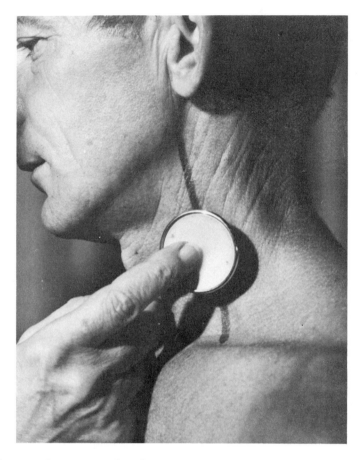

Figure 9.3 Auscultation for carotid bruit. The line marks the course of the artery in the neck.

down the midline into the thorax. Because it angles posterior-ly, the trachea lies several centimeters behind the sternal plate as it enters the thorax.

PHYSIOLOGY

Because of its musculature and structure, the face is normally quite mobile, producing familiar facial expressions indicative of an individual's physical and emotional state.

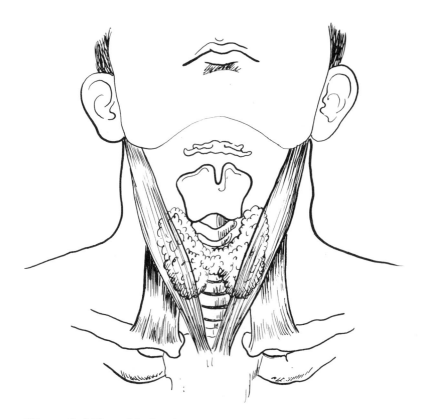

Figure 9.4 Thyroid gland.

The head moves on the cervical spine, which should be
flexible enough to allow the closed jaw to touch the chest in
flexion and to reach the plane of the ears in hyperextension.
In rotation, the jaw reaches laterally over the right and left
shoulders without difficulty, and in lateral flexion the head
tilts approximately 45° to either side (per JRS, RPT, DOM)
(Figure 9.5).

EXAMINATION

Head

The normal shape and size of the head vary considerably from individual to individual. Although there are no measurement guides for head size of the adult as there are for infants and children, the observer will have little difficulty in judging an abnormal variation simply because of a lifetime of experience.

Brief palpation of the scalp and underlying skull is ordinarily adequate to identify the presence of underlying tenderness and the character of the hair. Of course, if there is a history of persistent itching of the scalp, localized pain, or a history of old or recent head trauma, both inspection and palpation will be much more detailed.

Percussion is not performed routinely. If, however, the patient has given a history suggestive of sinusitis or of persistent headaches localized to a particular region, percussion should be done. Here, blunt percussion with the fingertip or a knuckle may elicit tenderness signifying some underlying pathology.

Auscultation is not performed routinely in the examination. Infrequently, patients may complain of a distinct humming somewhere in the cranium and in such circumstances, auscultation of the skull should be performed, preferably with the bell of the stethoscope. The presence of a *bruit* may indicate an underlying vascular brain lesion. Bruit literally means "noise" and the term generally refers to a vascular sound produced over an artery or aneurysm. The term *murmur* (see Chapter 14) is commonly reserved for a specific abnormal cardiac sound either heard over the heart or transmitted along the larger arteries to some distant location.

The Face

In addition to the general skin lesions described in Chapter 8, a few other items are of special interest in the facial area. Pallor, which may be seen elsewhere, is particularly prominent in the face, and cyanosis is readily seen in the mucous membrane of the lips. Flushing due to fever and blushing are best seen in the face. Observe the face for emotional

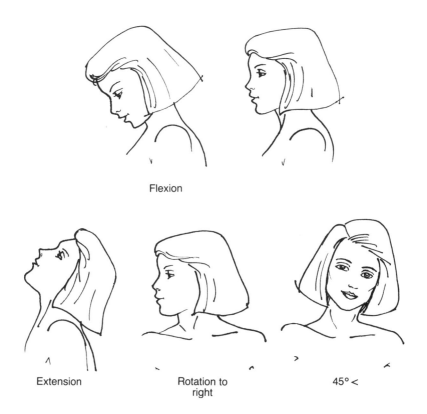

Flexion

Extension

Rotation to right

45° <

Figure 9.5 Rotation of head.

reaction, ability to sustain eye contact, expressions of anger, sadness, or inappropriate mood swings. Hypothyroidism, in addition to producing a coarse, thickened facial skin, often modifies the patient's countenance to a dull, sleepy expression (Figure 9.6). This is in contrast to the excited staring or startled expression often associated with hyperthyroid states. Another characteristic organic change of expression is the "masklike" face of the patient with Parkinson's disease.

The facial muscles should be carefully observed for significant asymmetry. Bell's palsy, a paralysis of the seventh (facial) cranial nerve, leads to smoothing out of the forehead and cheek, sagging of the lower eyelid, and drooping of the

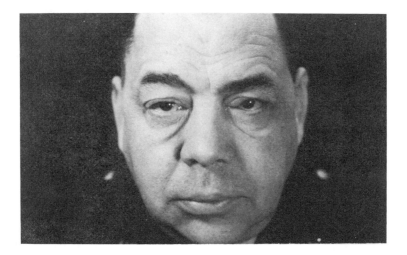

Figure 9.6 Myxedema facies. Note the dull appearance and the edema of the eyelids.

mouth of the involved side. Small degrees of paralysis may be present without much asymmetry when the face is at rest, so routinely the patient should be asked to shut his eyes, clench his jaw, and show his teeth. The presence of unilateral facial weakness will become obvious when only one side of the mouth can be raised or one eyelid does not fully close (Figure 9.7). (This technique of testing for weakness of muscles by having the patient put them into action is a general one and should be used whenever muscle groups are being examined.) Similar findings, although of lesser extent, may be seen in the facial muscles after a stroke involving the nucleus of the seventh cranial nerve.

Palpation of the face is generally reserved for the investigation of painful areas or swellings. Enlargement of one or both parotid glands, which occurs in mumps, is a common cause of swelling of the cheeks in children and young adults. The enlarged gland is palpably firm and tender. The face should be touched *lightly* in several places on both sides to be sure that the patient has no areas of anesthesia or significant differences in touch sensation from one side to the other.

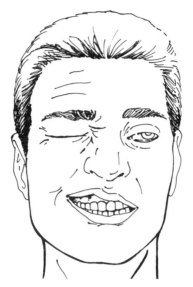

Figure 9.7 Bell's palsy.

The Neck

A complete examination of the neck must include inspection and palpation of the skin, cervical spine, muscles, blood vessels, thyroid area, and trachea. Masses in or under the skin should be searched for and carefully reported.

Skin. As elsewhere in the body, the skin is inspected and palpated for changes in color and texture, for scars, and for the presence of lesions.

Cervical Spine and Muscles. The curve of the cervical spine is inspected to see if it is exaggerated or absent. Active range of motion (ROM) is tested by having the patient move his head in flexion and hyperextension, in rotation, and in lateral flexion, as described earlier. Limitation of motion may be due to arthritis of the spine or to muscular stiffness or weakness. Evaluation of muscle strength is performed by having the patient attempt movements of the head against moderate resistance by the examiner's hand.

Blood Vessels. Veins of the neck ordinarily are not full except when the patient is recumbent, and they do not pulsate.

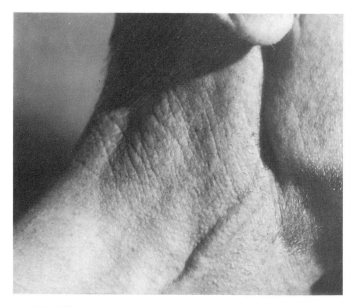

Figure 9.8 Dilation of neck veins with patient sitting up.

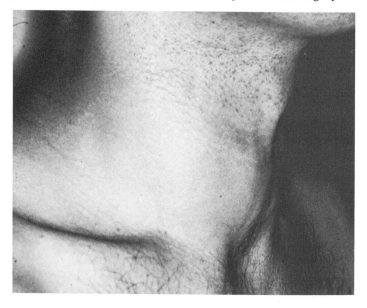

Figure 9.9 Enlargement of the thyroid gland. Note the position of the thyroid gland in relation to the prominence of the thyroid cartilage.

Engorgement of veins in the Fowler's or the upright position is evidence of increased venous pressure due to obstruction or to right heart failure (Figure 9.8). Pulsation of veins (be sure that this is not simply due to pulsation of the carotid artery) may be evidence of cardiac disease and *must* be reported. The carotid arteries should be palpated for forcefulness and for equality. Because some individuals have a particularly sensitive carotid sinus reflex, palpation should be done lightly on one side at a time to avoid production of bradycardia or, in rare instances, syncope. If carotid pulses are unequal, weak, or absent, auscultation should be done to check for a bruit (see Figure 9.3). Also, if certain cardiac murmurs are found, it is advisable to listen over the carotid arteries to see if the murmur is transmitted upward into the carotid arteries. Detection of an absent carotid pulse, with or without a bruit, is suggestive of partial or complete carotid artery occlusion, a most important finding.

Thyroid Gland. As is evident in Figure 9.4, the gland lies at the lower pole of the thyroid cartilage and the upper trachea. Gross enlargement (goiter) may be seen on inspection (Figure 9.9). Palpation is performed to evaluate a visibly enlarged gland for its consistency and for the presence of nodules, and palpation is routinely done to detect lesser enlargements. While there are several techniques for palpation of the thyroid gland, they all follow the principles of adequate exposure, comparison of one side of the gland to the other, and the use of motion of the gland through the fingers. A satisfactory technique is to press gently on one side of the gland, displacing the larynx and trachea laterally (Figure 9.10). The opposite side is then well-exposed and is palpated lightly. Then, keeping the fingers lightly in place, ask the patient to swallow. This motion will move the gland past the fingertips and will help to identify nodules, if present. The gland may be examined with the examiner standing behind (Figure 9.11) or in front of the patient. Both techniques should be learned. The normal thyroid gland is so soft that its lobes are hardly palpable. Thus, detection of tissue in the proper location, which moves on swallowing, is possible evidence of thyroid enlargement and should be reported. If one or both lobes of the gland are enlarged, auscultation over the enlarged area may detect a bruit due to the great increase in blood flow to an overactive gland.

Trachea. This is inspected and palpated primarily to determine if it lies properly in the midline and several centimeters behind the sternum (Figure 9.12). The trachea should be directly posterior to the suprasternal notch and far enough posterior to allow a fingertip to be inserted between it and the sternum. Displacement from this normal location must be reported, as it may be due to shifting of the lung, or to tumor.

Lymph Nodes. Nodes of the face and neck are grouped in four general areas, each of which should be carefully palpated for lymphadenopathy (Figure 9.13): under the jaw, in the anterior triangle of the neck, in the posterior triangle, and in the supraclavicular space. Occasionally, nodes may be found anterior or posterior to the ear lobe. If palpable, lymph nodes should be described using the criteria noted in the previous chapter.

RECORDING

Head: symmetrical, normocephalic; normal hair distribution

Face: no muscle weakness; appropriate facial expression; touch intact

Neck: full ROM; veins not distended; carotid pulsations equal and of good quality; thyroid not palpable; trachea midline; no lymphadenopathy

POTENTIAL NURSING DIAGNOSES

Self-concept, disturbance in

Body image, disturbance

Anxiety

Ineffective thermoregulation

PATIENT PROBLEM

Mrs. Jean R., a 25-year-old white mother of three young boys presents with a CC "sore throat for 3 weeks."

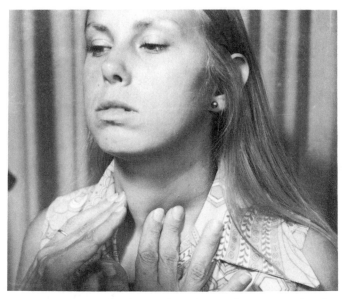

Figure 9.10 Palpation of the right lobe of the thyroid gland. The examiner is displacing the larynx to the right and palpating with his left fingertips.

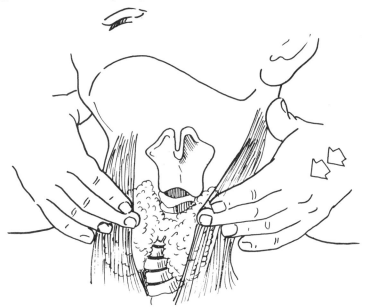

Figure 9.11 Thyroid exam posterior.

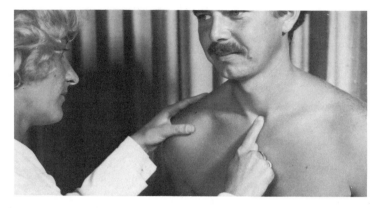

Figure 9.12 Palpation of the trachea. The trachea is felt directly posterior to the suprasternal notch and several centimeters behind the sternum.

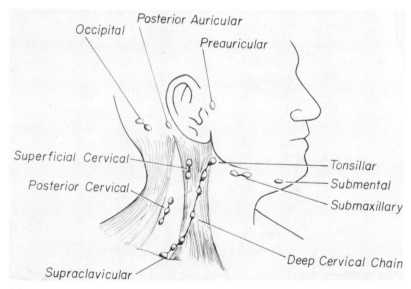

Figure 9.13 Lymph nodes of the face and neck.

Problem: Sore Throat

S: Three weeks ago noted cold symptoms; slight cough, sore throat, swollen glands, slight fever, aches, and fatigue. Since two of her youngsters were ill, she was unable to get rest. One week ago, when symptoms remained, she had CBC and throat culture by personal MD; both negative; has slept poorly, feels tired, depressed, irritable; appetite OK; has lost 6 lb in 2 wk; still has sore throat, thinks she had "palpitation of heart," has difficulty in swallowing, hoarseness, constant achy pain over anterior neck, radiating to both ears.

O: VS: Temp. 37.8°C (100°F); Pulse 130; Resp. 24; BP 120/80.

Insp: pale, thin, well-developed white woman who appears older than stated age; skin moist, nails bitten and ungroomed; hair thick and normally distributed; no eye changes; restless; poor eye contact.

Palp: neck: veins not distended; carotid pulsations strong, rapid and 'equal; ROM limited; unable to flex to chin, turn to shoulders, or hyperextend without pain; thyroid palpable, tender and generally firm to hard; no masses noted; cervical lymph nodes under jaw are palpable and tender; no other lymphadenopathy.

ASSESSMENT: In view of clinical manifestations of mild hyperthyroidism, negative throat culture with normal white count, thyroiditis is suspected.

Nursing Diagnosis: Nutritional, alteration in: less than body requirements, due to metabolic disturbance. Sleep pattern disturbance, due to metabolic disturbance.

PLAN: Goals: Diagnosis established.
Patient will be able to sleep and rest.
Patient will regain lost weight.
Nursing Orders:
Diagnostic: CBC, T_3, T_4, SMA-12; chest x-ray; consult with a physician.
Therapeutic: Complete bed rest, encourage fluids and high-vitamin, high-caloric diet with supplements, provide for family assessment by social services.
Referral to nutritionist.

Patient Education: Discuss need for period of bed rest and diet supplementation with patient and husband.

IMPLEMENTATION: Since no other family member available for assistance, referral made through social service for part-time homemaker.

EVALUATION: Diagnosis of thyroiditis confirmed. Plans made for child care by social services 4 hours per day.
Patient and husband met with nutritionist and understand dietary supplementation.

chapter 10

The Eyes

Topographical Anatomy

Physiology

Examination

Recording

Potential Nursing Diagnoses

Patient Problem

The eyes may readily reveal to the observer many clues to the physical and emotional status of the patient. They may, in their appearance or upon examination, reflect evidence of local or systemic disease processes. Any abnormal findings, or history of pain or loss of vision requires referral to a physician immediately.

TOPOGRAPHICAL ANATOMY

The eye is composed of the eyeball (Figure 10.1) and accessory structures, including the eyebrows, eyelids, conjunctivae, lacrimal apparatus, and extraocular muscles. These are set into the orbits, the bony sockets of the skull, which provide protection for this entire structure.

133

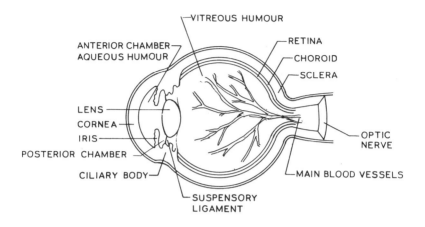

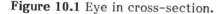

Figure 10.1 Eye in cross-section.

The Eyeball

The outer hard coat is the *sclera* (the white of the eye) to which the eye muscles are attached. The anterior portion of the sclera extends outward in the convex curve and becomes the transparent *cornea*. The middle coat includes the *choroid,* a muscular thickening extended from the choroid, and a suspensory ligament which supports the elastic capsule that encloses the lens of the eye. The ciliary muscle changes the shape of the lens and thus alters the refraction of light rays. The *conjunctiva* is a fine transparent membrane divided into two portions, the palpebral conjunctiva, which lines the inner lid surfaces, and the bulbar conjunctiva which covers the globe of the eye up to the *limbus* (the junction of the cornea and the sclera). Small blood vessels and nerves penetrate the sclera and may be visible as tiny dark dots about a 0.5 cm outside the limbus. These are more prominent in dark-complexioned persons. The *iris* is a round, pigmented disc, continuous with the ciliary body, containing the *pupil.* The innermost coat of the eyeball is the *retina,* a complex sensory organ. This will be described in association with the examination of the ocular fundus.

Accessory Structures

The accessory structures include the eyebrow and the upper and lower eyelids, which normally cover the eye completely when closed. When the eyelids are open and the patient is gazing straight ahead, the lower lid meets the iris, while the upper lid covers a small fraction (2-3 mm) of the iris. The free edges of the eyelids carry the eyelashes and lubricating glands (Figure 10.2).

PHYSIOLOGY

Mechanics of Vision

Vision depends upon light rays that enter the eye and, passing through the cornea and pupil, are then focused on the retina by the lens. Muscular activity of the iris regulates the size of the pupil, and therefore, the amount of light that enters the eye. The pupil will *constrict* in response to bright light and *widen* when looking from a near object to one in the distance (accommodation). The lens is pulled by the ciliary muscle to change its shape as needed so that the light rays will focus properly on the retina even though the object being viewed moves farther away from or nearer to the eye. Any event that interferes with the ability of light rays to focus on the retina will result in blurred vision.

In binocular vision, the light rays from an object normally strike corresponding points on the two retinas. The two somewhat differing images are interpreted by the brain as a single fused image. In the event that there are two images seen, for whatever reason, *diplopia* is said to be present.

Color blindness occurs in about 8% of the male population. It is due to the absence of certain color-receptive cones in the retina. It is an inherited recessive trait and sex-linked; color blindness occurs in less than 0.5% of the female population.

Tearing

Blinking, which normally occurs several times per minute, carries lacrimal gland secretions over the eye, bathing it continuously and carrying dust and foreign bodies to the inner

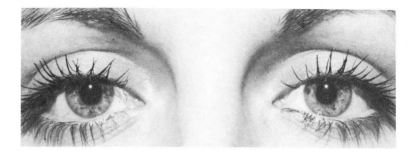

Figure 10.2 Note the normal palpebral fissures in which both lids are equally separated. The lids are in normal relationship to the iris. The pupils are perfectly round and are equally and moderately dilated.

or media angle (canthus), where they can be readily removed. The nasolacrimal duct opening on the lower lid margin at the inner canthus drains away the tears into the nasopharynx.

Extraocular Movements (EOM)

The motions of the eyeball are controlled by six pairs of extraocular muscles which are innervated by cranial nerves III, IV, and VI. Both eyes normally focus on the same point ard, at a distance (6 m or more), the visual axes of the eyes are essentially parallel. The eyes normally operate together, moving simultaneously in the same direction when tracking an object at a distance (conjugate movements), and moving symmetrically inward (nasally), when tracking an object nearing the nose (convergence). *Divergence* (strabismus) is an abnormal condition in which both eyes do not fix at the same point either at rest or while in motion (Figure 10.3).

EXAMINATION

The complete examination of the eye includes inspection of external structures, measurement of visual acuity, determination of visual fields, evaluation of extraocular

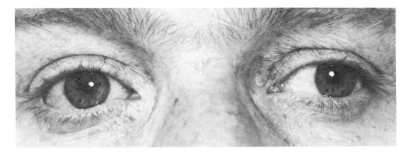

Figure 10.3 Strabismus or divergence. Note the increased amount of sclera visible in the left nasal angle, and the different positions of the spot of the reflected flash between the right and left eyes. Compare with the symmetrical positions of the light reflections in Figure 10.2.

motion, estimation of intraocular pressure, and exploration of the ocular fundus. Development of skill in estimation of intraocular pressure and exploration of the ocular fundus will require special instruction and a good deal of intensive practice.

Inspection of External Structures

Eyebrows and Eyelashes

The quantity, distribution, color, and texture of the eyebrow and eyelashes should be determined, keeping in mind the fact that tweezing, makeup, and false eyelashes are the rule rather than the exception for today's woman. The complete absence of eyebrows and lashes, however, may be due to disease, an inherited characteristic, or a manifestation of severe neurotic behavior in which the individual unconsciously removes the hairs.

Eyelash follicles can become infected, producing a painful red *sty* (hordeolum). A painless cystlike mass in the eyelid is usually a *chalazion* — a mass of collected debris due to an obstructed meibomian gland. When infected, it becomes uncomfortable and annoying, so the patient should be referred for treatment.

Eyelids

Very frequent or very infrequent blinking should be noted. Inspect the external surface of the eyelids for any abnormalities in color, lesions, superficial vascularity, or the presence of edema. Because the skin of the eyelid is very thin and loosely attached to underlying tissue, edema can readily occur as a result of a wide variety of systemic and local disturbances. For example, eyelid edema is a common sign in allergic reactions, glomerulonephritis, hypothyroidism, and cavernous sinus obstruction (see Figures 9.6 and 10.5).

Be certain to observe whether the eyelids close completely, for when this function is impaired, as in Bell's palsy, or in the unconscious patient, corneal drying occurs, leading to ulceration, scarring, and loss of vision, unless preventive measures are taken.

The palpebral fissure of each eye should be compared for symmetry (see Figure 10.2). Ptosis (drooping of the upper lid) may be a congenital condition or an early sign of involvement of the third cranial nerve (Figure 10.4). Observe the position of the lids for eversion (ectropion) and inversion (entropion). Lashes that are misdirected into the eye may cause corneal irritation.

Eyeballs

The globes are inspected to determine if they lie deep in the socket (enophthalmos) or if they project forward (exophthalmos or proptosis). Enophthalmos is often due to dehydration and is frequently associated with an abnormal softness or "mushiness" of the eyeballs to palpation.

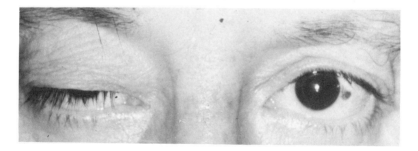

Figure 10.4 Ptosis of the right eyelid. The spot on the temporal side of the left eye is a subconjunctival hemorrhage.

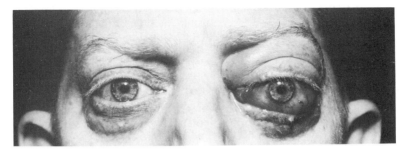

Figure 10.5 Unilateral exophthalmos. Note the edema of the upper and lower lids and the severe conjunctivitis of the involved eye.

Exophthalmos may be suspected if sclera can be seen between the upper lid and the iris. This may be due to actual protrusion of the eyeball, or to stare, in which the patient unconsciously raises the upper lid. Stare can usually be eliminated by asking the patient to gaze into the distance without focusing on any specific object. True early exophthalmos may be difficult to determine, but if it is suspected, the patient should be referred for accurate measurement. Greater degrees of exophthalmos, which do not allow for full closure of the lids, are dangerous since corneal drying may occur, as mentioned previously. Exophthalmos is also important to recognize because it is usually due to hyperthyroidism or to tumor behind the eyeball. Occasionally, the exophthalmos is unilateral (Figure 10.5).

Palpation for Ocular Tension

Abnormal hardness or softness of the globe is detected by gentle palpation. Softness, as noted above, is often related to dehydration and enophthalmos. *Glaucoma* is a serious condition in which there is increased resistance to aqueous humor outflow at the iridocorneal junction, resulting in the buildup of intraocular pressure. As the pressure rises, the retinal artery is compressed, reducing blood flow to the retina. Permanent progressive atrophy of the retina and optic nerve ensues, resulting in blindness if treatment is not instituted.

Although adequate examination for glaucoma (which should be done annually in all individuals over age 40) requires a tonometer, screening by simple palpation for eyeball tension can be performed (Figure 10.6). The patient is directed to look downward, moving the cornea down, and the tip of the examiner's middle finger is placed on the patient's forehead to steady his hand while the index finger is placed on the upper eyelid. *Gentle* downward pressure is applied on the eyeball with the index finger to feel for excessive hardness.

Conjunctivae

Examine both the palpebral conjunctivae lining the lids and the bulbar conjunctivae covering the sclerae. Adequate examination of the lower portions of the membrane can be obtained by pulling the skin below the lower lid downward and having the patient look up. If necessary because of symptoms, or conjunctivitis, the upper portions of the conjunctivae can be visualized by eversion of the upper lid. This may be accomplished by the following procedure:

1. With the patient looking down, grasp the upper lashes and pull downward gently; push down gently on the upper tarsal border with an applicator, finger, or tongue blade, and evert the lid by bringing the lashes to the brow.
2. When inspection is complete, remove the applicator and gently pull the lashes forward and downward as the patient is directed to look up.

Dilation of the small blood vessels (injection) causes the characteristic redness of *conjunctivitis* (Figure 10.7; also see Figure 10.5). A small degree of injection is normally seen at both angles of the eye.

Sclerae

Observe the sclerae for color change. Normally they are white; however, they may be yellow-tinged with jaundice or (rarely), if the sclerae are quite thin, they will be blue.

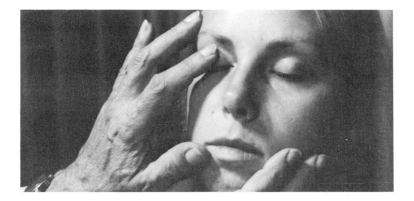

Figure 10.6 Palpation of the eyeball for ocular tension.

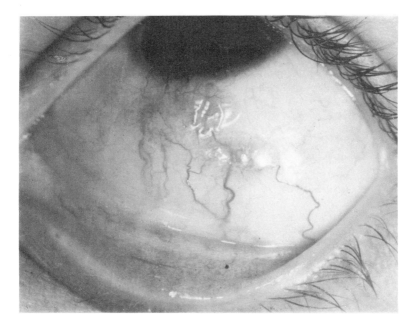

Figure 10.7 Severe conjunctivitis secondary to inflammatory disease of the iris, choroid, and sclera. Note the petechia in the lower lid.

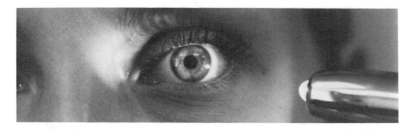

Figure 10.8 Examination of the cornea by lateral lighting.

Scleral color should always be reported, whether normal or not. Fatty deposits in the sclerae of dark-skinned patients may mistakenly lead the examiner to conclude that jaundice is present, since these deposits often take on a yellowish hue.

Cornea and Iris

The cornea is an organ that may be the site of abrasions that interfere with its transparency and subsequently affect the individual's visual capacity. The cornea should be inspected from the side with a flashlight for scars, irregularities, and for the presence of foreign bodies (Figure 10.8). Superficial irregularities create the appearance of a defect in the light reflection on the surface. A common finding in older persons is the deposition of an arc or circle of gray material in the cornea a few millimeters within the limbus. This is *arcus senilis* (see Figure 27.1), which may or may not be of clinical significance. Of distinct significance, however, is the presence of a ring of greenish golden pigment just inside the limbus. These are Kayser-Fleisher rings and are associated with a disorder known as Wilson's disease, in which there is serious neurologic and liver damage.

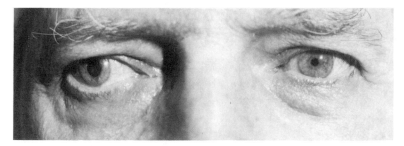

Figure 10.9 Inequality of pupil size. Note also the strabismus.

Pupils

Normally, the pupils are of equal size (see Figure 10.2) and, in a room of average illumination, will not be widely dilated or pinpoint in size. The inner margins should be smooth, forming a perfect circle. Significant inequality greater than 0.5 to 1 mm in difference is called *anisocoria* (Figure 10.9); 20% of the population has anisocoria. It does not always represent serious disease.

The test for *reaction to light* is performed by shining a bright light into each pupil and watching for pupillary constriction. The light is brought rapidly into the field of vision from the side to avoid having the patient looking at the light as it approaches. Shine the light into one pupil, and note the response of that pupil (direct reaction). The normal constriction should be prompt, not sluggish or absent. Repeat this procedure in the same eye, this time watching the other pupil, which should also constrict, although to a lesser degree (consensual reaction). It is important to test for this direct and consensual reaction in *both* eyes. Pupils constrict with accommodation, a result of contraction of the ciliary body, which relaxes the zonules and increases the lens size. This clears the image from distant focus to near focus.

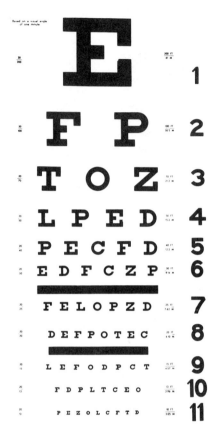

Figure 10.10 The Snellen chart. The bar below the letters of line 6 is colored green and that below line 8 is red. Asking the patient to "read the letters over the red line" will quickly identify the patient's color perception, and if he reads the letters correctly, he has 20/20 vision in the tested eye.

Visual Acuity

Distant visual acuity and color vision are best tested with the familiar eye chart (Snellen chart, American Optical Company, Figure 10.10). If the patient uses corrective lenses for distant vision, he should wear them for this examination. Test one eye at a time by having the patient cover the other eye with a card, not his hand, to avoid peeking. The patient

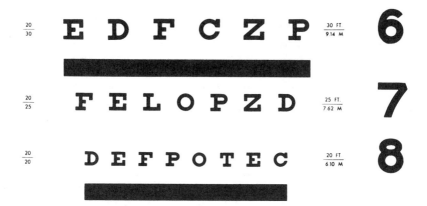

Figure 10.11 The Snellen chart, lines 6 through 8. Note distance in feet and meters in the border to your right, and visual acuity for each test line on the left.

is placed at the test distance just 20 ft (6.1 m) from the chart and is asked to read lines of smaller and smaller letters until he can no longer read almost all the letters in one line.

The recording system is expressed in relative fraction form. Until the metric system comes into general use, record visual acuity by the common system, in feet. The chart is so constructed (Figure 10.11) that the number in feet or meters in the right margin represents the theoretical distance from which a person with normal distant vision could have read that line accurately. Thus, if the patient can read all (or almost all) of the letters in the test line 8, vision in the tested eye is normal, or 20/20. He has read, from a distance of *20 ft,* what a normal eye should be able to read at *20 ft.* If, however, the patient can read the letters of line 6 but not line 7, vision in the tested eye is 20/30, since he has read at 20 ft what the normal can read at the greater distance of 30 ft.

Record vision in each eye separately, viz.: Right eye (OD) 20/70, left (OS) 20/40. If either eye tests *below* 20/20, the patient should be asked to read the smallest letters he can with both eyes open; (viz.: Both eyes [OU] 20/40). If no Snellen (or similar) chart is available, the examiner should try to test distant vision with anything at hand. Large letters in newspaper headlines, textbook titles, labels on equipment boxes, etc., may be used for a crude test.   Place the object at any distance at which you can just read the letters clearly and compare the patient's ability to read from the same distance.   While such a test cannot *measure* the patient's distant vision, it can give a clue as to the patient's need for referral for a proper examination.   Since the Snellen chart tests distant vision, the use of a small commercial pocket card is useless for this purpose.   Near vision may be tested readily by use of the small print in a newspaper or magazine.   Newsprint should be able to be read at 15-30 cm (6-12 in).   If the patient uses reading glasses, they should be worn for this test.   Inability to read clearly at less than 30 cm warrants referral for refraction.   The term myopia means near-sightedness and means simply that, without glasses, the myope sees better at near than at far.

Visual Fields

These are superficially tested by comparing the patient's peripheral vision with your own, by noting when both you and the patient can see an object as it enters into the field of vision.   Place yourself about 1 m from the patient and at about the same height, so that your eyes are at the same level.   Test one eye at a time by having the patient close one eye (i.e., his left) while you close the opposite eye (i.e., your right).   Instruct the patient to keep his eye on yours so that you are both looking straight forward.   Then extend your arms wide apart, placing your hands and raised index finger on a line midway between yourself and the patient (Figure 10.12).   Now move your hands slowly together, asking the patient to notify you as soon as he sees either finger.   Wiggling the index finger may assist in being certain that both of you actually see the target.   The procedure is then repeated to test the horizontal fields of vision by moving a finger from above and from below the head (Figure 10.13).   This technique is known as gross *confrontation* and any significant reduction of the patient's fields must be confirmed by a specialist.

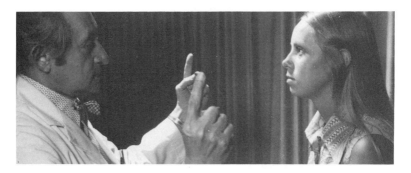

Figure 10.12 Testing of horizontal fields of vision by gross confrontation. The fingertips must be midway between the examiner and the patient.

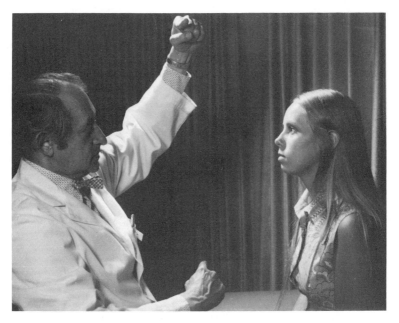

Figure 10.13 Testing of vertical fields of vision. Notice that the patient and the examiner are both looking directly at each other's eyes.

Extraocular Movements (EOM)

The positions of the eyeballs are examined both at rest and in motion. Simple inspection may detect strabismus (see Figure 10.3) but a better test is examination of the corneal light reflection (or reflex). Stand about 1 m in front of the patient, and direct the beam of a small flashlight or penlight into the patient's eyes. The corneal light reflection should be seen in almost the same location in each of the patient's eyes (see Figure 10.2). If the patient's visual axes are not parallel, the corneal light reflex will not be symmetrical and will indicate strabismus (see Figures 10.3, 10.5, and 10.9). If this condition is of recent origin, the patient may have complained of diplopia. In longstanding divergence, the patient will have learned to suppress the vision in one of his eyes.

If the history has elicited a complaint of diplopia, one additional test for minor degrees of strabismus should be performed. This is the *cover* test. The patient is instructed to look at a fixed point (a mark on the wall, small light source, etc.) and the examiner then covers one eye with a card or his hand. Watch the uncovered eye for movement, for if it does move, it was not looking straight at the fixed point. Repeat the test, covering the other eye. Any move of either eye suggests a small degree of strabismus. The eyeballs should then be examined in motion. With the examiner directly in front of the patient, ask the patient to follow the movement of a fingertip or point of a pencil without turning his head (Figure 10.14). A simple rapid test can be done by tracing an imaginary circle in front of the patient, large enough to move the eyes to their full range of motion, horizontally and vertically. A more precise technique is to trace a large letter H. Move the target finger horizontally to the left, until the patient's eyes are at extreme gaze in that direction. From that position, trace upward and downward. Next, move the finger horizontally to the extreme right, and then move it up and down on that side. This maneuver will test all of the six extraocular muscles of each eye, separately.

Failure of either eye to follow any of these movements smoothly and symmetrically should be carefully recorded. Watch for *nystagmus* — a rhythmic jerking motion of the eyes — when the eyes are in extreme lateral or upward gaze. Lesions of any of the pertinent cranial nerves may result in divergency, convergence, or diplopia. Test for *convergence*

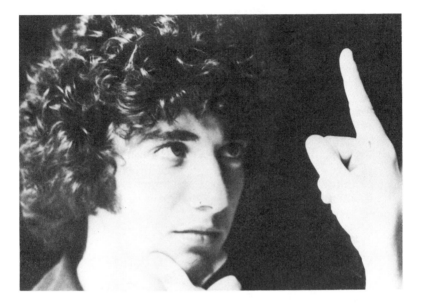

Figure 10.14 Test for extraocular motion.

by bringing the fingertip toward the patient's nose. The normal individual should be able to keep both eyes fixed on the target as it is brought to within 15 cm of the eyes.

Ophthalmoscopy (Fundoscopy)

There is no doubt that ophthalmoscopic examination presents one of the greatest challenges to the student whose aim is skill in physical assessment. Certainly no textbook can provide the beginner with adequate preparation for this objective. Only through the assistance of an instructor and continuous practice can some degree of competence be attained. Practice with specially designed models is useful.

Inspection of the interior of the eye through the ophthalmoscope is of importance in evaluation of local disorders (e.g., cataract, retinal detachment) or of systemic diseases (e.g., diabetes mellitus, hypertension). In the ocular fundus, the examiner can directly see a nerve (the optic disc), arterioles, venules, and the retinal pigment epithelium since the retina is a transparent structure.

The Ophthalmoscope

This is basically a simple instrument that projects a narrow beam of light and has a small aperture through which the examiner can look along the beam (Figure 10.15). There is a set of about 22 lenses (depending on the model) that can be rotated into the aperture. Usually, there are about 11 convex lenses, identified by black numerals ranging from +20 diopters (D) to +1 D, one zero (plano) lens with no correction, and about 10 concave lenses (red numbers) from -1 D to -20 D. The lenses are used to focus on different parts of the patient's eye, and to adjust for myopia or presbyopia in either the examiner's or the patient's eye. Many models have a small wheel below the lens wheel that modifies the projected beam. There are settings for a narrow light beam, a wider light beam, a grid, a very narrow slit, and a red-free filter. The beginning practitioner is advised by most experts to ignore all but the wide light beam.

Technique of Examination

Introduction. The student should understand the principles of the examination at this point, although examination should not actually be tried until one is familiar with the structures of the ocular fundus and some of the major abnormalities. This familiarity should be obtained by examining color photographs or color slides. There are several atlases available that provide excellent photographs and descriptions. The light beam from the ophthalmoscope passes through the cornea, aqueous humor of the anterior chamber, lens, vitreous humor, and strikes the retina (see Figure 10.1). Light is then reflected through the transparent structures to the examiner's eye. In this way the clinician can evaluate the clarity of the media through which the light must pass, and also can see the structures that make up the fundus of the eye. The image of the optic disc, blood vessels, and retina (the fundus or eyegrounds) is greatly magnified by the lens of the patient's own eye.

The Question of Eye Glasses. If the examiner wears glasses or contact lenses for moderate correction of distant vision, he may either learn to do the examination wearing these, or he must find the appropriate correction with the ophthalmoscope lenses. Once having determined the proper setting allowing him to be in sharp focus on the retina of pa-

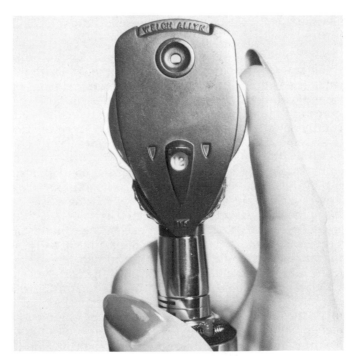

Figure 10.15 The ophthalmoscope. The examiner's index finger is on the lens disc and a black +12 diopter lens has been set in the small viewing aperture above.

tients with no refractive error, he uses this setting each time an examination is begun. However, if the examiner's glasses correct for astigmatism, or for a large error of refraction, he should wear glasses.

Dilation of the Pupils. A more thorough and careful examination can be done through dilated pupils, and dilation should be done if there is no contraindication. If there is *no* scarring of the iris, or evidence of *glaucoma* (i.e., previous diagnosis, history of seeing colored rings when looking at lights, acute attacks of eye pain, or hard eyeballs on palpation), it is safe to dilate the pupils. A drop or two of tropicamide (Mydriacyl) in 1% strength or phenylephrine (Neo-

Synephrine) 2.5% solution will produce adequate dilation in most cases.

General Conditions. The examiner should position himself and his patient so that their eyes are approximately at the same level. One convenient technique is for both to be seated on adjustable stools. The room should be dimly lit — not totally dark. The patient should be instructed to stare straight ahead at some distant spot at about eye level — a light switch, thermostat, etc., or at a mark or tape specifically placed on the wall at the proper location. Holding the ophthalmoscope in his *right* hand, the clinician examines the patient's *right* eye; he reverses this procedure for examination of the left eye. The index finger should be on the lens wheel, so that different lens settings can be made during the examination. With the head of the scope steadied against his brow or nose, and his free hand stabilizing the patient's head, the examiner begins by directing the beam of light into the patient's eye from a distance of about 30-60 cm (Figure 10.16). Here he should pick up the red reflex. Following this reflection, the examiner then moves in until the hand holding the scope nearly touches the patient's cheek. If the patient blinks too frequently, the thumb can be used to elevate the upper lid (Figure 10.17).

If one keeps the red reflex in sight and moves in at about 15° to the patient's line of sight, the optic disc should

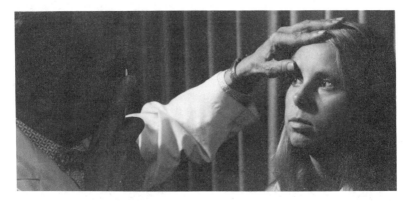

Figure 10.16 Ophthalmoscopy. Examination of the red reflex.

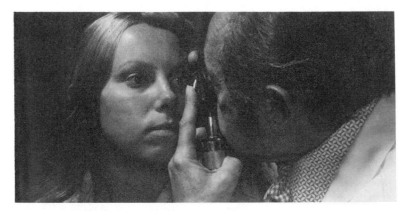

Figure 10.17 Ophthalmoscopy. Examination of the ocular fundus.

come into view. If only retina and vessels are seen, the examiner should track vessels back to the disc to start the examination. If the disc and vessels are not in sharp focus, the lens wheel should be turned in one direction or another until the proper setting is found. Under normal circumstances, all of the fundus should be in sharp focus at one lens setting (Figure 10.18).

The clinician should learn a pattern of examination in which he examines and notes one portion at a time. The sequence of the following descriptions is a recommended pattern, i.e., red reflex, disc, vessels, and retina (including the macula) in all quadrants.

Examination of the Fundus

Red Reflex. If the cornea, anterior chamber, lens, and posterior chamber are all clear, the examiner should see a red reflection filling the pupil. The color will vary somewhat, depending on the amount of pigment in the fundus, but should be a reddish orange and bright in intensity (Figure 10.19).

Anything that interferes with light transmission or reflection will change the red reflex. For example, a cataract will produce dark lines or black spots; other opacities, such as inflammation or hemorrhage, will produce local cloudiness of the reflection or spots in the reflection. Should such objects be seen interfering with the red reflex, a more detailed

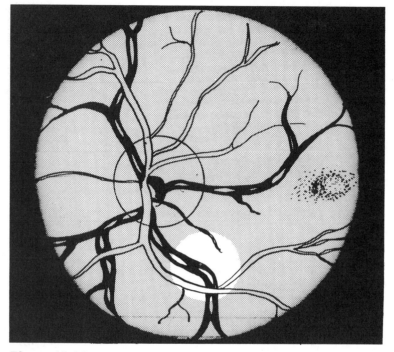

Figure 10.18

view of the opacity may be obtained by using the lens system of the ophthalmoscope. A +20 or +15 lens (black numbers) will enlarge and focus well on lesions of the *cornea, anterior chamber,* and *lens.* Lens settings from +10 to +4 will focus at different portions of the vitreous, while, as noted earlier, a zero lens should focus on the *retina,* if both examiner and patient have normal vision or are wearing corrective lenses. The presence of opacities anywhere in the red reflex warrants referral of the patient for special examination.

   Disc. The flat optic disc (see Figure 10.18) is the head of the optic nerve and is a prominent landmark. It is round or oval, with a disc diameter (DD) of about 1.5 mm. The temporal margin is quite sharp, while the nasal margin is often less clearly defined. The disc is a pale reddish yellow in color, a bit darker on the nasal half, and has a small depression near its center, the physiologic cup.

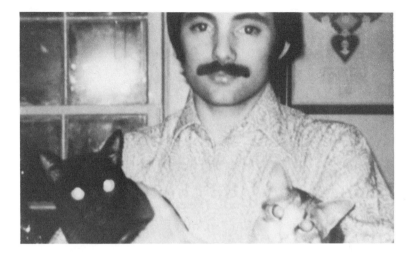

Figure 10.19 Red reflex. An unplanned red reflex resulting from a photoflash bulb. Note also the large "green" reflex from the eyes of the black cat, sometimes seen when car headlights are reflected from the retina of an animal on the road at night.

The cup may not be seen in all patients, but is usually present, is lighter in color than the rest of the disc, and should occupy much less than half of the disc diameter. The relationship between the cup and disc diameters is conveniently expressed as a ratio (Figure 10.20). When the cup enlarges so that the cup/disc ratio is 0.5 or greater, the possibility of glaucoma must be considered, and the patient should be referred to a specialist promptly.

Another significant abnormality of the disc is *papilledema* (see Figure 10.22), caused by increased intracranial pressure (often due to brain tumor). As the name suggests, there is edema of the optic disc, causing it to be raised above the level of the retina, and therefore the disc will not be in sharp focus compared to the retina. The margins of the disc are blurred, the disc itself is hyperemic, and the cup may not be clearly visible. Papilledema represents a sign of current danger, requiring immediate referral.

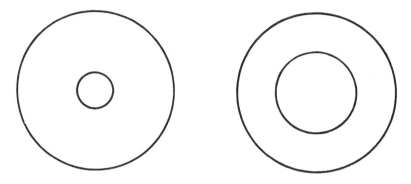

Figure 10.20 Cup/disc ratios. The diagram on the left has a normal ratio (0.2:1.0), while that on the right is suggestive of a glaucomatous cup with a ratio of 0.5:1.0.

Vessels. The central retinal artery arises from the cup and spreads out in smaller and smaller branches to all quadrants of the fundus. These branches are *arterioles.* Venules run roughly parallel to arterioles and reach the retinal vein at the cup. Close observation will often reveal a pulsation of the retinal vein, a normal phenomenon. Arterioles are smaller in diameter and brighter red in color than venules, which are wider and of a purplish red color. In the normal state, an arteriole and venule, at the same distance from the cup, will have an arteriole/venule (A/V) ratio of about 2:3 (see Figure 10.18).

The reflection of light from arterioles generally produces a narrow light streak, while similar reflections from venules are often patchy. Both arterioles and venules spread across the fundus in wide curves and taper down, more or less evenly, until their caliber is so small that they can no longer be seen. There are frequent crossings, most often with the arteriole crossing above the venule. In a normal crossing, the venule is not kinked, and its outline is not changed; there is no indentation of the venule.

Pathology of the vessels is suggested by changes in size and shape of the vessels and by deformity of the venule at a crossing. In hypertension, the arterioles become spastic; they narrow and become tortuous. With narrowing, the A/V ratio, instead of being about 2:3, changes to about 1:2 or 1:3

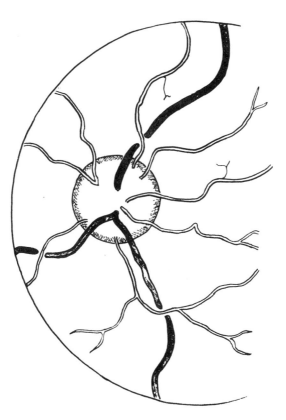

Figure 10.21 Ocular fundus in moderate arterial hypertension. Note the narrowed, somewhat tortuous arteries compared to the veins and the severe compression of the veins at crossing points.

(Figure 10.21). Also, the light streak becomes more prominent so that only a small portion of the arteriole can be seen on either side of the light streak. If narrowing becomes extreme, only the light streak may be seen. As pressure in the arteriole increases, the vessels become more tortuous and, occasionally, they seem to be segmented rather than smoothly tapered.

Kinking or indentation of the venule at a crossing is also abnormal and is referred to as AV nicking. It may become so

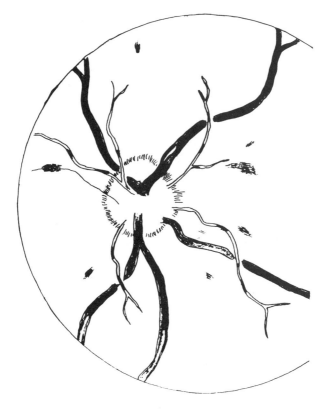

Figure 10.22 Ocular fundus in severe arterial hypertension. Here, the arteries are extremely narrow, are tortuous, and compress the veins. The edges of the optic disc are blurred, indicating bulging of the disc due to increased intracranial pressure. There are numerous flame-shaped hemorrhages visible on the retina.

extreme that a portion of the vein seems obliterated (Figure 10.22). AV nicking is considered to be abnormal only if it occurs at least 1 DD outside the optic disc. This crossing phenomenon is characteristically seen in hypertensive vascular disease and in generalized arteriosclerosis.

   Retina. The color of the retina arises from the blood in the underlying choroid vessels and is modified considerably by melanin pigment of the choroid and retina. Thus, the retinal color may vary from a pink yellow in a light-skinned blonde, to nearly brown in a dark-skinned black individual. The pigment is usually evenly distributed, but occasionally it may be patchy, giving an uneven appearance of the color of the retina. Cyanosis may produce a purplish color, and anemia is a paler red tint.

Hemorrhage into the fundus may appear as flame-shaped deep red spots (see Figure 10.22), as round red spots, or, if there is hemorrhage into the vitreous humor, it may produce a hazy medium that partly obscures the normal sharp appearance of the retina. There are many other variations in the appearance of hemorrhage, depending on the amount and specific location of the bleeding site.

Exudates are grayish white patches on the retina and are classified simply by appearance. "Soft" exudates are often called cotton wool exudates, since they appear to be fluffy and fuzzy in outline. "Hard" exudates are somewhat smaller, lighter in color, and have more discrete borders. Both indicate damage to the retina and must be reported, if present. They occur in various types of diseases such as hypertension, diabetes, and renal disease and, although not diagnostic for any disease, are evidence of general or local abnormalities.

Macula. The macula is a portion of the retina in which the cones are collected in greater number, so that this is the area of maximal visual acuity and of central vision. Due to increased pigmentation, the macula appears darker than the rest of the retina, with even distribution of the pigment throughout. It lies about 1.5 DD from the temporal margin of the disc and is about 1 DD in diameter.

During the examination, when the patient is asked to look directly at the ophthalmoscope light, the macula comes directly into the field, and a tiny pinpoint of bright light can be seen near the center of the macula. This is a reflection from a small depression in the macula, the fovea (see Figure 10.18). Damage to the macula may appear as a patchy increase in pigment with loss of the foveal reflex, hemorrhage, or scar, obliterating some or all of the area. These are always serious because they interfere with central vision.

Eyegrounds in Hypertension. Hypertension is a common problem and much useful information about this disorder can be obtained through fundoscopy. While the level of blood pressure is quite variable from hour to hour or day to day, the retinal changes are relatively permanent. A direct relationship exists between the retinal changes and the severity of the disease. These changes are graded by the criteria of Keith, Wagener, and Barker (often abbreviated as K-W) as follows:

K-W grade 1: arteriolar constriction, increased tortuosity of arterioles

K-W grade 2: grade 1 changes *plus* AV kinking or nicking (see Figure 10.21)

K-W grade 3: grade 2 changes plus retinal hemorrhages or exudates

K-W grade 4: grade 3 changes *plus* papilledema (see Figure 10.22)

Both morbidity and mortality from hypertension are increased as the K-W grade increases. Treatment of severe (i.e., K-W 3 or 4) hypertension may result in slow disappearance of the papilledema and of the exudates and hemorrhages. The arteriolar changes, however, are more or less permanent even with adequate control of the blood pressure.

As indicated at the beginning of the section, fundoscopy is a difficult, complex portion of the physical examination. This section must be considered to be only a brief introduction to the subject and must be pursued by much reading, practice, and instruction. The references at the end of this chapter are recommended for the student who wishes to develop competence in this examination.

RECORDING

Eyes: Lashes and brows present; no stare or ptosis; normal ocular tension; conjunctivae clear; sclerae white; no defects of cornea or iris; pupils equal, round, react to light and accommodation (often abbreviated as PERRLA). Snellen: right eye (OD) 20/20; left eye (OS) 20/20;

color vision intact for red and green; fields normal by confrontation; extraocular movements (EOM) normal; no nystagmus or strabismus

Fundi: Red reflex: clear
Discs: flat with sharp margins; cup normal

Vessels: Arterioles and venules normal; no AV nicking

Retina: No hemorrhages or exudates; macula normal; foveal reflex present

POTENTIAL NURSING DIAGNOSES

Injury: potential for

Mobility, impaired

Sensory-perceptual alteration: visual

Social isolation

PATIENT PROBLEM

An 18-year-old woman presents in college infirmary, brought in by roommate because of severe bilateral eye pain and visual disturbances.

Problem: Eye Pain

S: Has been wearing glasses for distant vision since age 12 and hard contact lenses for past 2 yr, with no previous difficulty; because of social commitments, kept lenses in over 18 hr; awakened from sleep tonight with severe "scratching" pain in both eyes, unable to keep eyes open.

O: Injected conjunctivae; with exam under fluorescein, multiple abrasions noted over both corneas; excessive lacrimation; PERRLA.

ASSESSMENT: Corneal abrasion due to excessive use of contact lenses.

Nursing Diagnosis: Alterations in comfort related to corneal irritation.
Sensory deficit related to "inability to keep eyes open."
Knowledge deficit of contact lens hygiene.

PLAN: Goals: To express relief from discom-
                       fort and be able to resume visual
                       activities.
                       To verbalize importance of following
                       medical regime and hygienic use of
                       contact lenses.
                       Nursing Orders:
                       Diagnostic: None further.
                       Therapeutic: Per protocol: tetra-
                       caine 1% ophthalmic ung. OU;
                       flush with Dacrasol and normal
                       saline Neosporin ophth. ung. OU
                       patch both eyes; refer to ophthal-
                       mologist promptly.
                       Patient Education: Review procedures
                       for wearing contact lenses; reassure
                       re: prognosis; discuss resumption
                       of use only following consultation
                       with ophthalmologist.

IMPLEMENTATION: Follow treatment regime per protocol.
                       Call ophthalmologist for appointment
                       immediately.
                       Discuss medical regime, prognosis,
                       and hygienic care for lenses.

EVALUATION: Patient visited ophthalmologist in after-
                       noon. To return to infirmary in one week.
                       Able to describe appropriate hygienic
                       care of lenses.

chapter 11

The Ear, Nose, Mouth, and Pharynx

The Ear

The Nose

Mouth and Pharynx

Recording

Potential Nursing Diagnoses

Patient Problem

The examination of the ear is principally an inspection of the eardrum, while examination of the nose, mouth, and pharynx is primarily of the mucosa and architecture. Brilliant illumination is essential for viewing these areas which may reflect signs of numerous local afflictions. In addition, the functions of all of these parts must be evaluated carefully.

THE EAR

Topographical Anatomy

The ear is divided into three parts: the external, middle, and inner ear. The external ear consists of the *auricle* (or pinna) and the *external auditory canal* (Figure 11.1). Auricles vary widely in shape and size, but unless very tiny or absent, these variations are usually of no clinical significance. The external auditory canal is about 2.5-3 cm in

163

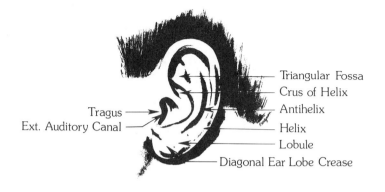

Triangular Fossa
Crus of Helix
Antihelix
Tragus
Ext. Auditory Canal
Helix
Lobule
Diagonal Ear Lobe Crease

Figure 11.1 External ear. The diagonal ear crease is ordinarily not present, but it may be found on one or both lobules.

length; it narrows toward the midportion and widens near the eardrum. Of particular importance is the fact that the first portion of the canal is directed nearly straight into the head, while the remainder of the canal angles medially, anteriorly, and inferiorly. This curve requires the examiner to position the speculum carefully in examination of the eardrum. (It is also the reason that stethoscope earpieces must be tailored to each examiner's external auditory canal.)

The *middle ear* consists of the tympanic membrane (eardrum), the tiny ear bones (ossicles), and an air-filled bony chamber which is connected to the pharynx by the *eustachian tube.* The *inner ear,* which is not accessible to direct examination, is composed of organs that translate sound waves from the outer world into the language of the "upper world" — nerve impulses — carried by the *acoustic branch* of cranial nerve VIII. Also here are the semicircular canals that provide the sense of balance, conducted by the *vestibular branch* of the eighth cranial nerve.

Examination

The auricles are inspected for abnormally small size or absence, malpositioning, skin lesions, and the presence of

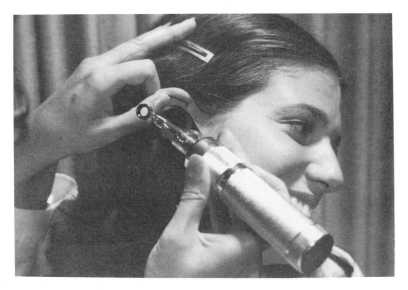

Figure 11.2 Otoscopy. The examiner's left hand is used to position and to hold the patient's head steady, while the thumb and index finger pull the auricle. Holding the otoscope in the fingers prevents too much force from being applied as the speculum is inserted.

nodules. The auricle should also be palpated for nodules; in particular for *tophi* which are hard, pale, nontender nodules usually found in or near the outer fold (helix) or near the lobe of the auricle. These tophi are collections of urate crystals associated with gout. Occasionally these tophi rupture, in which case the examiner will see the chalk-like crystals that make up these nodules. Crystals should be taken for laboratory examination since gout may be diagnosed definitely if uric acid is identified.

Occasionally, a diagonal earlobe crease (Figure 11.1) may be present on one or both ears. If present, it should be reported.

The external auditory canal should be carefully inspected for the presence of blood or discharge of pus or serous fluid *before* using the otoscope. If present, such discharge should be carefully collected on a cotton-tipped applicator and its character recorded.

For examination with the otoscope (Figure 11.2), the patient's head should be tilted and the otoscope held firmly between the thumb and fingers of one hand. The auricle is held by the thumb and index finger of the other hand, with the remaining fingers placed on the patient's head. This latter positioning allows the examiner to steady the patient's head and to pull on the auricle upward and backward.

Pulling the auricle serves two purposes: it tends to straighten the curve of the external auditory canal, making insertion of the otoscope speculum easier, and it may produce tenderness in the ear. The presence of tenderness will alert the examiner to the possibility of infection in the canal or the middle ear. The speculum is then inserted slowly and carefully in the direction of the axis of the canal while the examiner "watches his way in." Blind insertion of the speculum *always* is to be avoided. Cerumen in the external canal, which often appears to be red under the bright light, is a common and normal finding. Unless the wax obstructs too much of the canal for adequate visualization, it may be ignored. Unless you have had special instruction, do not attempt removal of hard, impacted cerumen: simply report that the examination was incomplete.

Watch for the presence of blood, tumors, or foreign bodies as the speculum is pushed gently toward the eardrum. If difficulty is found in inserting the speculum through the canal, pulling slightly more or less on the auricle and varying the angle of tilt of the patient's head may assist in passage.

Only a portion of the tympanic membrane (TM) may be seen from one position, so the angle of the otoscope will need to be changed, being rotated so that the entire drum and annulus can be visualized completely. The drum normally appears as an oval, thin, partly transparent, gray membrane (Figure 11.3). There are three important landmarks of the TM: the annulus, the malleus, and the light reflex. The *annulus* forms the outer border of the drum and is normally much paler in color than the membrane itself.

At the superior portion of the *malleus,* a bright, small knob is readily seen. This is the short process of malleus. The handle of the malleus—largest of the ear bones—angles downward and posteriorly from the annulus to a point (the umbo) at the center of the tympanic membrane. From the umbo a bright cone shaped reflection of light can be seen — the *light reflex.* In cases where the membrane is quite

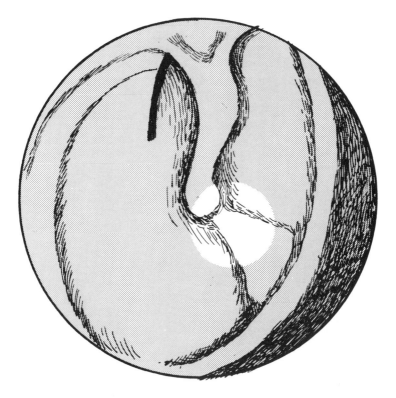

Figure 11.3 Major landmarks of the oval tympanic membrane as seen through the speculum. The dark crescent seen at the right is the wall of the auditory canal.

transparent, a portion of another bone, the incus, may be seen extending downward from the annulus, slightly posterior to the malleus.

Inspection of the Eardrum

Some common abnormal findings are listed in Table 11.1.

Table 11.1 Some Abnormalities of Otoscopy

Finding	Interpretation	Examples
Bright red drum	Inflammation	Acute middle ear infection (otitis media)
Yellowish drum	Pus or serum behind drum	Acute or chronic otitis media
Bluish drum	Blood behind drum	Skull fracture
Bubbles behind drum	Serous fluid in middle ear	Chronic otitis media
Absent light reflex	Bulging of drum	Acute otitis media
Absent or diminished landmarks	Thickening of drum	Chronic otitis media or otitis externa
Oval dark areas	Perforation	Recent or old rupture of drum
Malleus very prominent	Retraction of drum	Obstruction of eustachian tube

Hearing Tests

Despite the fact that the examiner has had much conversation with the patient up to this point, he should perform one specific clinical hearing test. Some patients with hearing loss will, consciously or unconsciously, deny such a loss, or may have been able to compensate for a unilateral loss by a combination of use of the good ear and some basic lipreading.

Clinical tests to evaluate the patient's ability to hear are rather crude in that they can give evidence of a hearing loss but are not adequate to measure the degree of loss. It is our opinion that if the patient has difficulty with any of these simple, nonquantitative, clinical tests, he should be referred for further examination. All of these will test hearing somewhere in the conversational range of hearing (roughly 80-2000 cps), and a defect here may definitely impair a patient's daily life-style. Any one of the following is an adequate screening test but the examiner should become familiar with all of them so that he can select one, depending upon the circumstances. All should be done in a quiet environment, however.

Simplest is the *watch test,* if the examiner carries a watch that ticks loudly enough. Here, the examiner tests one ear at a time by moving the watch toward the patient's ear and estimating the distance at which the ticking begins to be heard. Knowing the distance at which the normal can just hear the ticking, the examiner can judge the presence or absence of hearing loss. Simply record normal or diminished hearing for each ear.

Another method is to use your tuning fork as the sound source. Stand at the patient's side, set the fork vibrating *gently* and hold it at an equal distance between your ear and the patient's. Testing each ear separately, ask the patient to let you know when he no longer hears the sound. Should you still be able to hear the hum distinctly when the patient no longer hears it, you have identified some degree of loss for the tested ear. One the other hand, if you no longer can hear the sound and the patient still has not signalled that the sound is gone, it may suggest that the patient is not being truthful. Of course, this test assumes that you have normal hearing.

The *whispered voice* test is somewhat better than the others and is useful if no suitable watch is available, or if the examiner's own hearing is not normal. Position the patient about 6 m (20 ft) away, turned so that one ear is facing the examiner and have the patient plug the other ear with a fingertip; whisper a few words slowly and clearly, asking the patient to repeat each word as he hears it. Use two-syllable words such as "baseball," "forty-six," "hot dog," and "textbook." Two or three such words are adequate. Have the patient face in the opposite direction and test the other ear in similar fashion, using different words. If the patient hears these words well, his hearing can be reported as normal. If he cannot hear at that distance, simply report a loss for the affected ear, or ears. Do not waste time by continuing to repeat this test by moving closer and closer to the patient, as this is still a rough, clinical test for the *presence* of enough hearing loss to warrant referral.

It is obviously necessary for the examiner to practice on a normal subject so that he learns just how loudly to project his voice to be heard clearly at about 6 m, but not much further. It also is obvious that hearing should be tested after otoscopy, for if a patient has one or both canals completely obstructed by cerumen, no proper evaluation of hearing function in a blocked ear can be performed.

The *Weber test* is routinely performed. Strike the tuning fork, hold it by its stem, and press the stem firmly against the skull or forehead in the midline (Figure 11.4). The sound should be heard equally well in both ears, or nearly so; a distinct difference is abnormal. The Weber test should be reported as normal if the sound is equal in both ears, and as "heard best in the _____ ear" or "lateralized to the _____ ear," if abnormal. A defect in hearing by the watch or whispered voice test, and/or a lateralization in the Weber test is sufficient to determine that the patient has a hearing defect, and therefore should be referred for further examination. Vestibular function is not tested in this examination, as specialized equipment is required.

THE NOSE

The functions of the nose are to serve as an organ of smell, as a passageway for air into the sinuses and the respiratory tract, as an accessory organ in speech production, and as part of the disposal system for tears which reach it via the lacrimonasal duct. In addition, the nose, as the most prominent feature of the face, is extremely important to the individual's appearance. Deformities, supposed deformities, or disfigurements, are therefore frequently disturbing to the person's self-image.

Topographical Anatomy

Internally, the nasal septum divides the nose into right and left nasal cavities. The septum, which is composed of a lower cartilaginous portion and a superior bony portion, is frequently not perfectly straight. Septal deviations are of little importance unless they obstruct the flow of air through the cavity. The lateral wall includes three bony structures: the inferior, middle, and superior turbinates. The septum and outer walls are covered by a specialized mucous membrane often of a slightly redder color than the oral mucosa. The frontal, maxillary, ethmoidal, and sphenoidal sinuses all open into the nasal cavity.

Examination

Simple inspection of the external nose is generally adequate unless there has been recent facial trauma or a complaint of pain, in which case palpation for tenderness should be performed.

Before use of the nasal speculum, a brief check for patency of each nasal passage should be performed. Obstruct

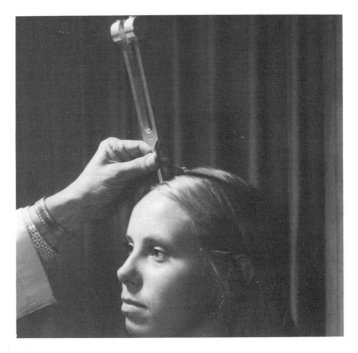

Figure 11.4 The Weber test.

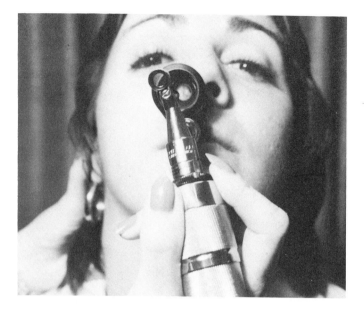

Figure 11.5 Use of nasal speculum. The patient's head is tilted backward to allow for easy viewing of the nasal passage.

one nostril, have the patient exhale with the mouth closed, and feel the puff of air with the fingertips several inches away from the other nostril. Significant degrees of obstruction can be detected and will alert the observer to identify the cause of the obstruction as he inspects the nasal cavities.

The examination of the nasal cavities is carried out with a nasal speculum (Figure 11.5). This instrument, like the ear speculum, is inserted gently while the examiner "watches his way in." The presence and character of any discharge should be noted. The septum is inspected for perforation, tumor, and significant deviation. On the lateral wall, the large inferior turbinate is readily seen and the middle turbinate should ordinarily be seen. Difficulty in visualizing the cavity up to the level of the middle turbinate is often due to swelling of the mucosa of the inferior turbinate — a common finding in our modern environment. No attempt should be made to push the speculum past a swollen turbinate. The upper or superior turbinate is almost never seen since it is small and lies in the deep posterior portion of the wall.

The color of the mucosa varies from the bright, fiery red of inflammation to normal pink to a pale grayish color often associated with allergic rhinitis.

If the patient's history or the finding of pus in the nasal cavity suggests sinusitis, palpation over the sinuses may produce useful information. Here, palpation is in the form of firm pressure on the right and left sides simultaneously to detect tenderness — just above the supraorbital ridge (frontal sinuses) and just below the orbits and across the cheek bones (maxillary sinuses). Percussion over the frontal or maxillary sinuses may elicit pain in the presence of acute sinusitis.

With his eyes closed, the patient should be able to identify the odor of a common substance such as alcohol, chocolate, or tobacco.

MOUTH AND PHARYNX

The oral cavity and pharynx, with their associated structures, are highly complex organ systems that function in numerous important somatic and psychic activities. The mouth is only rarely used as a weapon of offense, but serves to bite, chew, taste, mix, and propel food; it is used constantly to express emotions; and together with the pharynx, it is a major passageway for respiratory air and for speech. In such a complex system there is much for the practitioner to examine.

Early detection of malignant lesions is of critical importance because of the tendency for rapid spread of squamous cell carcinomas of the tongue, floor of the mouth, and tonsils.

Anatomy

The roof of the mouth consists of an anterior, pale, *hard palate,* and a smaller, pink, mobile, *soft palate* posteriorly. The *uvula* hangs downward in the midline from the posterior border of the soft palate (Figure 11.6).

The floor is made up of the tongue and underlying muscles. Posterolaterally, on either side, the anterior and posterior *tonsillar pillars* frame the passageway to the oropharynx (Figure 11.7). Between these pillars lie the *palatine*

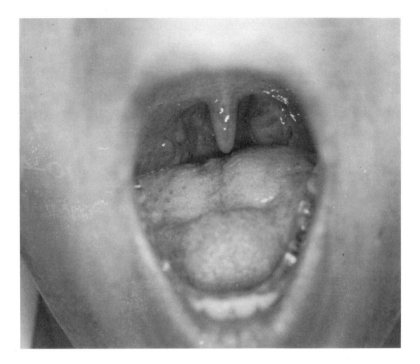

Figure 11.6 View of the mouth showing the uvula hanging in the midline from the soft palate, the tongue, and enlarged tonsils.

tonsils. At the back of the oropharynx is the *posterior pharyngeal wall.*

The tongue is a muscular organ with small taste buds in the anterior two-thirds of its surface, and larger taste buds, the circumvallate papillae, posteriorly (Figure 11.8). When the tongue is raised, a fold of oral mucosa called the *frenum* can be seen, attaching the lower surface of the tongue to the floor of the mouth (Figure 11.9). It is congenital shortening of this frenum that causes tongue-tie. The ducts of both the sublingual and the submandibular salivary glands open into the mouth along the frenum. Lateral to the frenum near its attachment to the tongue, the sublingual veins can be seen.

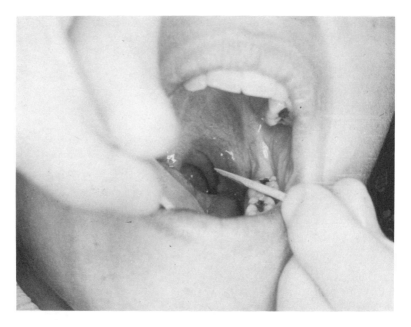

Figure 11.7 Tonsillar area. The pointer is on the anterior pillar, and the posterior pillar is seen directly behind it. The space between the pillars is the tonsillar fossa. The patient has had a tonsillectomy.

The openings of the ducts of the main salivary glands, the *parotids,* can be seen on the lateral (buccal) surfaces of the cheeks opposite the upper second molar teeth. These ducts usually open on a small raised pad on the buccal surface.

The mouth contains 32 teeth in the adult with complete dentition. These are set in spongy tissue, the *gingivae* (gums).

Examination

The external portions of the mouth and lips are inspected for color changes (i.e., cyanosis, pallor), for clusters of darkly pigmented freckles, for ulcerative lesions, or incomplete fusion (i.e., cleft lip), and for symmetry. The corners of the mouth are observed carefully for cracks or fissures.

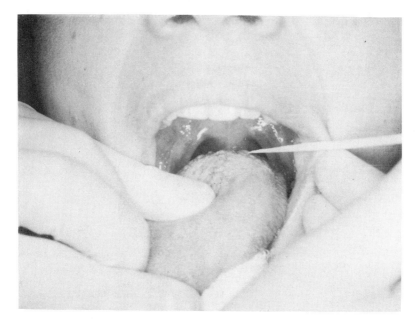

Figure 11.8 The large, circumvallate papillae of the tongue are indicated by the pointer.

If present, the condition is called *cheilosis,* commonly due to poor dental hygiene, ill-fitting dentures, or vitamin deficiency.

An acute vesicular eruption, referred to as fever blister or cold sore, may be found on or around the lips. Known as *herpes simplex,* this condition is due to a viral infection, and is frequently associated with prolonged exposure to the sun, the common cold, menstruation, or high fevers in bacterial infections.

If any drooping of one side of the mouth is noted on preliminary inspection, it may be evidence of paralysis of the seventh cranial nerve. Since major degrees of paralysis may not be evident, all patients should be asked to clench the teeth tightly together while opening the lips as wide as possible. Seventh nerve weakness may become evident with distinct asymmetry of the corners of the mouth (see Figure 9.7). Failure to be able to clench the teeth tightly is evidence of weakness of the jaw muscles or of the motor nerve to those

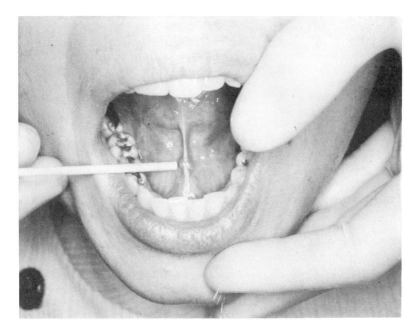

Figure 11.9 The frenum of the tongue (lingual frenum). The pointer indicates the location of the outlets of the ducts of the sublingual and submaxillary salivary glands.

muscles. The upper and lower teeth should be aligned when the jaw is clenched. Free movement of the jaw is expected, and the temporomandibular joint should be pain-free when palpated or moved.

In dark-skinned patients, the oral mucosa may be hyper-pigmented, unevenly distributed, or spotted.

With the tongue blade and a penlight, or other good source of light, inspect the teeth and gums, including the biting and chewing surfaces of the teeth, and both the buccal (cheek) and lingual (tongue) aspects of all of the teeth and gums. The teeth are inspected for obvious defects such as large cavities, cracks or chips, looseness in their sockets, discoloration, or loose appliances such as bridges or crowns on the teeth. The gums are examined for bleeding, swelling, pus, or discoloration. Then the oral mucosa of the floor of the mouth, cheeks, and palate is gently dried with a gauze applicator to absorb saliva. Then the examiner is better able to inspect for changes in color, pigmented spots, vascular lesions such as telangiectases, ulceration, firm white plaques, tumors or erythroplasia. The erythroplasic lesion, the earliest sign of oral cancer, may appear as either a smooth, nongranular lesion primarily red in color, or as a granular red lesion with patchy areas of white keratin. In either case the overlying mucosa will appear atrophic and abraded. The lesion will have poorly defined borders and blend into the surrounding normal mucosa.

Any lesions of the lip or buccal mucosa seen on inspection should be palpated (Figure 11.10). The floor of the mouth is routinely palpated. This is best done bimanually with one finger in the mouth and the other hand outside; masses or tenderness are reported in detail.

The tongue is inspected by having the patient stick it out as far as he can. It should protrude in the *midline,* and there should be no tremor. The upper surface, the sides, and the undersurface of the tongue should then be inspected for color, texture, size, symmetry, and the presence of lesions. The color of the tongue is ordinarily not much different from that of the oral mucosa, and its surface is slightly irregular due to taste buds and small furrows. Its size must be evaluated in proportion to the mouth. Only experience will teach the student what represents an enlarged tongue, but the presence of deep furrows running from the back toward the front of the tongue is a sign of reduced size of that organ. This frequently is due to dehydration of the patient. Palpation of the tongue should then be performed to detect masses or tenderness.

Since the lateral posterior third of the tongue at the junction with the floor of the mouth cannot be seen readily, and since it is a location in which squamous cell carcinoma can remain hidden, it is necessary to pull the tongue aside for a proper view. A recommended technique is to fold a 4 x 4 gauze pad into a 1 x 4 strip and have the patient place his tongue on the middle of the strip (Figure 11.11). The gauze is then wrapped around the tongue, firmly but not tightly, making a thick, nonslippery, protective pad. This pad is then grasped by one hand, and the tongue can be pulled gently outward and laterally, exposing the lateral posterior portion

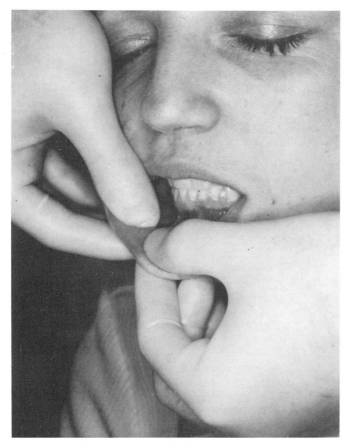

Figure 11.10 Bimanual palpation of the lip. Note that both hands of the examiner are gloved.

of the tongue (Figures 11.12 and 11.13). A tongue blade or gloved finger can then pull the cheek outward to provide a good view.

Prompt referral to a dentist is indicated for any significant abnormalities noted on the inspection or palpation of the oral cavity.

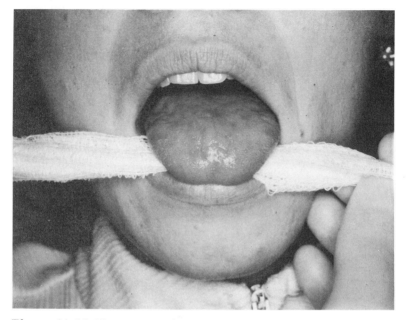

Figure 11.11 Placement of gauze pad.

After this, the pharynx is examined. Since many patients gag readily, it is often easier to examine one side at a time. Have the patient protrude his tongue and breathe rapidly. Place the tongue blade on the right or left half of the tongue, with its tip no further back than the level of the uvula, and press downwards and medially. This will give good exposure of the tonsillar pillars, the tonsil, and a portion of the posterior pharyngeal wall of one side. The presence of pus or large amounts of mucus on the posterior pharyngeal wall is evidence of inflammation or infection of the nasopharynx or sinuses. After repeating this procedure on the other side, ask the patient to say a prolonged "ah." This act of phonation should cause the soft palate to elevate, providing a better view of the posterior pharyngeal wall. Both sides of the soft palate should rise equally, carrying the uvula upward in the midline. Deviation of the uvula to one side or the other is evidence of probable involvement of the ninth or tenth cranial nerve on one side (Figure 11.14).

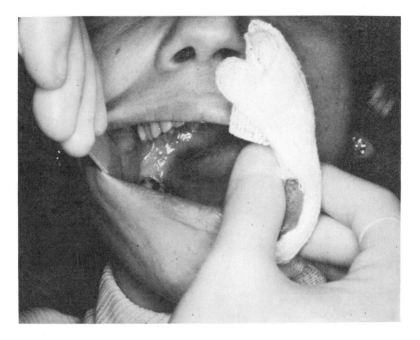

Figure 11.12 View of the posterolateral portion of the tongue.

Absence of upward motion of the soft palate is indicative of probable damage to these nerves bilaterally. As a final test, touch the tonsillar pillar on each side to produce a gag reflex. Watch carefully to see if both sides of the soft palate rise equally.

RECORDING

Ears: no masses or lesions of auricles or canals; no discharge; both TM pearly gray, no perforations; light reflex present; watch ticking heard bilaterally; Weber test normal

Nose: patent bilaterally; no septal deviation or perforation; mucosa pink; can identify alcohol

Mouth: can clench teeth; mucosa and gingivae pink, no lesions or masses; teeth in good repair; tongue protrudes in midline, no tremor

Pharynx: mucosa pink, no lesions; tonsils absent; uvula rises in midline on phonation; gag reflex present bilaterally

POTENTIAL NURSING DIAGNOSES

Airway clearance, ineffective: due to trauma

Nutrition, alteration in: less than body requirements due to inability to ingest food

Oral mucous membrane, alteration in: due to trauma from dentures

Communication, impaired: Potential

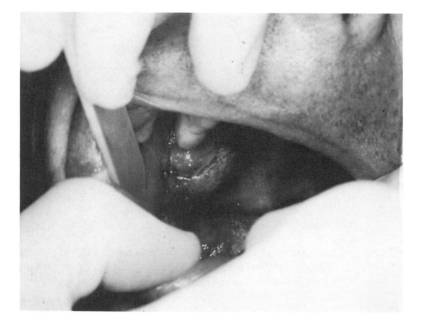

Figure 11.13 Carcinoma of the posterolateral portion of the tongue. This is a large lesion, seen late in its growth.

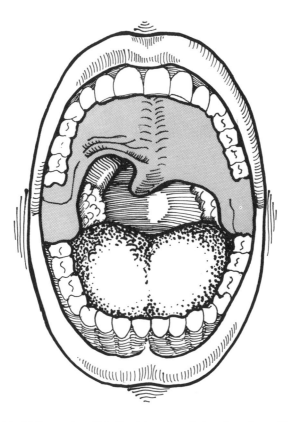

Figure 11.14 Paresis of left side of palates (uvula pulled to right).

PATIENT PROBLEM

Mr. T.A. is a 55-year-old production supervisor who came to the plant health office requesting "something for this hoarse throat." He had sore throat and cold 6 months ago with laryngitis.

Problem: Hoarseness

S: Has had repeated episodes of hoarseness; treated self with hot fluids, steam and aspirin gargles; throat feels tired and achy with slight cough; smokes 1 1/2 packs per day for 40 yr; has noticed change in appetite; unable to eat as before; lost 5-6 lb recently; father died of CA of prostate; mother, 75, diabetic and hypertensive.

O: Tall, thin, tired-appearing grey-haired male, appearing older than stated age; voice harsh and breathy; temp. = 38.0; pulse = 100; resp. = 26.

Ears: No masses or lesions of auricles or canals; unable to visualize tympanic membrane due to wax; watch ticking heard better in right than left; Weber test normal.

Nose: Patent on right; mucosa grey pink; septum deviated on left.

Mouth: Mucosa and gingivae pale; no lesions or masses; teeth stained yellow brown; tongue protrudes in midline, slight tremor.

Pharynx: Mucosa pale and slightly injected; tonsils on right enlarged and irregular; uvula rises in midline on phonation; gag reflex +4 bilaterally; full physical exam refused by patient.

ASSESSMENT: Acute laryngitis; risk factors of family history of CA, smoking, age, repeated laryngitis, may indicate CA larynx; immediate evaluation by ENT specialist necessary.

Nursing Diagnosis: Communication, impaired verbal.
Alteration in nutrition status related to inability to eat and change of appetite.
Alteration in health maintenance related to smoking and self care procedures.

PLAN: Goals: To establish medical diagnosis. To reestablish speech. To be interested in and able to eat.
Patient verbalizes understanding of need to stop smoking.

Nursing Orders:
Diagnostic: Nose and throat culture,
CBC, refer to ENT specialist.
Therapeutic: Recommend warm fluids,
cold stream inhalation; increase
fluid intake until evaluation by MD.
Patient Education: Explain need to
consult with specialist.
Stop talking and increase fluids;
stop smoking.

IMPLEMENTATION: Appointment made for ENT consultation.
Discuss need for consultation and importance of increase in fluids and avoidance of smoking and speaking.
Discuss alternative blended fluids—high calorie, high protein foods as liquid supplements.
Provide menu of nonirritating soups and drinks.

EVALUATION: Verbalizes understanding of full liquid menu and supplements.
Verbalizes acceptance of plan for stopping smoking.
Patient visited ENT specialist.

chapter 12

The Thorax and Lungs

Topographical Anatomy

Physiology

Examination

Recording

Potential Nursing Diagnoses

Patient Problem

Although x-ray study of the chest is considered a major tool in health screening and evaluation of respiratory problems, it is not intended to replace careful physical examination. Both of these types of examination contribute to the total examination of the chest wall and its contents, since each can detect abnormalities that the other cannot pick up. Certain abnormalities of respiratory disease may be detected only by physical examination (i.e., asthma), while deep-lying tumors can be found only by x-ray examination.

Within the bony framework of the thorax lie the bronchi, lungs, and heart. The domes of the right and left portions of the diaphragm rise high into the thoracic cage, so that the upper abdominal contents are also enclosed within the chest (see Figure 12.18). Although all of these structures, as well as the breasts, eventually will be examined as a unit, this chapter will consider only the examination of the thorax and lungs.

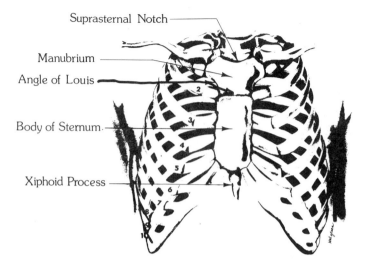

Suprasternal Notch

Manubrium

Angle of Louis

Body of Sternum

Xiphoid Process

Figure 12.1 Bony thorax. The second ribs articulate at the junction of the manubrium and body of the sternum where the angle of Louis is formed.

TOPOGRAPHICAL ANATOMY

The bony thorax (Figure 12.1) includes 12 pairs of ribs and 12 thoracic vertebrae.

Anteriorly the sternum is seen in the center of the chest as a vertical flat bone consisting of a manubrium, body, and xiphoid cartilage. At the superior edge of the manubrium is a depression that is referred to as the suprasternal notch. The junction of the manubrium and the body forms a slight angle protruding forward, which is known as the *angle of Louis* or sternal angle. Since the second ribs articulate at this angle, it serves as a reference point for counting the ribs.

The shape of the thorax is essentially elliptical in adults with a wider diameter at the base than at the top, but in infants it is cylindrical with a more nearly equal diameter from top to base.

The anteroposterior (AP) diameter of the thorax is clearly smaller than the transverse diameter in normal individuals. Each rib is a flattened arched bone, arising at

approximately a 45° angle from its junction with the verte-
bra, and continuing as a costal cartilage in its attachment
anteriorly to the sternum. It is separated from the next rib
by an intercostal space that takes its number from the rib
above. There is a downward and forward slope of each rib
that increases progressively, so that the width of the intercostal spaces increases toward the inferior edge of the rib
cage.

The thorax includes this bony cage, the scapulae, and
the soft tissues. For purposes of reference, several vertical
lines are used (Figures 12.2 and 12.3). The *midsternal line*
passes from the suprasternal notch to the xiphoid and the
midclavicular lines are drawn from the centers of each clavicle. The *anterior and posterior axillary lines* are dropped
vertically from the anterior and posterior axillary folds,
respectively, and a midaxillary line lies between these.
Posteriorly, the *midspinal line* runs vertically down through
the spinous processes of the vertebrae. The space between
the medial borders of the scapulae is referred to as the interscapular area (see Figure 12.16). Imaginary horizontal lines
are not necessary, since the ribs and interspaces are used as
reference lines.

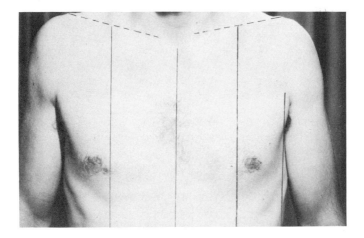

Figure 12.2 Reference lines. From the left of the picture
these are the right midclavicular line, the midsternal line,
the left midclavicular line, and (barely visible) the left anterior axillary line.

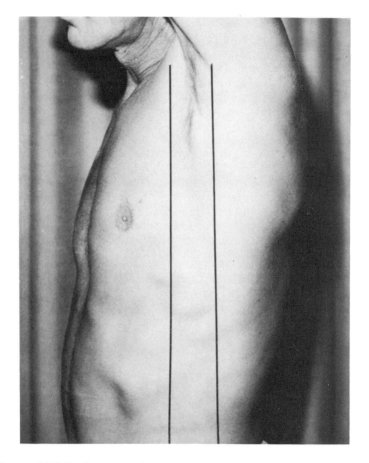

Figure 12.3 Reference lines. Anterior axillary line and posterior axillary line are shown. The midaxillary line falls midway between these.

The trachea, as mentioned in the section on neck examination, should be in the midline directly posterior to the suprasternal notch. It bifurcates into the right and left mainstem bronchi at about the level of the angle of Louis. Thus, physical findings related to the major bronchi occur in the upper midportion of the chest.

Figure 12.4 illustrates the projection of the right and left lungs as they appear in different phases of respiration.

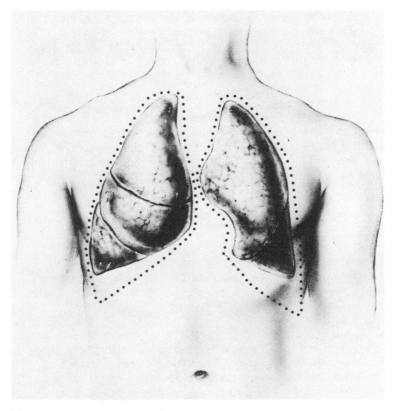

Figure 12.4 Projection of the lungs on the chest wall. The dotted lines show the lung expansion during inspiration. The right lung is seen to be divided into a right upper, and right middle, and a right lower lobe. The left has only an upper and lower lobe.

PHYSIOLOGY

In the normal adult, the resting rate of respiration is approximately 16-20 cycles per minute, regular in rate and rhythm. The normal respiratory cycle consists of an inspiratory phase requiring muscular activity, and a shorter, passive expiratory phase.

During inspiration the ribs are elevated primarily by action of the intercostal muscles. This serves to increase

the anteroposterior diameter of the chest. Also during inspiration the diaphragm descends. This coordinated action
increases the volume of the thorax, allowing for the free
entry of respiratory air into the lungs. Expiration, on the
other hand, is a passive and more rapid action in which the
air is expelled by a recoil of the expanded thoracic cavity
in a return to its resting state.

Normally the entire chest wall moves together and
expands equally with a 5-8 cm expansion from maximum
expiration to maximum inspiration. Males characteristically
use the chest wall less than females in normal respiration,
depending more on diaphragmatic breathing.

EXAMINATION

Adequate examination of the thorax requires that the
patient have all clothing removed to the waist and that, if
possible, he be sitting on an examining table or standing.

Axilla

The axilla is a pyramid-shaped space in which the
examination is directed toward the sebaceous glands of
the apex and the lymph nodes of the apex and thoracic wall
of the pyramid. The patient's arm should be raised to allow
for inspection. Lymph nodes may be enlarged enough to be
visualized, and occasionally the development of infection of
the sebaceous glands will be evidenced by reddening and
edema of the skin near the apex.

Following inspection with the patient's arm still raised,
the fingertips are placed at the apex. When the patient's
arm is lowered, the muscles of the area are relaxed and deep
palpation of the apex can be accomplished (Figure 12.5).
Lymph nodes should be felt for here and down the thoracic
side of the pyramid. If nodes are palpable, they should be
described as masses using the criteria described in Chapter 8.

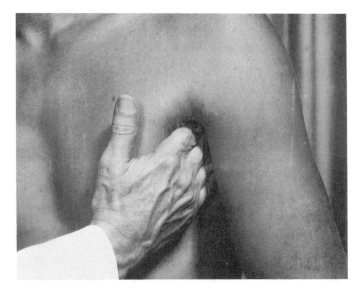

Figure 12.5 Palpation of the left axilla. Note the examiner's hand flat against the chest wall and the relaxed arm of the patient.

The Thorax and Lungs

General

The thorax and lungs are examined as a unit because of the intimate relationship between the bony cage of the thorax and the chest motions in ventilation of the lungs. For purposes of clarity, the breast and the heart are described separately. The sequence of examination of the chest should be inspection, palpation, percussion, and auscultation.

Inspection

Consideration should be given first to posture, contour, general development, and motion of the thorax. It is important to note the patient's posture, since individuals with chronic obstructive lung disease often sit up and prop themselves on their arms (Figure 12.6, or lean forward with their elbows on a desk, in an attempt to fix their clavicles and gain greater ability to expand the chest.

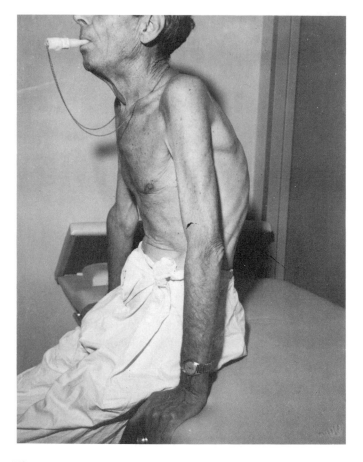

Figure 12.6 Patient with chronic emphysema. Note the use of his arms to fix the clavicles and the increased anteroposterior thoracic diameter (barrel chest). He is using an "emphysema whistle," which assists in controlling his forced expiration.

The contour of the chest is often abnormal due to an increase in the AP diameter so that it approaches the transverse diameter. The sternum appears pushed forward and the ribs are more horizontal. The patient seems to be in a constant state of full inspiration with little motion during the respiratory cycle. This is called *barrel chest* and is characteristic of advanced chronic obstructive pulmonary disease (see Figure 12.6).

Other deformities of the chest contour may be caused by unilateral lung disease or structural deformities of the bony framework. *Pigeon breast* or *chicken breast* is a permanent deformity, usually caused by rickets, in which the AP diameter is increased, the transverse diameter is narrowed, and vertical grooves are formed on the line of the costochondral junctions.

Funnel breast (pectus excavatum) is the reverse of pigeon breast. The softened ribs of the lower part of the sternum sink posteriorly, creating a pit or depression which decreases the AP diameter (Figure 12.7). Other thoracic deformities include bulges on the chest wall caused by cardiac enlargement, aortic aneurysm, neoplasm, or depressions caused by retractions due to underlying fibrosis, or surgical removal of ribs.

Inspection of the profile of the thoracic wall from the side and from the back may identify several spinal deformities

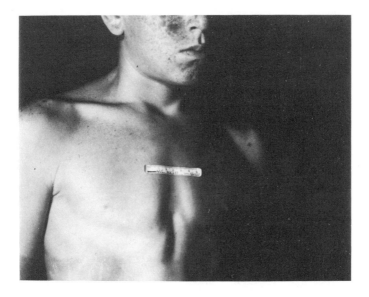

Figure 12.7 Young man with moderate degree of pectus excavatum.

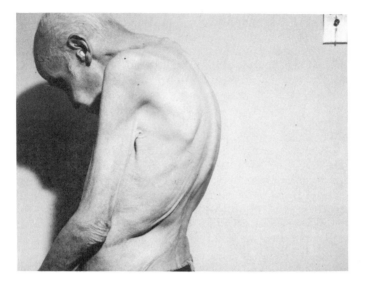

Figure 12.8 Elderly man with severe degree of thoracic kyphosis.

that modify the contour. In the long thoracic spine, several abnormalities are of importance. Both an increase in the normal curve, or *kyphosis* (Figure 12.8), as well as straightening of the normal curve with rigidity *(poker spine),* interfere with free movement of the ribs and thus with good ventilation. If either deformity is observed, the patient's chest expansion should be measured to determine the degree of limitation of motion of the chest wall. *Scoliosis* (Figure 12.9) or lateral curvature, of significant degree, will cause one side of the chest to be compressed and the other to be abnormally expanded, thus also interfering with normal respiratory motion. (See Chapter 16 for specific screening examination.)

Respiratory Motion

The motion of the thoracic wall should be observed during quiet normal breathing and then during deep inspiration. It is important to note the type, rate, rhythm, and depth of the respiratory effort, as well as the use of accessory

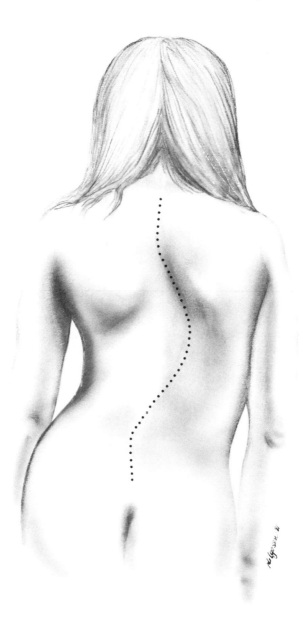

Figure 12.9 Diagram of severe scoliosis with the concavity toward the right.

respiratory muscles of the neck. The rhythm of a single
respiratory cycle should have a longer inspiratory phase and
a shorter expiratory phase (see Figure 12.14, upper diagram).
Irregularities in rhythm should be noted, such as *Cheyne-
Stokes* breathing in which there are alternating periods of
apnea and respiration with variable rate. The depth of
respiration is as meaningful as the rate, for it may help to
distinguish between pulmonary, metabolic, or neurologic
causes of rapid or slow breathing. Rapid, deep respirations
may indicate *Kussmaul* respiration of diabetic acidosis,
while rapid, *shallow* breathing may signify obstructive or re-
strictive lung disease. The duration of inspiration versus
expiration is important in determining whether or not there
is airway obstruction. In patients with obstructive lung disease, expiration is prolonged and requires the use of muscular effort, an important diagnostic sign.

The chest should also be observed for symmetrical expansion. Unilateral diminished expansion may be due to
acute pleurisy, pleural fibrosis, or massive atelectasis. A
pulmonary embolus, pneumonia, pleural effusion, pneumothorax, or any cause of chest pain (such as fractured ribs)
may lead to diminished chest expansion. In addition, general
chest expansion may be limited in ankylosing spondylitis,
since the ribs cannot rotate at their joints with the spine.

A comparison should be made of expansion of the upper chest to that of the lower chest. If the examiner suspects
that there is a significant difference, he should use the tape
measure to verify his suspicions.

The examiner should also look for bulging or *retraction*
of the interspaces. Bulging of interspaces may occur in a
massive pleural effusion, with tension pneumothorax, or during the forced expiration of the patient with emphysema or
asthma.

Palpation

Although palpation may be conducted together with inspection in the process of examination of the chest, the
beginning student should approach the technique as a separate entity. Initially, he will be concerned with validating
the data found upon inspection, particularly in relation to
symmetry of expansion of the chest wall during respiration.

Symmetrical areas of the thorax should be palpated
with the fingertips and the palms. With the patient upright,

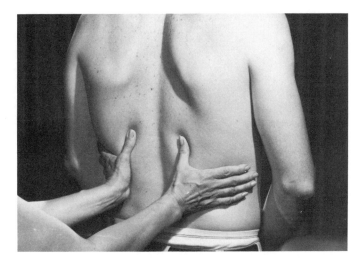

Figure 12.10 Palpation for equality of lower posterior chest expansion. Note the positions of the thumbs and fingers.

the anterior, lower lateral, and posterior thorax can all be examined for symmetry of onset and depth of inspiration. The movement of the chest can be seen particularly well by placing the hands on the lower portion of the posterolateral wall with the thumbs adjacent near the spine (Figure 12.10). During deep inspiration the thumbs should move apart at the same time and equally in distance from the midspinal line.

General palpation of the chest wall should also give attention to the temperature, moisture, and general turgor of the skin, as well as to the presence of edema. Any evidence of masses or tenderness should receive special consideration.

In the event that the patient complains of chest pain, bones and joints of the thorax should be palpated for presence of tenderness.

Fremitus

Speaking produces vibrations in the larynx that are transmitted through the respiratory system to the chest wall. These vibrations, known as *fremitus,* can be felt with the hands (tactile fremitus) or heard with the stethoscope (vocal resonance). Fremitus varies from individual to individual,

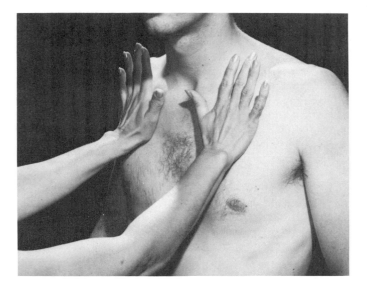

Figure 12.11 Palpation for equality of lower posterior chest expansion. Note the positions of the thumbs and fingers.

being better transmitted in males and in thin-chested persons. Fremitus is also better felt or heard in the upper portion of the chest wall than near the base.

Feel for fremitus with the palms, or the ulnar aspect of the hands (Figure 12.11) and ask the patient to say, "1, 2, 3" or "99." A mild purrlike sensation should be felt, similar to the sensation one would feel if hands were placed on the sides of a cat while it was purring. Fremitus should *not* be palpable unless the patient is vocalizing. A satisfactory technique is to use both hands simultaneously on corresponding areas of the chest so that comparison of one side to the other can be made. Since, in general, only large lesions of the chest produce changes of fremitus, one can examine about three areas anteriorly, two laterally, and three areas of the back for fremitus; each square centimeter need not be tested.

A solid medium of uniform consistency will conduct vibrations from the larynx to the chest wall better than one containing air, such as normal lung tissue. Therefore, one can expect increased fremitus in conditions such as pneumonia, where there is consolidation of the lung, especially when that consolidation is close to the lung surface. When a major bronchus is obstructed, vibrations cannot be transported, and fremitus will be absent over the lung area served by that bronchus.

Decreased fremitus will occur when abnormalities involving the pleura interfere with the normal transmission of laryngeal sounds. Thus fibrous thickening of the pleura, pleural effusion, or pneumothorax all will lead to either decreased or absent fremitus.

An unusual finding on palpation of the neck or chest is *crepitation* (crackling), produced when the fingertips press on and move tiny air bubbles in the subcutaneous tissues. This is most often secondary to trauma, which allows escape of air from the lung and pleural space. Such trauma may arise from a fractured rib, a chest wound, or following surgery. Crepitation infrequently may be felt in the abdomen or in an extremity — and in rare instances it may be due to gas gangrene. The term is also used to describe the grating sensation when a damaged joint is moved, or when the rough ends of a fractured bone are moved against each other. Some authors describe fine rales as crepitant rales. Thus, the student may be prepared to understand that when the term appears it means crackling or grating either on palpation or auscultation from any source.

Percussion

The general procedure for percussion described in Chapter 6 assumes special significance during examination of the chest.

The normal percussion note, heard as a result of the vibration of underlying chest wall and organs, varies with the thickness of the chest wall, the muscular development, and the location of underlying organs, as well as the force applied by the examiner. The clear, long, medium-pitched sound usually heard over the normal lung is called *resonance*. The sound can be appreciated fully only through the experience of percussion of many normal chests.

Where the air content of the underlying tissue is decreased and its solidity increased, such as over the heart, *dullness* is heard. This is a short, higher-pitched, soft thud that fails to demonstrate the vibratory quality of a resonant

sound. The high pitched, clear, longer drumlike sound over
the air-filled stomach or over any hollow intestine is a musical note referred to as *tympany.* Naturally, the changes in
sounds from one area to another are gradual so that there
are zones of transition.

Proceed to percuss the anterior and lateral chest in a
systematic manner from top to bottom. At each level, parallel areas of both sides are percussed, each interspace being
compared with the corresponding space, keeping in mind the
normal changes in sound expected over the heart, the liver,
and the stomach and colon (Figure 12.12).

On the right chest, percussion down the midclavicular
line will identify the location of the upper edge of the liver.
The transition is quite distinct here between lung resonance
and liver dullness. The upper border of the liver is ordinarily
found at about the fourth or fifth intercostal space. With the
patient's head flexed forward and the forearms crossed at
the waist to separate the scapulae, the posterior chest should
be percussed starting at the apices and continuing downward
to the bases where the location and range of motion of the
diaphragm are determined (Figure 12.13). The method used
to locate and measure the respiratory excursion of the diaphragm requires instructing the patient to take and hold a
deep breath. The lowest level of resonance is identified by
percussing downward until the tone changes to dullness. The
patient is then instructed to exhale and hold, while the procedure is once again accomplished. The range of motion of
the diaphragm is determined by the distance between the two
levels, which is normally about 3-5 cm in females and 5-6 cm
in males. Reduced movement of the diaphragm is often seen
in pleurisy or emphysema.

Abnormal findings identified through percussion are
created when there is an increased amount of air or when
fluid or pleural thickening is present in the underlying structure. For example, in emphysema and in extensive pneumothorax, increased air creates a "booming," well-sustained,
and easily heard sound referred to as *hyperresonance.* When
there is a considerable amount of fluid in the lung, dullness
will be located where there should normally be resonance.
Consolidation or filling of alveolar spaces by fluid, pus, or
blood due to pneumonia, tuberculosis, tumor process, lung
abscess, infarction, and pulmonary edema are examples of
situations that produce dullness. The presence of some fluid
in the pleural space over underlying air-containing lung will

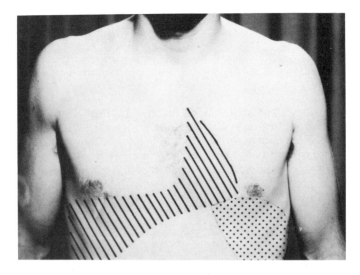

Figure 12.12 Normal percussion areas. Dullness will normally be found in the hatched areas. On the patient's left, dullness is due to the underlying heart while the area on the right represents liver dullness. The dotted area, somewhat variable in actual size, is tympanic. This is Traube's space, lying over air in the stomach and splenic flexure of the colon. See also Figs. 12.18 and 14.1.

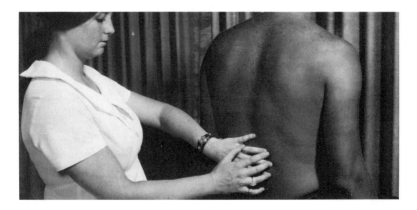

Figure 12.13 Percussion of the diaphragm.

also create abnormal dullness. Absolute dullness or flatness will occur when there is a large amount of fluid over an area, with little underlying aircontaining lung remaining, as with pleural effusion.

Auscultation

Much of what has been learned through inspection, palpation, and percussion of the chest, as well as from the history, can be appreciated further when the examiner goes one step beyond and uses the stethoscope. Auscultation determines the character of the breath sounds, the character of the whispered voice, and the presence of abnormal (adventitious) sounds heard over the chest wall during respiration.

Breath Sounds. As a result of the movement of air through various portions of the respiratory system during respiration, soft audible vibrations are produced — the breath sounds. The quality and intensity of the sounds depend upon the location of their production and the tissues through which they are transmitted to the examiner's stethoscope. There are three types of *normal* breath sounds (Figure 12.14).

1. *Vesicular sounds:* soft, low-pitched (100–300 cps) fine rustling or swishing sounds, like a sigh, heard from early inspiration to early expiration. In quiet respiration the expiratory portion may not be heard at all. These sounds are produced by air movement in the terminal bronchioles and alveoli and are heard over most of the chest (see Figures 12.15 and 12.16).
2. *Bronchial sounds:* loud, high-pitched (over 500 cps) "tubular" sounds, louder and longer in expiration with a brief pause between the inspiratory and expiratory components. These are normally heard only anteriorly over the trachea and major bronchi (see Figure 12.15).
3. *Bronchovesicular sounds:* a combination of the above two sounds, since they represent a mixture of sounds being produced by both bronchial and alveolar air vibrations. Note that there is no pause between the inspiratory and expiratory sound. These are characteristically heard over portions of the chest where a bronchus is near lung parenchyma, i.e., over the upper anterior chest, the apex of the right lung, and in the interscapular space (see Figures 12.15 and 12.16).

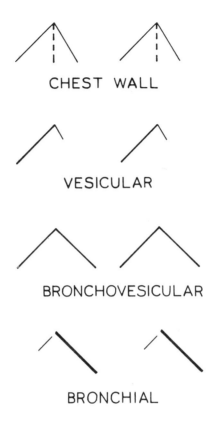

CHEST WALL

VESICULAR

BRONCHOVESICULAR

BRONCHIAL

Figure 12.14 Diagrammatic representation of two breaths. The upper diagram represents chest wall motion during inspiration (upstroke) and the shorter expiratory period (downstroke). For purposes of clarity, bronchovesicular sounds are illustrated between vesicular and bronchial sounds to show the mixed character of these sounds.

If ever the beginning practitioner needs a quiet room, it is when learning to listen for breath sounds. The patient should be as comfortable as possible to avoid any unnecessary movement. With the diaphragm of the stethoscope (warmed, if necessary), placed firmly against the chest wall, the patient is directed to breathe quietly with his mouth open. Concentrate first on the quality of the breath sounds. Once again,

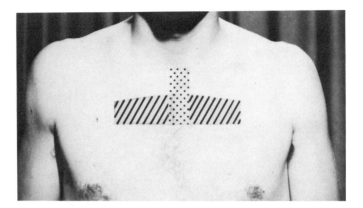

Figure 12.15 Location of normal breath sounds. Bronchial breathing may be heard in the area over the trachea and major bronchi (dotted area). Bronchovesicular sounds may be heard normally within the hatched area. Elsewhere, the predominant sounds are vesicular.

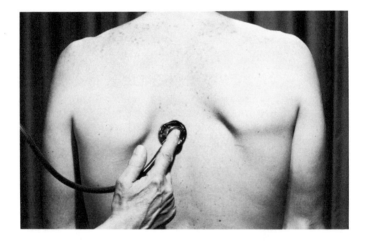

Figure 12.16 Auscultation in the interscapular space where bronchovesicular sounds are normally present. Vesicular breath sounds are normally present in the remainder of the posterior thorax.

as in palpation and percussion, corresponding regions of each side of the anterior chest from the apex to the base of the lung are auscultated. Symmetrical regions should be compared in relation to pitch, intensity, quality, and duration of breath sounds, and the presence of abnormal sounds noted. Figures 12.15 and 12.16 illustrate the areas in which the three types of breath sounds are heard in the normal person. Note again that vesicular breathing is heard over most of the chest.

It should be noted well that deep breathing will convert the fine vesicular sounds into bronchovesicular sounds, so a portion of the auscultation should be done with quiet respiration on the part of the patient. Breathing through the mouth will avoid the production of sounds in the nasopharynx and nares and is, therefore, preferred.

In pathologic conditions, such as early pneumonia or minimal pulmonary edema, fluid begins to fill some of the alveoli, converting vesicular sounds into bronchovesicular sounds. Thus, the presence of bronchovesicular sounds is *abnormal* in an area where only vesicular sounds should be heard. This finding will be detected in the early stage of disease when the chest x-ray is still unchanged. As larger amounts of fluid collect, such as in lobar pneumonia, the involved area becomes much more solid, no vesicular component is present, and the sounds produced by underlying bronchi are well transmitted, producing bronchial sounds in an abnormal location (see Patient Problem). This is a classical sign of consolidation of the lung.

If a large bronchus becomes obstructed, no air will pass in or out of a portion of the lung. Listening over such an area, the clinician will hear no breath sounds of any type.

The absence of breath sounds, in addition to indicating obstruction of a bronchus, may also be found over an area of lung collapse such as in pneumothorax. In both situations, no air is passing to the area under the stethoscope; therefore, no breath sounds are produced. Conditions in which there is very little air moving (severe emphysema, fractured ribs with a splinted chest, etc.), will cause the breath sounds to be diminished or absent. Another reason for diminished sounds is the presence of air or fluid in the pleural space that separates the underlying lung from the stethoscope. Thickened pleura will also prevent good transmission of breath sounds.

Whispered Voice Sounds. As noted earlier, speaking produces vibrations in the respiratory system that are transmitted to the chest wall. Place the stethoscope on the chest in various locations and ask the patient to whisper a few words or numbers. In the normal situation, the examiner should hear the sounds as a muffled hum with the words not clearly distinguishable. Increased transmission, which makes the whispered voice sound louder and the syllables clear, is evidence of consolidation of the underlying lung. This abnormality may be detected quite early in the course of pneumonia or other diseases causing the lung to become more solid. Increased transmission of the whispered voice is referred to as *whispered pectoriloquy.* This is a more sensitive index of consolidation than *bronchophony* in which the spoken voice is transmitted more loudly than normally.

Adventitious Sounds. These are abnormal sounds superimposed on the basic breath sounds. They consist of *rales, rhonchi, wheezes* and *rubs.* Unfortunately, there are several definitions and classifications, leading to some confusion in terminology.

Rales (crackles) are clusters or showers of sounds produced by the bubbling of air through fluid in the alveoli, bronchioles, or bronchi. In general, they vary in quality, depending upon the location of the abnormal fluid. Thus, *fine rales* are produced by bubbling in the alveoli and terminal bronchioles. They are not loud, are high-pitched, and seem to the listener to be heard quite close to the ear. A classical analogy is that fine rales sound somewhat like the sound of several strands of hair being rubbed between the fingers close to the ear. Rales are heard mainly on inspiration.

Course rales result from air passing through larger amounts of fluid in larger air passages, usually the bronchioles. They are lower pitched and crackling, not unlike the bubbling sound of a freshly opened bottle of a carbonated beverage.

When showers of rales are heard, the patient should be instructed to cough. If the rales do not disappear, or if they are accentuated by the cough, they are significant and are evidence of fluid in the lung due to left heart failure (pulmonary edema), pneumonia, or other inflammatory diseases such as tuberculosis. Deep breathing may help to accentuate rales.

Rhonchi are coarser sounds, probably produced in the larger bronchi by passage of air through mucus or through a narrowing of the air passage. *Coarse (or sonorous) rhonchi* are low-pitched, "snoring" sounds resulting from vibrations of mucus strands in the bronchi. They are generally continuous through one or both phases of the respiratory cycle, are often variable in pitch and loudness from one breath to another, and tend to change in character after a cough. These are typical of bronchitis with accumulation of mucus.

Wheezes are musical, whistling, or hissing sounds, of distinctly higher pitch than coarse rhonchi. Wheezes are produced by narrowing of bronchioles (as in asthma) or by partial obstruction of larger bronchi due to edema of the mucosa, a tumor, or other lesions that reduce the normal diameter of the bronchi. A *unilateral* wheeze is highly significant, suggesting localized compression or obstruction of a bronchus. This is often the first sign of carcinoma of the lung or of obstruction due to aspiration. Wheezes may be heard during inspiration or expiration.

If rales, rhonchi or wheezes are detected, the observer should report where they are heard in the respiratory cycle. This is an important distinction since they have quite a different significance in the inspiratory phase from those heard during expiration. A sketch may be drawn to illustrate the examiner's findings. Figure 12.17 shows several examples.

Friction rub is a coarse, grating sound that results from two inflamed surfaces of pleura rubbing against each other, as in pleurisy. It is similar to the sound elicited when the palm of one hand is placed over the ear and the finger of the other hand is used to rub the back of the hand. Most of the time it is heard over the anterolateral chest throughout the respiratory cycle. The practitioner should hold the stethoscope firmly over the chest so that sliding on the skin does not artificially produce sounds similar to a rub.

Table 12.1 is a brief summary of major findings on auscultation and percussion.

Table 12.1 Common Findings on Physical Assessment of Thorax: Auscultation and Percussion

Sound Name	Description	Incidence and Location	Caused by	Probable Indications
Percussion				
Resonance	Long, clear medium-pitched	Over most of chest	Aerated lung tissue	Normal functioning
Hyperresonance	Booming, well-sustained		Increased air content	Emphysema; extensive pneumothorax
Dullness	Shorter, higher-pitched soft thud	Over liver and heart	Decreased air content	Normal
		Over lungs	Fluid, pus, or blood; consolidation of lung	Pneumonia; TB; tumor; abscess; infarct; pulmonary edema
Flatness			Fluid in pleura over aerated lung	Pleurisy
Absolute dullness			Fluid in pleura over nonaerated lung	Pleural effusion

Auscultation

Vesicular	Soft, low-pitched rustle or sigh	Early inspiration to early expiration, over most of chest	Air movement in terminal bronchioles and alveoli	Normal functioning
Bronchial	Loud, high-pitched "tubular"	Louder and longer in expiration; pause between inspiration and expiration; anteriorly over trachea and major bronchi	Air movement in bronchi	Normal functioning
Broncho-vesicular	Combination	No pause between inspiration and expiration; areas where bronchus is near parenchyma	Air movement	Normal functioning
Diminished breath sounds		In vesicular areas	Fluid in alveoli	Lobar pneumonia; consolidation of lung
			No air movement	Severe emphysema; fractured ribs with splinted chest

Table 12.1 (*continued*)

Sound Name	Description	Incidence and Location	Caused by	Probable Indications
Absence of breath sounds			Obstruction	Lung collapse; pneumothorax
Whispered pectoriloquy	Whispered words distinguishable	Various areas	Consolidation	Pneumonia
Increased fremitus	Vibrations when patient speaks	May also be palpated	Consolidation	Pneumonia
Decreased fremitus			Bronchial obstruction; abnormality of pleura	Pleural thickening; pleural effusion; pneumothorax
Adventitious Sounds				
Rales	"Rubbing hair between fingers"; "Carbonation"	Various areas heard mainly on inspiration	Bubbling of air through fluid; fluid in lung	Pulmonary edema; pneumonia; inflammation (as in TB)

Rhonchi coarse (sonorous)	"Snoring," variable in pitch and loudness	Change after coughing	Passage of air through mucus; mucus accumulation	Bronchitis
Wheezes	Whistling, hissing high-pitched	Inspiration or expiration	Narrowing of bronchioles; Partial obstruction of bronchi	Asthma Edema of mucosa; tumor; lesion which decreases diameter of bronchi
Rub	Coarse grating, "finger rubbing on hand placed over ear"		Two inflamed surfaces of pleura rubbing; friction	Pleurisy

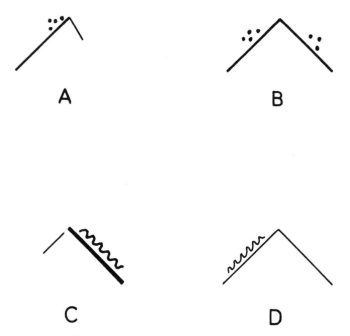

Figure 12.17 Sketches of breath sounds and adventitious sounds. (a) Vesicular sound with rales at the end of inspiration; (b) bronchovesicular sound with rales in midinspiration and midexpiration; (c) bronchial sound with rhonchi in expiration; and (d) bronchovesicular sound with inspiratory rhonchi.

RECORDING

Thorax

Insp: symmetrical; full expansion equal bilaterally; AP diameter not increased
Palp: no axillary adenopathy

Lungs

Palp: fremitus equal bilaterally
Perc: lung fields resonant throughout
Ausc: breath sounds normal; voice sounds normal; no rales, rhonchi, wheezing or rubs

The Thorax and Lungs   215

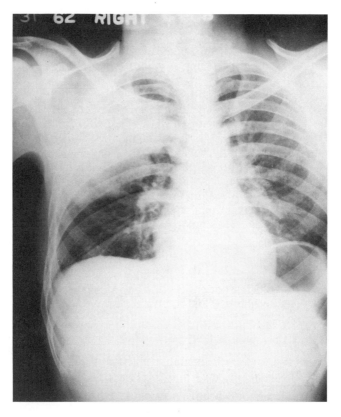

Figure 12.18 Chest x-ray showing characteristic consolidation due to pneumonia of the right upper lobe. The relationships of the heart to the chest and the diaphragm are well illustrated. Note that the left leaf of the diaphragm is above the gas bubble of the stomach.

POTENTIAL NURSING DIAGNOSES

Activity intolerance: due to exertional dyspnea

Airway clearance, ineffective: due to tracheobronchial obstruction (or others)

Breathing pattern, ineffective: due to decreased lung expansion or others

Gas exchange, impaired: due to altered oxygen supply

PATIENT PROBLEM

Mr. L.A., 36-year-old construction laborer with CC of chest pain, cough, chill and fever of 6 hours duration (Figure 12.18).

S: Four days ago pt. noted mild sore throat and "sniffles," for which he took aspirin with some relief. He continued to work 12 hour shifts because his foreman insisted. At about 6 a.m. today, awakened by a severe shaking chill that lasted for about 20 min. Felt sick but was able to fall back to sleep. Awakened about 2 hours later with right chest pain, began coughing, produced small amounts of "rusty" sputum and wife brought him to HMO emergency center. Major complaint now is chest pain, malaise, and chills.

O: Temp. 39.4 C (103 F); pulse 120; resp. 26, BP 140/60.

Insp: Face flushed; skin hot and sweaty; labored respiration; right chest splinted.

Palp: Confirms splinting of R chest; increased fremitus R chest above 4th ICS.

Perc: Diminished resonance R chest from clavicle to 5th ICS, from midaxillary line to sternum.

Ausc: Bronchial breath sounds, crackling rales, whispered pectoriloquy over R chest over involved area; remainder of chest clear.

ASSESSMENT: These findings on History and PE are characteristic of lobar pneumonia. Patient is acutely ill.

Nursing Diagnosis: Potential injury: infection of respiratory system. Breathing pattern: ineffective due to pain.

PLAN: Goals: Diagnosis established. Patient understands and complies with treatment plan. Medical therapy initiated. Patient asymptomatic.

Nursing Orders:
Diagnostic: Stat PA x-ray, CBC with
differential, sputum for culture;
present to MD at once.
Therapeutic: Escort to resting area,
provide blanket and pitcher of fluids.
Patient Education: Advise patient
and wife that he probably has infection of lungs, possible pneumonia,
that hospitalization may be necessary.
Advise wife to contact husband's
employer regarding sick time needed.

IMPLEMENTATION: Blood drawn and sent to lab.
Chest film taken in E.R. x-ray room.
Physician examined patient.
Hospitalization ordered.
To return to HMO after discharge.

EVALUATION: Pneumonia confirmed.
Transferred to St. Luke Hospital.

The Breast

Despite marked progress in prolonging lives and the development of new methods of treatment, breast cancer continues to strike women with relentless force. One of 11 women in the United States will develop breast cancer during her lifetime, more than 120,000 new cases will be detected this year, and almost 40,000 will die.

Meanwhile, the basic method of examination of the breast can reveal the presence of the disease in its early stages when it is 80–90% curable. It is essentially a simple technique, easy enough for women to learn themselves. For primary health practitioners, the mastery of this technique and subsequent teaching to large groups, as well as individual patients, may become one of the most important tasks for which they can assume responsibility. In any event, the significance of careful, thorough, systematic inspection and palpation of the breast in all patients cannot be overemphasized.

TOPOGRAPHICAL ANATOMY

The breasts, or mammary glands, two highly specialized glands, are located on either side of the anterior wall of the chest between the third and the seventh ribs, from the edge of the sternum to the anterior axillary line with an extension to the anterior axillary fold. Each organ is divided into 15-20 lobes which are separated from each other by fibroelastic tissue. The external surface is made up of a soft area of skin extending from the circumference of the gland to the areola, which is a pigmented circle surrounding the nipple. The areola, which has a pinkish hue in blondes, a darker rose color in brunettes, and darkens after childbirth, has a more or less roughened surface with small fine papillae, known as the glands of Montgomery.

The nipple is composed of sensitive, erectile tissue and forms a large conic projection in the center of the areola, its summit holding multiple openings of the milk ducts.

The breasts are particularly well supplied with lymphatic channels, especially toward the axillae, which are included in the examination of the breast.

PHYSIOLOGY

The breasts lie close to the skin between the superficial and deep layers of the superficial fascia supported by the suspensory ligaments.

During the developing years and in young women, especially those who have not borne children, the breasts are soft and almost homogenous in consistency despite their lobular characteristic, but as the years progress and pregnancies occur, their consistency becomes more nodular and stringy.

Since the breasts are the organs of lactation, they change during pregnancy in anticipation of lactation. In the early months, the changes are similar to those that occur monthly under cyclic influence of pituitary and ovarian hormones: tenderness and slight enlargement. As pregnancy continues, the breasts themselves enlarge, while the Montgomery glands, particularly, become more marked, the areola becomes darkened, and the nipples become larger and more mobile. A yellowish secretion, colostrum, is formed and is maintained until several days following delivery, when milk is formed. During lactation, the breasts continue in their enlarged state and, in addition, present multiple prominent vascular markings.

Breast development and function is under the complex control of many endocrine substances, particularly ovarian estrogen and progesterone. During the normal menstrual cycle both of these hormones lead to breast engorgement and sensitivity in the premenstrual period. The blood levels of these hormones fall just prior to menstruation, allowing for decongestion of the breast over the next few days. The ideal time for examination, therefore, is in the few days immediately after the menstrual period is finished, while the hormone levels have not yet risen to a significant degree. While the clinician must often examine the patient at other than ideal times, if there are questions about the presence of small masses or excessive tenderness, the examination should be rescheduled to be repeated after the next period. As noted later, instructions for self-examination should include explanation of this optimum time for such examination.

RISK FACTORS FOR BREAST CANCER
(See Table 13.1)

The breast is the most common site of cancer in women (although each year more women in this country die of lung cancer, as it is more lethal than breast cancer). Women who are at the greatest risk for breast cancer are those with a previous history of breast cancer. Other major factors are:

1. Age: over 50 years
2. History of cystic breast disease
3. Discharge from nipples
4. History of some types of disease requiring breast surgery
5. Family history of breast cancer

Table 13.1 Breast Cancer Risk Factors

1. Maternal family member with premenopausal breast cancer: risk 3 times that of the general population

2. Maternal family member with postmenopausal breast cancer: risk 1 1/2 times that of the general population

3. Maternal family member with bilateral breast cancer at diagnosis: risk 5 1/2 times that of the general population

4. Maternal family member with premenopausal and bilateral breast cancer at diagnosis: risk 9 times that of the general population

5. Early menarche or late natural menopause: risk more than twice that of the general population

6. Nulliparous woman: risk 4 times that of the general population

7. Woman older than 30 at her first pregnancy: risk 5 times that of the general population

8. Woman with benign breast disease: risk 4 times that of the general population. (This risk appears to continue for 30 years after diagnosis)

9. North American and Northern European women: risk 5 times that of Asian and African women, and 2 1/2 times that of South American and Southern European women

10. Ionizing radiation reaching more than 100 rads: risk significantly increased

11. Hypothyroidism: believed to increase risk slightly

12. Obesity (only in postmenopausal women): risk statistically increased

13. Estrogen therapy in women: risk slightly but inconsistently increased (No increased risk is seen with use of combination-type oral contraceptives)

Source: Hatfield HA, Guthrie TH: Breast Cancer Concepts. *Am Fam Physician* 1984,30(2):195-199, by permission.

Minor risk factors are:

1. Menarche before age 12
2. Late menopause
3. No live births before age 30

Specific recommendations regarding screening for breast cancer that effectively reduce mortality in women aged 50-59 vary among authorities. The American Cancer Society recommends breast self-examination monthly in women over 20, and practitioner-provided examination every 3 years from age 20-40, and annually beyond age 40.

EXAMINATION TECHNIQUE

To conduct a thorough examination of the breast, the patient's gown must be removed and a good light and screen provided.

Despite the Madison Avenue attention given to the female breast in the United States, and the fashionable acceptance of the bikini on the beaches around the world, it must be remembered that, perhaps because of its role as a sexual organ, many women, both young and old, respond to the need for this examination and its possible pathologic implication with fear and anxiety. Certainly, the examiner's approach must be gentle, supportive, and reflective of such understanding.

The breasts, nipples, and lymph nodes in the axillary and supraclavicular region should be carefully inspected and then palpated first with the patient sitting, hands at the sides and then over the head, and later, in the supine position. The details to be noted are included in the next sections under the specific technique. Characteristics of breast masses are described in Table 13.2.

Inspection

Since the size, shape, and position of the breasts vary markedly depending upon age, heredity, endocrine function, and presence of adipose tissue, it is impossible to provide data here classifying normal breasts in relation to these factors beyond the illustrations we have included. Even the beginning practitioner should have little difficulty in

Table 13.2 Characteristics of Breast Masses

Characteristic	Fibrocystic disease	Fibroadenoma	Breast Cancer
Borders	Usually distinct	Distinct	Often indistinct
Consistency	Rubbery	Hard	Hard
Response to menstrual cycle	Fluctuates	Rarely fluctuates	Rarely fluctuates
Fixation to underlying tissues	No	No	Yes
Tenderness	Yes	No	Rarely
Growth pattern	Stable over time	Stable over time	Progressive
Associated lymphadenopathy	No	No	Yes
Fluid aspirate	Clear, rarely bloody; cytology normal	No fluid	Clear, often bloody; cytology abnormal
Mammogram	Consistent with benign disease	Consistent with benign disease	Highly diagnostic of malignancy

Source: Hatfield HA, Guthrie TH: Breast cancer concepts. *Am Fam Physician* 1984, 30(2):195–199, by permission.

recognizing deviations from normal once a variety of breasts have been examined.
    The examination should begin by inspecting and comparing both breasts for (1) size, (2) shape, (3) symmetry, and (4) position. Asymmetrical development is not uncommon, but may be a source of emotional distress to the patient. It is also important to consider that any unilateral increase in size may indicate cyst formation, inflammation, or tumor, as well as congenital anomaly.
    The position of breast and nipple should be observed and then compared by having the patient raise her arms above her head, making note of any unilateral shift in position.
    Edema may be noted upon inspection when there is an underlying disease process. This causes the hair follicles and their openings to be more pronounced and is usually due to obstruction of lymphatic drainage (lymphedema), or leakage of serum into intercellular spaces (inflammatory carcinoma). This condition is commonly referred to as "orange peel" or "pig skin" (Figure 13.1).

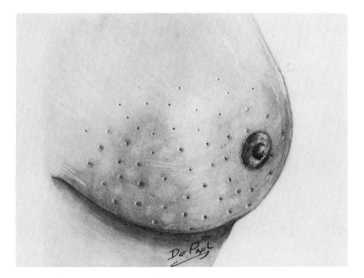

Figure 13.1 "Orange peel" defect of skin of breast due to edema or carcinoma.

Attention should then be paid specifically to the nipples themselves. The areola and nipple are carefully inspected for pigment change, erosions, crusting, scaling, discharge, and edema. Although many women have inverted nipples without evidence of disease, any retraction should be noted, especially when it is unilateral. *Paget's disease,* a malignant condition of the breast, may give rise to unilateral ulceration of one nipple, while bilateral ulceration may be a benign process. Any discharge from the nipple should, of course, be described according to color, amount, and consistency.

Skin retraction is one of the most significant findings to note in examination of the breast (Figure 13.2). Any disease process may infiltrate the tissue enough to apply abnormal traction on the suspensory ligaments, pulling with it a portion of the skin overlying the lesion and even the nipple itself, usually toward the side of the lesion.

The examiner should first inspect for retraction with the patient's hands at her side and then overhead. Since contraction of the pectoral muscles will exaggerate any retraction, it may be better seen when the patient presses her

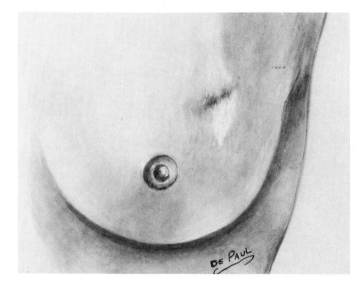

Figure 13.2 Skin retraction, or "dimpling" of the breast. An early sign of underlying carcinoma that has invaded the skin.

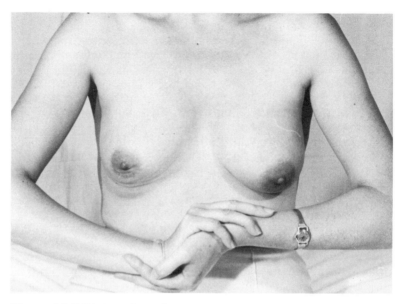

Figure 13.3 Tightening of the pectoral muscles to bring out possible dimpling of the skin of the breast.

palms together or applies pressure to both hips (see Figure 13.3).

It is important to remember that even when evidence of acute inflammation is not present, skin retraction may be one of the earliest physical findings of malignant tumor.

Inspection is not complete, however, unless attention is given to the axillary and supraclavicular regions where retractions, bulging, discoloration, and edema may also provide clues to underlying disease processes. Each arm should be put through a full range of motion, to fully visualize problem areas.

Palpation

The examiner should now proceed to palpate the dependent breast with the patient still sitting up, first with the arms at the side, and then with the arms raised over the head.

For purposes of examination and identification of location of lesions, the breast may conveniently be divided into
quadrants: the upper outer, upper inner, lower inner, and
lower outer quadrants. It is extremely important to recognize the fact that breast tissue of the upper outer quadrant
extends laterally upward to the anterior axillary fold. This
portion must not be neglected in the examination of the
breast.

With the fingers and thumb, the areola and nipples are
examined and then gently compressed in order to elicit the
presence of tenderness, nodules, and nipple discharge. Then,
each quadrant is carefully examined for consistency, elasticity, tenderness, and masses. A preferred technique is to
place the palmar surface of the fingers gently but firmly
against each quadrant of the breast, and to move the hand
in a rotary motion, pressing the breast tissue against the
chest wall (see Figures 13.4 through 13.6).

Another useful technique is bimanual palpation, in
which one hand raises the breast and the other presses breast
tissue between the two sets of fingers (Figure 13.7). This
may detect small dimples or mobile masses not picked up
by other techniques.

The presence of a mass should be described according
to criteria outlined in Chapter 8 and the patient immediately

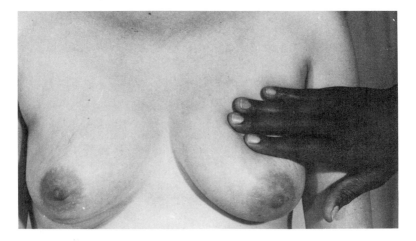

Figure 13.4 Examination of the breast. Palpation of the
breast in the upright position.

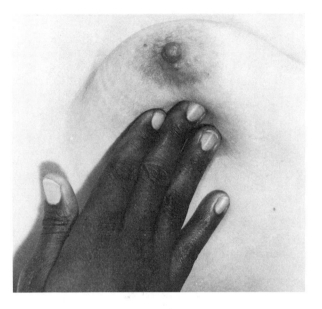

Figure 13.5 Examination of the breast. Palpation of the lateral breast in the supine position.

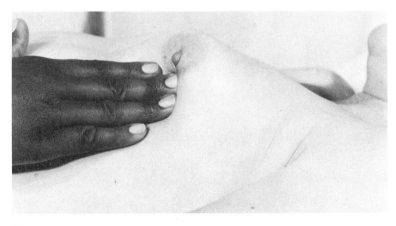

Figure 13.6 Examination of the breast. Palpation of the inferior portion.

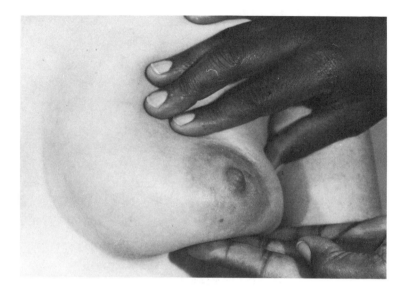

Figure 13.7 Bimanual palpation of the breast.

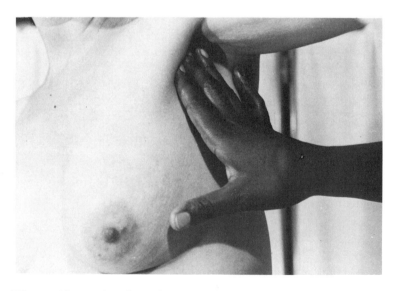

Figure 13.8 Palpation of the upper outer breast quadrant into the axilla.

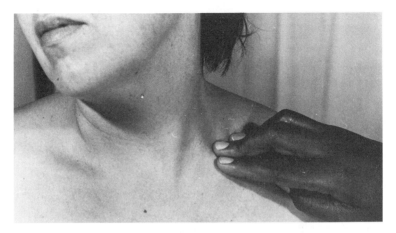

Figure 13.9 Palpation of the supraclavicular regions of lymph nodes.

referred to a specialist.   Since all masses are not malignant, the patient should not be unduly frightened by such a referral, but must be impressed with the importance of prompt consultation.

Once the breast and nipples themselves have been palpated, attention must be given to the axillae (Figure 13.8), the supraclavicular area (Figure 13.9), and the neck, in a search for lymph nodes, if these areas have not been examined up to this point.

SELF-EXAMINATION

As health educators as well as practitioners, we have obligations for teaching self-examination to all women past their menarche.   It is reliably estimated that almost 120,000 new cases of breast cancer will be discovered each year, and many should be first detected by the woman herself.   This will enable early detection and can have the important result of initiating diagnosis and treatment soon enough to prevent unnecessary death from this epidemic disease.

For the development of a common technique that should be taught to all American women, there is no better source than the brochure entitled "How to Examine Your Breasts," published in 1984 and distributed free of charge by the American Cancer Society. Provision of one technique to all will avoid confusion on the part of the female population, who otherwise might get several sets of instruction from different practitioners. All practitioners should obtain copies of this brochure, and should advise their female patients to perform the examination as specified in the brochure. The technique should be reviewed with the patient, who should then perform the examination under observation, so that the clinician can evaluate the patient's ability to do it fully and properly, even if she claims to know the technique.

Advise the patient to examine her breasts at a regular time each month, preferably after her menstrual period. Figures 13.10 through 13.15 are offered to illustrate the appropriate self-examination technique.

EXAMINATION OF THE MALE BREAST

Although significant lesions of the male breast are rare compared to those of the female breast, this organ must not be neglected. The normal male breast is flat and smaller than the female breast. If slightly or moderately prominent, it is usually because there is underlying fat, not breast tissue.

Inspection and palpation may be much more brief in the male, but discharge from the nipples, swelling, tenderness, or masses must be searched for. If the breast is prominent, palpation should be used to distinguish between the soft, mushy feeling of fat and the presence of true breast tissue underneath the nipple with its firmer, slightly nodular, and stringy characteristics. If true *breast tissue* is present, the condition is referred to as *gynecomastia* and may represent an endocrine disorder.

RECORDING: FEMALE

Breasts: symmetrical; contour and consistency appropriate for age and parity; no retraction, no nipple discharge; no masses or tenderness

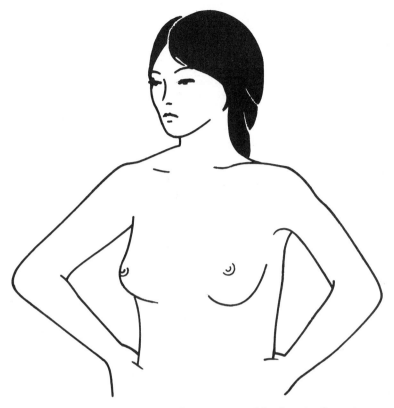

Figure 13.10 Advise the patient to stand in front of a mirror with her hands at her sides and look for any changes in size, shape, and position, as well as for areas of indentation or dimpling, redness, or irritation.

RECORDING: MALE

Breasts: symmetrical; no nipple discharge, masses or tenderness; no breast tissue

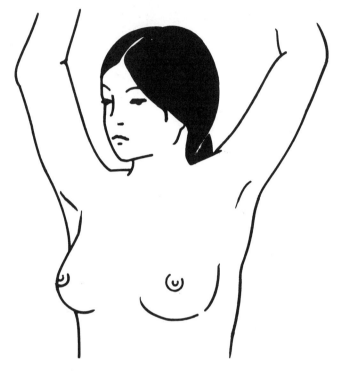

Figure 13.11 Tell her then to inspect with her hands raised over her head. Have her do a self-examination in front of a mirror under your directions so you can point out what to look for, as well as the technique of examination.

POTENTIAL NURSING DIAGNOSES

Anxiety: due to threat to self-image and threat of death

Grieving, dysfunction due to potential loss of sexual organ

Sexual dysfunction due to altered body structure

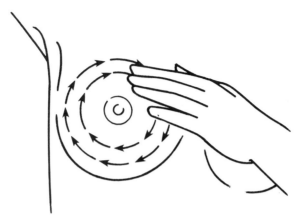

Figure 13.12 She should systematically palpate all four quadrants of the breast with the palmar surfaces of her fingertips.

PATIENT PROBLEM

Mrs. J., a 75-year-old alert, well-developed, well-nourished black woman, is brought to the health center by her daughter, who is concerned that her mother may have cancer of the breast.

Problem: Breast Lesion

S: Mrs. J. has been generally well, except for mild hypertension, and has been able to care for herself in her own apartment in another city. She is now visiting her daughter for the summer. While assisting her mother to dress, Mrs. J.'s daughter noted that the nipple of Mrs. J.'s right breast was deeply retracted. Mrs. J. said she noticed it several months ago but thought it was due to age.

O: *Insp:* Breasts are pendulous and not symmetrical. Right breast is larger than left, with nipple deeply retracted. Areola of right nipple is darker than left, with crusting at 9 o'clock. Surrounding skin is reddened, with increased vascular markings.

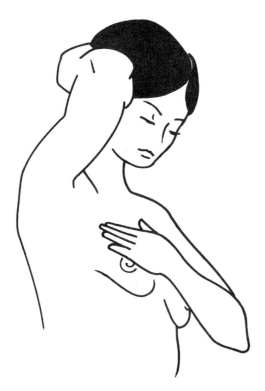

Figure 13.13 Show her how to examine the axillary area for any sensations of tenderness, nodules, or masses. Have her palpate while you observe her technique. Explain what she is feeling.

Palp: Hard, irregular, slightly tender mass 2 cm x 2 cm, about 3 cm deep behind the retraction. Mass is mobile within the breast but skin is adherent to mass; several matted lymph nodes palpable in right axilla; no other masses palpable in left breast or axilla.

ASSESSMENT: Mass of right breast with retraction, apparently carcinoma.

Nursing Diagnosis: Knowledge deficit of breast self-examination and need for early medical evaluation. Fear related to possible cancer of breast. Anxiety related to pending definite diagnosis, treatment, and outcome of present illness.

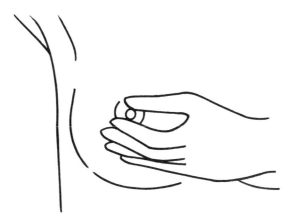

Figure 13.14 Demonstrate how to compress the nipples for discharge.

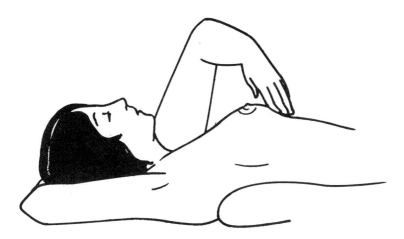

Figure 13.15 Show her how to examine all areas again while lying down so the breast is spread against the chest wall.

PLAN: Goals: To keep appointment for further
                         medical diagnosis and treatment.
                         To decrease fear and anxiety.
                         Nursing Orders:
                         Diagnostic: Refer to MD immediately.
                         Therapeutic: None at this time.
                         Patient Education: Mother and daughter
                         advised that there is need for medical
                         evaluation and psychologic counsel-
                         ing; discussions of strong possibility
                         that mass is carcinoma and that
                         surgical intervention will be necessary;
                         appointment made for consultation
                         today to avoid prolonged delay in
                         evaluation; will follow up after medical
                         consultation to provide continued sup-
                         port and counseling to both mother
                         and daughter.

IMPLEMENTATION: Assist with keeping appointment with
                         physician.
                         Inform of diagnostic procedure.

EVALUATION: Appointment made.
                         Patient visited in hospital and coping
                         effectively with diagnosis.

chapter 14

The Heart

Topographical Anatomy

Physiology

Examination

Recording

Potential Nursing Diagnoses

Patient Problem

This chapter deals with direct examination of the heart, for the sake of concentrating the student's attention on this facet of physical diagnosis. However, the student must be aware that full appreciation of the state of the heart's function must be obtained by combining what is found here with all that is learned elsewhere. Thus, peripheral cyanosis, edema of the eyelids, dilation of neck veins, splinter hemorrhages of the fingernail beds, clubbing, cough, shortness of breath, enlarged liver, ankle edema, and many other findings on history and physical examination all may provide evidence of cardiac disease.

TOPOGRAPHICAL ANATOMY

The heart lies in the thorax as if it were hung from the top, as, in fact, it is (Figure 14.1). The aorta, pulmonary arteries, and great veins all are at the upper (superior) portion of the heart, called the *base,* while the lower portion,

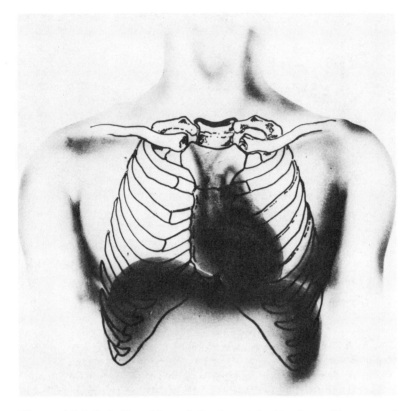

Figure 14.1 Relationships of the heart to the bony thorax and the diaphragm. On the right, the liver lies just beneath the heart, under the diaphragm.

the *apex,* hangs free. The organ is a wedge-shaped muscle with its base (the right and left atria) facing backward and to the right, and its apex (formed by the left ventricle) pointing forward and to the left. In the average adult, the base extends slightly to the right of the sternum while the apex comes into contact with the anterior chest wall at or near the fifth left intercostal space (ICS), usually just medial to the midclavicular line.

The right ventricle is anterior and thus lies directly under the sternum while the left ventricle is posterior and lateral, making up a large portion of the left cardiac border and the apex. The area of the chest overlying the heart bears the name *precordium.*

Except for the portion of right ventricle that lies against the sternum, the heart is separated from the chest wall by lung. The deeper portions of the heart are therefore covered by more lung tissue than the more superficial parts. Thus in doing percussion and auscultation over the precordium, the examiner will elicit signs from both organs to a greater or lesser degree.

Pericardium

The heart is encased in a tough, double-walled fibrous sac — the *pericardium* — which protects the heart from trauma. The outer layer of pericardium is firmly attached within the thorax to the esophagus, the aorta, the pleura, the sternum, and the diaphragm. A few cubic centimeters of fluid are present between the inner and outer layers of pericardium.

PHYSIOLOGY

As William Harvey said in 1628, "When the ventricle is full, the heart raises itself, forthwith tenses all its fibers, contracts the ventricles, and gives a beat." This single event, and the relaxation that follows, is the source of the point of maximum intensity, sternal heave, thrills, and the first and second (and other) heart sounds. Murmurs, clicks, snaps, pericardial friction rubs, as well as the pulse, the systolic blood pressure, and venous pulse waves all are related to this event.

Keep firmly in mind that the normal heart sounds are produced principally by *valve closure.* There is much argument still going on today about exactly what events contribute to heart sounds, but for a clear understanding of physical findings, remember that *valve closure produces the first and second heart sounds.*

For convenience, the cycle of events will be described beginning with blood flowing into the atria. Venous blood from the systemic circulation and oxygenated blood from the

lungs flow into the atria and through the open atrioventricular valves (mitral and tricuspid) into the relaxed ventricle
under very low pressure. When the atria are stimulated to
contract, they squeeze the blood in them into the ventricles,
which are then filled. Now the ventricles become tense and
the pressure, rising rapidly, snaps the atrioventricular (AV)
valves shut (Figure 14.2). Although both AV valves do not
snap shut simultaneously, the closures occur so closely together that the result is ordinarily heard as a single sound —
the first heart sound (S_1).

As pressure continues to rise rapidly in both ventricles,
the semilunar (aortic and pulmonic) valves are forced open

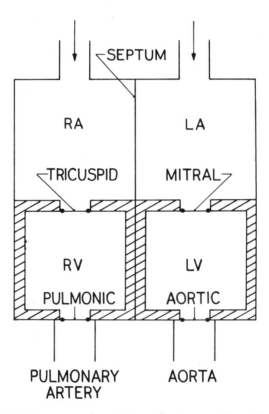

Figure 14.2 Diagram of position of valves. The AV valves
have just shut, producing the first heart sound. This is the
beginning of systole.

(A) (B)

38.97	Rm
8.75	lunch
5.00	admission
1.50	snacks
14.75	dinner
1.16	snacks
.75	newspaper
1.00	snacks
5.00	admission
1.46	A lunch
3.75	snacks
14.20	dinner
96.39	
5.00	gas T
1.56	card

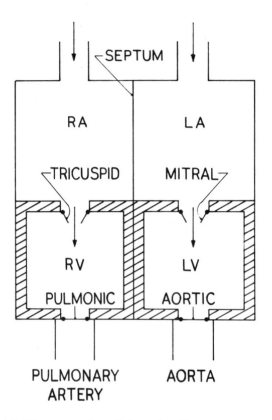

Figure 14.3 Diagram of position of valves. The semilunar valves, which opened during systole, have just snapped shut producing the second heart sound, marking the end of systole.

and blood begins to flow into the aorta and pulmonary artery. When the ventricles have emptied themselves of blood, the pressure in the aorta and pulmonary arteries forces the semilunar valves shut (Figure 14.3). This shutting of the valves produces the *second heart sound (S$_2$)*.

Blood then flows through both the systemic and pulmonary systems, the ventricles relax, blood returns through the veins, and the AV valves open, letting blood flow again into the ventricles, completing a single cardiac cycle. The entire sequence just described takes 1 second at a heart rate of 60 beats per minute, or 0.5 second at 120/minute. Pause for a moment in awe as you review this remarkable phenomenon before going on!

Systole begins with the first heart sound and ends at the second heart sound. During this period the ventricles have contracted and the apical portion of the heart has swung forward and upward, striking the anterior chest wall. *Diastole* is the period beginning with the second sound and ending at the next first sound. This is the period of relaxation of the ventricles and it is usually longer than systole (see Figure 14.6).

EXAMINATION

The cardiac examination is carried out in the same sequence used for the thorax and lung — inspection, palpation, percussion, and auscultation. While the examiner often is in a hurry to get his stethoscope on the chest, he should not do so. Auscultation is deliberately done last so that the clinician will have had time to obtain clues from other modes of examination. He frequently will have a considerable amount of diagnostic information before listening, so that he can listen with more understanding.

Inspection

The principal purpose of inspection is to see the effect of ventricular contraction on the precordium. The normal findings are an apical impulse and slight retraction medial to this impulse. These occur synchronously with cardiac systole and may be timed by palpating the carotid pulse while watching the chest.

Apical Impulse

The apical impulse may be found somewhere in the fourth, fifth, or sixth left intercostal spaces, normally at or medial to the midclavicular line. An apical impulse will *not* be seen (or palpated) in nearly half of the normal adult population.

When present, the apical impulse identifies an area very near the cardiac apex and is the *best* index of cardiac size on physical examination. Report its location carefully by interspace and relationship to the midsternal line (MSL) or midclavicular line (MCL) (see Figure 14.1). Both methods of reporting the horizontal location of the apex are used. Normally, the apical impulse is no more than 10 cm to the left of the MSL. However, considering the great variation in body build, our preference is to use the MCL for reference, since this line lies approximately halfway across the left chest wall no matter what the patient's size or shape. The apical impulse is normally found at or medial to the MCL, and if the heart is enlarged — or displaced — the impulse may be found lateral to that line. Thus, a normal location might be described as follows: "Apical impulse in fifth LICS at the MCL." If laterally displaced, the location should be reported by measurement, viz., "Apical impulse in sixth LICS 4 cm lateral to MCL."

Retraction

If an apex impulse is seen, look just medially to see if slight retraction of the intercostal space occurs. This, too, is a normal phenomenon. It is not normal, however, to have actual retraction of rib. Rib retraction commonly is due to pericardial disease and occurs because the pericardium is bound firmly to the chest wall.

Lift or Heave

When cardiac action is abnormally forceful, the sternum, or ribs, may be seen to lift with each heart beat. This is referred to as a *lift* or *heave* and should be confirmed by palpation. Both terms mean the same thing, but some authors refer to a slight movement as a lift and a more vigorous movement as a heave.

Palpation

Point of Maximum Intensity

If the apical impulse is not seen, try to locate the cardiac apex by locating a point of maximum intensity (PMI). The fingertips should be placed over the area where the apex usually is located and moved about to see if a pulsation can be felt. Having the patient lean forward may assist in identifying the apical impulse. If one is located, report the PMI as described earlier for apical impulse, i.e., by interspace and relationship to the MCL. Should it not be found easily, do not spend much time in searching since, as noted previously, the apex cannot be located in about half of the patients examined.

Lift or Heave

The precordium should be felt by placing the palm over the entire area to detect a movement of the chest wall with each systole. Heave, due to increased pressure or enlargement of the right ventricle, usually will be found in the sternum or near it, while overactivity or hypertrophy of the left ventricle will often produce motion of the chest wall near or lateral to the apex.

Thrill

A thrill is a palpable heart murmur or rub that is best described as a vibration. The sensation of a thrill may be reproduced by palpating the larynx while an "M" sound is being made. Thrill should be felt for across the entire precordium with the palm of the hand. Any murmur associated with a thrill is considered pathologic.

Percussion

The major objective of percussion of the heart is to detect the location of the left cardiac border (Figure 14.4). Usually, the left border will be found at or medial to the MCL. If located outside this line, the lateral distance from the MCL should be measured and reported as for the PMI.

Since the heart is much more dense than the lung, percussion over the organ will produce dullness. This cardiac dullness is best detected by percussing in the fourth LICS from the anterior axillary line toward the midline.

Although it is more awkward to perform, percussion should be done, where possible, with the patient sitting or standing, rather than lying down. In the supine position, the patient's heart sinks away from the chest wall so that dullness is detected in a smaller area than it would be with the patient upright. The preferred technique is to percuss as lightly as possible, barely producing resonance over lung tissue, so that

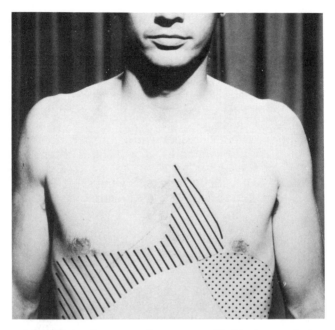

Figure 14.4 Normal percussion areas. Dotted area is tympanitic and hatched area is dull, being over the heart and liver.
See Figure 14.1.

when the cardiac border is reached, the sound will disappear
because of the dullness.

The left border of cardiac dullness (LBCD) should be
percussed first in the fourth interspace, as suggested. Percussion should be repeated in the fifth and sixth interspaces
to identify and report the location where the cardiac border
is most lateral. Thus "LBCD 2 cm lateral to MCL in fifth
LICS" means that this is the place where the cardiac border
is furthest to the left.

The right cardiac border ordinarily cannot be percussed adequately. At the base (refer to Figure 14.1), the
heart lies too deep beneath lung to produce dullness, while
the remainder of the right border is underneath the sternum.
A brief percussion may be made about 1 cm to the right of
the sternum to be sure that the heart does not project further

than this, but this is not a mandatory portion of the examination, unless one fails to find a left border. (Congenital dextrocardia occurs in about one person in 10,000, so it is great one-upmanship to be the first to detect this rare abnormality in the patient.)

The student should try to see chest x-ray films of patients whom he has examined to see how close he has come to the actual border. The two methods of examination will not locate the border in exactly the same place, but they should not be far apart.

Enlargement of displacement of the left ventricle, which makes up most of the left border, will often produce the findings of the LBCD lateral to the MCL, and although such a finding suggests cardiac enlargement, it is not a reliable enough technique to be diagnostic by itself.

Auscultation

General

While the two heart sounds are heard all over the precordial area, there are locations where the sounds produced at each of the valves are transmitted best to the chest wall, and therefore heard loudest. Thus, the portion of the second sound produced by aortic valve closure is ordinarily heard best in the right second intercostal space near the sternal border. This is referred to as the *aortic* area. Similarily, the *pulmonic* area is in the left second interspace at the sternal border, the tricuspid area near the lower end of the sternum, and the *mitral* area at the cardiac apex (Figure 14.5). The examiner should listen at these general locations, moving the stethoscope around to find the place where these sounds are loudest on a particular patient's chest.

However, auscultation will not be limited to these four valve areas, but must include the entire precordium for an adequate examination. It is useful to vary the patient's position to see if sounds (and murmurs) can be better heard. Listening with the patient leaning forward while seated, and then again, when the patient is supine, may assist in the process of complete auscultation.

As indicated in the brief review of physiology, at the slow heart rate of 60 beats per minute, all of the events of a single cardiac cycle occur within a single second. Thus,

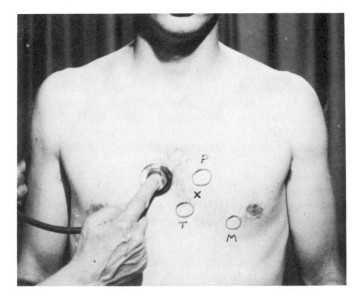

Figure 14.5 Cardiac auscultation at the aortic area. Circles mark the valve areas. According to the old poem, "Aortic right, Pulmonic left, Tricuspid's 'neath the sternum, Mitral's at the apex beat, and that is how we learn 'em." Erb's point is marked by an X.

everything seems to be happening at once. To interpret what one hears, there must be a high degree of concentration, which the student must discipline himself to learn, and which he must practice to achieve.

The student must learn to "tune in" on specific events — to concentrate his full attention on one feature at a time. Since there are normally two sounds and two intervals, a logical method is to "tune in" on the first heart sound (S_1). Concentrate on this *alone* to the exclusion of all else, for enough cardiac cycles to be certain of its characteristics. Then shift attention to S_2 and listen to it *alone*. After this, listen to the systolic interval between S_1 and S_2. Try to hear nothing else. Lastly, fix on the interval between S_2 and the next S_1 — diastole.

Such concentration is not easily learned, but only by continued discipline will the examiner begin to develop competence in cardiac auscultation. Listening to recordings of heart sounds and murmurs is helpful in learning and practicing this technique of specific "tuning in." One must learn and train oneself to *listen for* sounds rather than just *listening at* heart sounds or murmurs.

It is important to keep in mind the facts relevant to heart sounds — that the first sound (S_1) is produced by closure of the AV valves (mitral and tricuspid), that the second sound (S_2) arises with closure of the semilunar valves (aortic and pulmonic), and that these two sounds are heard over the entire precordium.

It is absolutely necessary to be able to identify the first sound and the second sound during all of cardiac auscultation. At heart rates of 90 or below, systole is distinctly shorter than diastole, so that identification of S_1 and S_2 is quite easy. However, as heart rates become more rapid, diastole begins to approach systole in duration, making timing a less certain technique for identification of the two sounds. At the aortic area, both S_1 and S_2 are better heard than in other locations on the chest. Here, also, S_2 is distinctly *louder* than S_1, enabling the examiner to distinguish one from the other in almost all cases (Figure 14.6). Confirmation may be obtained by palpating the apex beat (PMI) while listening. The apex beat is synchronous with S_1. If the apex beat is not palpable, the *carotid* pulse (but not the radial or femoral) may be palpated, as it rises just as S_1 ends.

By auscultation, S_1 is heard as a duller, lower-pitched, and slightly longer sound than S_2. S_2 has a higher pitch and is snappier and shorter than the first sound. Figure 14.6 is a sound recording (phonocardiogram) of normal heart sounds, which illustrates some of these features.

Technique

The examiner routinely should place himself at the patient's right side. This will assist him in developing a regular pattern of examination and in keeping the earpieces of his stethoscope in proper location in his auditory canals.

Certain sounds and murmurs are heard better with the patient upright or leaning slightly forward, while others are brought out in the recumbent position. The student should, therefore, make a habit of examining patients in at least two positions.

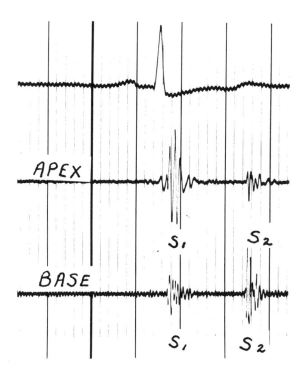

Figure 14.6 Phonocardiogram of normal heart sounds. The upper tracing is an electrocardiograph recorded for purposes of timing. The middle line was recorded at the apex (mitral area) and the lower tracing was taken at the pulmonic area. Note the fact that at the apex the first sound is louder, while at the base, the second sound is louder.

The clinician will listen to the characteristics of the heart sounds first in his examination to determine if they are normal. Obviously, such a judgment must be made on the basis of what one has heard in many normal hearts. Intensity (loudness) is graded as normal, louder or fainter than normal, or absent. Quality has to do with the character of the sound, i.e., sharp, snapping, full, or booming. Another feature of the character of a heart sound is whether it sounds like a pure single sound or a "split" sound. This must be heard to be appreciated but it is a distinction that can be readily made once learned (see Splitting, later in this chapter).

Remember that the diaphragm chestpiece amplifies sound and transmits higher-pitched sounds and that the bell transmits low-pitched sounds much better and is critical in certain portions of the examination.

Clinical Auscultation

The examiner should be at the patient's right side and auscultation should begin at the *aortic* area, using the diaphragm of the stethoscope. Identify S_2, which is the louder sound here, and then begin the examination by concentrating your full attention on S_1. Listen to its loudness, pitch, and quality. Next, fix attention on S_2 and evaluate *this* sound. Only when the characteristics of S_1 and S_2 are determined and compared in your mind with the expected normal characteristics should you proceed.

Concentrate next on systole, the normally silent interval between S_1 and S_2. Any sounds heard in systole are to be described as accurately as possible. Then listen to the diastolic interval between S_2 and the next S_1. Here, too, there should be no sounds, normally.

Having completed this examination in the aortic area, shift the diaphragm of the chestpiece to the *pulmonic* area and repeat the entire sequence of auscultation: the S_1, then S_2, then to the systolic interval, and lastly to diastole. You will note that, as in the aortic area, the S_2 is louder than S_1 and that S_2 is a shorter, snappier, higher-pitched sound than S_1. Splitting of S_2 is often heard in this area, and may or may not be abnormal.

Before leaving the base of the heart, compare the loudness of S_2 in the *aortic* area to S_2 in the *pulmonic* area. You may need to shift the stethoscope rapidly between the aortic and pulmonic areas several times to make this comparison. S_2 generally is louder in the pulmonic area in children and young adults. By age 30, most adults will have an S_2 louder in the aortic area than in the pulmonic area. The loudness of S_2 (aortic) is roughly related to the arterial blood pressure in the systemic circulation, while loudness of S_2 heard in the pulmonic area is influenced by pulmonary artery pressure. Thus, for example, arterial hypertension will cause S_2 (aortic) to be even louder than normal. Factors that increase pulmonary pressures, such as chronic obstructive pulmonary disease, may lead to an increase of loudness in S_2 (pulmonic).

The finding of S_2 (pulmonic) louder than S_2 (aortic) in an adult over age 40 is abnormal. The relationship between S_2 (aortic) and S_2 (pulmonic) should always be established and recorded. Use of mathematical symbols is a convenient way to record this relationship. Thus, in the normal adult S_2 (aortic) is louder than S_2 (pulmonic) and would be symbolized as: S_2 (aortic) $>$ S_2 (pulmonic).

The examiner now "inches" his stethoscope down from the pulmonic area toward the lower end of the sternum. The first sound (S_1) at the tricuspid area may be normally louder than S_2, or both may be equal. Shift to the bell of the stethoscope since the lower-pitched sounds are heard better than with the diaphragm. As before, examine S_1, S_2, systole, and then diastole, evaluating the sounds and then the intervals for any abnormalities.

From this area, move the bell slowly toward the cardiac apex. The point at which sounds are loudest is called the mitral area, the cardiac apex. The examination of heart sounds and intervals in repeated at this location. Normally, S_1 will be louder than S_2 here, although the sounds may be of about equal intensity.

If there is significant emphysema present, with an increase in AP diameter of the chest, either or both sounds may be difficult to hear at the tricuspid and mitral areas. Having the patient lean forward may help to bring these sounds out better.

Splitting

As noted earlier, the valves of the right and left sides of the heart snap shut almost simultaneously so that the sound produced is heard as a single sound. Should enough delay in one of the closures occur, the heart sound will be heard with two distinct components and it is said to be *split* (Figure 14.7). Splitting is more often heard in first heart sounds at the apex, and in second sounds at the base.

It is important to be able to identify a split so as not to confuse it with other sounds that may occur during cardiac auscultation. This distinction will be made principally on quality and timing: the split sound still has the same general quality (i.e., pitch, loudness, and character) as the unsplit sound, but is made up of two distinct components, one occurring immediately after the other. A crude representation of this may be produced by saying aloud the

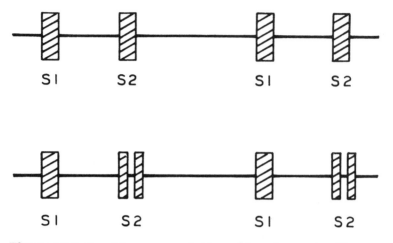

Figure 14.7 Graphic representation of heart sounds. The upper line is normal. The lower represents a split second sound. Note the closeness of the two components of the split sound. Systole is the interval between S_1 and S_2; diastole occurs between S_2 and the next S_1.

sound, "spit-spit-spit" to represent a single heart sound; then at the same speed, pitch, and loudness, say "split-split-split." Pronouncing the extra letter gives the word a split quality.

If a split sound is heard, the examiner should note and record variation in the split, with respiration. A split may occur in perfectly normal hearts or under abnormal situations. The *physiologic split* of the pulmonic second sound will be heard to appear and *widen* during *inspiration* and to disappear on *expiration.* Such a split is a normal phenomenon. If the split does not vary with respiration, it is called a *fixed split;* if it becomes wider and more pronounced on expiration, it is called a *paradoxical split* since it varies in an opposite way from the physiologic split. Both the fixed split and the paradoxical split have different causes and are generally evidences of cardiac disease.

There are several other sounds that may be heard on cardiac auscultation, only two of which will be described here (Figure 14.8).

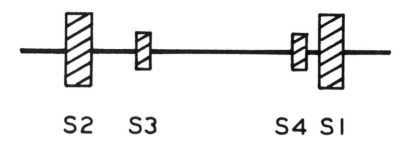

S2   S3   S4 SI

Figure 14.8 Third and fourth heart sounds. Note that both occur during diastole.

Third Heart Sound (S₃)

In some normal patients, particularly in those under age 30, a third heart sound (S_3) may be heard. The third sound has the following features:

1. Heard best near the apex, not at the base of the heart.
2. May be accentuated by left lateral decubitus position
3. Has a low-pitched sound (use bell of stethoscope)
4. Occurs early in diastole
5. May become louder with expiration
6. May be more prominent with tachycardia
7. May be associated with pulses alternans

These features should suggest several maneuvers for the examiner to use to find or identify an S_3.

The exact cause of S_3 is not fully agreen upon by all authorities, but it is commonly accepted that while S_3 may be normal in young adults, it is to be considered abnormal in patients over 40 years of age, and should always be reported when found.

Fourth Heart Sound (S₄)

A fourth sound may occur at the time of atrial contraction. It was noted, in the section on physiology that, when the atria contract and fill the ventricles, ventricular contraction begins. Since this occurs before the beginning of the first heart sound, the fourth sound (S_4) will be heard at the end of the diastolic interval — or before systole begins (see

Figure 14.8). This is more often heard near the apex or left sternal border, but it may be heard in any location. However, since S_4 is a low-pitched sound, like S_3, it will be picked up more distinctly by the bell and can be distinguished from S_3 by the time of its appearance. S_4 is generally an abnormal finding.

Although other sounds do occur, their description will not be discussed in this text. When the student is sufficiently competent to be certain of the identification and characterization of these four heart sounds and of murmurs, he should then, by reference to other sources, expand his knowledge of sounds such as the opening snap, systolic ejection clicks, and pericardial knocks. He must, however, describe all sounds even if he is unclear about identification.

Triple Rhythm (Gallop)

A triple rhythm refers to one consisting of three distinct heart sounds: S_1, S_2, and another of varied origin. This triple rhythm often resembles the sound of galloping hoofbeats, particularly when the heart rate is increased. There are several varieties of triple rhythm that are distinguished by the timing of the extra sound. It is very important to determine whether the extra sound occurs during systole (systolic gallop) or in diastole (diastolic gallop). Systolic gallops may be heard in normal hearts, whereas a diastolic gallop rhythm is almost certain to indicate heart disease.

Since, by definition, there will be three distinct sounds making up a gallop, the two normal heart sounds must be identified to know where the third component falls in the cardiac cycle. The major reference point for identification of the normal sounds is in the aortic area, where S_2 is loud, crisp, and distinct.

Triple rhythm is usually best heard with the patient supine, and most often is picked up at or near the cardiac apex. Once the examiner hears the triple rhythm of a gallop, he should begin to inch the chestpiece of his stethoscope toward the aortic area, using either the bell or diaphragm, depending on which allows him to hear all three sounds best.

As he approaches the base of the heart, the examiner will hear S_2 becoming louder and clearer. S_1 will also become more distinct and the extra sound will fade in intensity or actually disappear. This maneuver should identify which

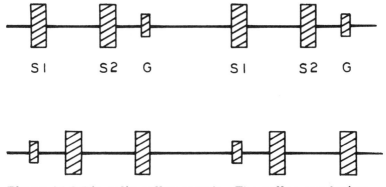

Figure 14.9 Diastolic gallop sounds. The gallop-producing sound is labelled G. The upper line shows an S_3 gallop rhythm sounding somewhat like the word "Ken-*tuck*-y." The lower line represents an S_4 (presystolic) gallop, with a "Ten-ne-*see*" rhythm.

of the three sounds is "gallop-producing" and, therefore, in which phase of the cardiac cycle it appears.

There are, in fact, two types of diastolic gallop frequently referred to as S_3 gallop and S_4 gallop, depending upon whether the extra sound occurs early in diastole where S_3 usually is heard (Figure 14.9) or late in diastole, where S_4 is generally present. If this distinction can be made, it should be reported, but this distinction is *far* less important than the determination that a gallop is systolic or diastolic.

As noted earlier, the presence of either an S_3 or S_4, whether they produce a gallop rhythm or not, must be assumed to be abnormal and should be carefully described as to timing, location on the precordium, quality of sound, and change in respiration or patient's position. The distinction between an abnormal and a normal third or fourth sound should be left for the consultant.

Murmurs

Cardiac murmurs are the result of turbulent blood flow within the heart, produced at the valves, or through abnormal passages, such as openings between atria (atrial septal defect), ventricles (ventricular septal defect), or a patent ductus arteriosus. Ordinarily the term *bruit* is reserved for a similar sound heard over arteries distant from the heart. Murmurs have a greater duration than heart sounds.

Turbulence at a valve generally arises from narrowing of the valve opening (stenosis) or from blood flowing backward through a defective closed valve (insufficiency or regurgitation).

The timing of murmurs is based upon the time of the murmur in relation to the first and second heart sounds. The identification of the defect is not easy, for it is not always true that the murmur will be loudest at the named area on the chest identified earlier. Thus aortic valve murmurs are generally transmitted toward the apex and may be at maximum intensity at the left sternal border or at the apex itself. Also, murmurs may be due to defects other than to damaged valves. The task of the examiner, therefore, is to establish the exact timing of the murmur, and then to describe carefully the location of maximum loudness, the quality, loudness, pitch, radiation, and change during exercise, respiration, or movement of the patient.

It must be remembered, in cardiac auscultation, that all murmurs do not indicate disease and conversely that some cardiac defects do not produce murmurs. In general all diastolic murmurs are to be considered pathologic.

By definition, systolic murmurs occur betweem S_1 and S_2. If the murmur is loudest in midsystole, it is referred to as an *ejection murmur* and is called diamond-shaped because of its appearance on the phonocardiograph (Figure 14.10). The other common type of systolic murmur is one heard throughout systole and is more or less equal in loudness from beginning to end. This is called a *pansystolic* or *holosystolic* murmur. Occasionally, a murmur is heard only in early or late systole and would be described in those terms.

Similarly, diastolic murmurs must be described in terms of onset, duration, and "shape." True pandiastolic murmurs are less common than are pansystolic. More often they are heard early or late in diastole. Early murmurs generally begin immediately after the second sound and fade out in late diastole (decrescendo); late murmurs begin near middiastole and become louder (crescendo) as they merge into the first sound. These are sometimes referred to as presystolic murmurs. Figure 14.11 illustrates some characteristic forms or shapes of murmurs.

Murmurs must be described by the location of the point on the chest where they sound loudest. As noted earlier,

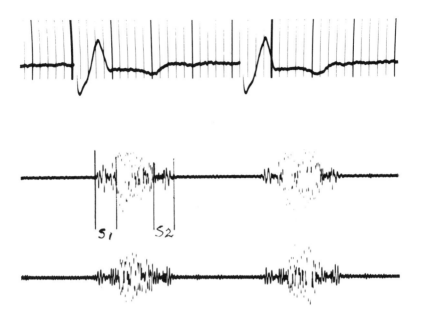

Figure 14.10 Phonocardiograph of a systolic murmur. The upper line is an electrocardiograph. The middle and lower tracings were recorded with different electronic filters but both show the "diamond" shape of the systolic murmur.

these locations may or may not correspond to the valve sites because of transmission of the sounds. This is particularly true for murmurs of the aortic valve, which are so frequently radiated to the third left interspace at the sternal border that this area is called the *secondary aortic area,* or Erb's point (see Figure 14.5).

When listening for murmurs at the cardiac apex, it is a good practice to examine the area with the patient supine, and then to have him move to a *left lateral decubitus* position, while listening. This maneuver occasionally will exaggerate a faint diastolic murmur not heard in any other position.

In addition to recording the point at which the murmur sounds loudest, the clinician should describe the radiation of the murmur. Such radiation is often characteristic of a

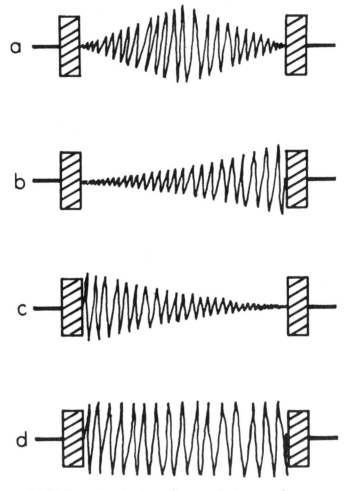

Figure 14.11 Representation of several shapes of murmurs as seen on phonocardiography. These may be either systolic or diastolic in time. (a) Diamond-shaped; (b) crescendo; (c) decrescendo; (d) pansystolic or pandiastolic.

particular lesion and may be quite helpful in diagnosis. Thus, the murmur of aortic stenosis often can be tracked into the carotid arteries, that of mitral insufficiency into the axilla, while that of mitral stenosis hardly radiates at all from the apical area.

The pitch of a murmur is an important feature to describe. The terms *low, medium,* and *high* are used; the student will learn to define these terms by experience. The examiner must also describe the quality of any murmur by descriptive terms. Commonly used words are blowing, rough, harsh, rumbling, or musical. Other fanciful terms may be used if they provide a good description. Thus, for example, the murmur of aortic stenosis with calcification of the valve is often perceived and described as a "sea gull" murmur.

Descriptions of murmurs require inclusion of many features: timing, location, radiation, pitch, and quality. Additionally, the loudness or intensity of a murmur must be described and recorded. This is so subjective and so much related to the experience of the observer that it is difficult to evaluate and to agree on. Fortunately, it is not nearly so critical an item as timing or location for purposes of diagnosis or evaluation. Two systems are in general use for grading the intensity of murmurs, one based on four and one on six grades. The six grade system is as follows:

Grade 1: the faintest murmur you can hear; often not heard at first

Grade 2: faint, but heard without difficulty

Grade 3: soft, but louder than grade 2

Grade 4: loud, but less loud than grade 5

Grade 5: loud, but not heard if stethoscope is lifted just off the chest (thrill will be present)

Grade 6: maximum loudness; heard even if stethoscope is lifted from chest

Obviously, the difference between grades 3 and 4 is not exact, but the other criteria are rather easy to define. In recording the intensity by this system the observer must identify that he is grading on the basis of six, e.g., "grade 4 (of 6) murmur," or "grade 4/6 murmur." The four grade system is simpler and perfectly adequate. Here the criteria are:

Grade 1: faintest murmur you can hear

Grade 2: soft

Grade 3: loud

Grade 4: very loud

Table 14.1 Typical Characteristics of Several Common Murmurs[a]

Area	Timing	Heart Sounds	Quality of Murmur	Transmission of Murmur	Probable Lesions
Aortic or Erb's pt.	Systole	S_2 normal or decreased, S_4 may be present	Medium pitch, harsh, ejection	Vessels of neck	Aortic stenosis
	Diastole	S_1 normal or decreased	High pitch, blowing, decrescendo	Left sternal border	Aortic insufficiency
Pulmonary	Systole	S_2 normal or decreased, S_2 split	Medium pitch, harsh, ejection	Little to none	Pulmonary stenosis
	Diastole	Generally normal	Medium pitch, blowing, decrescendo	Little to none	Pulmonary insufficiency
Mitral	Systole	S_1 normal or decreased, S_3 may be present	Medium pitch, blowing, pansystolic	Toward axilla	Mitral insufficiency

Location	Timing	Additional sounds	Murmur character	Radiation	Lesion
Left sternal border, 4th interspace	Diastole	"Snapping" accentuated S1, "opening snap"	Low pitch, rumble, crescendo	Little to none	Mitral stenosis
Left sternal border, 4th interspace	Systole	S3 may be present	Medium pitch, variable harsh, holosystolic	Variable	Ventricular septal defect
Left sternal border, 2nd interspace	Systole and Diastole	May not be heard	Variable pitch, harsh, crescendo-decrescendo	Precordium	Patent ductus arteriosus

aThe features listed are generally present, but vary according to the severity of valve damage and dynamic factors such as pressure. Also, where there is both stenosis and insufficiency of one valve, or damage to more than one valve, the characteristics of murmurs are modified.

Reporting by this system would be identified as follows: "grade 2 (of 4) murmur," or "grade 2/4 murmur."

If deep inspiration or deep expiration changes the intensity of a murmur, this should be noted. If variations in heart sounds also occur, these should be noted to complete the description.

Table 14.1 is a condensed outline describing several common murmurs. Only a few descriptive terms are used and the student is cautioned to recognize that this is only a brief and incomplete starting point for interpretation of murmurs.

Friction Rub

In pericarditis, a friction rub may develop that can often be heard over the lower sternum. It is not usually related to systole or diastole, but may be heard during various parts of the cardiac cycle often beginning in late diastole and going through systole. Sounds may vary with respiration since the pleura may be involved where it attaches to the pericardium. The pericardial friction rub is typically transient and may change in character from time to time.

RECORDING

Heart

Insp.:   no heave; apical impulse in 5th LICS medial to MCL

Perc.:   LBCD at MCL in 5th ICS

Palp.:   no heave; thrill or rib retraction

Ausc.:   rate 80/min regular, sounds normal S_2 aortic > S_2 pulmonic, S_2 split at pulmonic on inspiration; no murmurs, gallop, rubs

POTENTIAL NURSING DIAGNOSES

Activity intolerance: due to imbalance between oxygen supply and demand

Cardiac output, alteration in: decreased due to alteration in i.e. rate, rhythm, or conduction

Fluid volume, alteration in: excess due to compromised regulatory mechanism

Tissue perfusion, alteration in: cardiopulmonary due to hypervolemia

PATIENT PROBLEM

Mrs. T.F., a 65-year-old widow with CC short of breath this a.m., felt "faint, weak."

Problem: Cardiac Murmur and Left Heart Failure

S: Good general health; no history of rheumatic fever; had systolic murmur noted at age 38 but no symptoms until 1 year ago; had episode of "feeling faint" upon exertion this a.m.; has never had ankle edema.

O: BP, LA 180/80; pulse 100, vigorous beat.

RA 170/80 sitting and lying.

Insp: Carotid pulse visible and pulsation noted in suprasternal notch; apical impulse in 6th LICS, 2 cm lateral to MCL.

Palp: PMI forceful at location of apical impulse, slight lift at apex; liver not enlarged.

Perc: No pulmonary dullness; LBCD maximal in 6th LICS, 2 cm lateral to MCL.

Ausc: Few bilateral basal rales, posteriorly; S$_2$ accentuated; blowing, high-pitched decrescendo grade 2/6 murmur, heard best at Erb's point, radiating up to aortic area and carotid vessels, downward to apex; no gallop.

ASSESSMENT: Probable aortic insufficiency with minimal early left heart failure.

Nursing Diagnosis: Alterations in cardiac output related to cardiac murmur and left heart failure.

Activity intolerance related to shortness of breath and weakness.
Potential for injury related to episodes of feeling "faint and weak."

PLAN:
Goals: To verbalize increased knowledge of diagnostic procedures during appointment with cardiologist.
Diagnosis confirmed and Medical Therapeutic regimen initiated.
Health maintenance routines implemented.
Nursing Orders:
Diagnostic: ECG: chest x-ray; sed rate; CBC.
Therapeutic: Appointment with cardiologist for consultation, promptly.
Patient Education: Health status discussed regarding murmur, significance of SOB; advised as to necessity for consultation and further tests, diet control, drugs, and activity.

IMPLEMENTATION: Discussed functions of the heart in relation to "breathing and faintness."
Discussed diagnostic tests.
Discussed home safety.
Discussed regime of activity and rest.

EVALUATION:
Appointment made with cardiologist.
Verbalized knowledge of diagnostic tests without evident anxiety.
Verbalized that she planned to remove scatter rugs from home and not climb on chairs to reach out-of-the-way cupboards.
Stated that activity and rest regime presented no problems.

The Abdomen

The abdomen may be thought of as a shallow bowl containing the stomach, intestines, liver, spleen, kidneys, and other organs and blood vessels. The bowl is made up of the spine and muscles of the back and is covered by the anterior abdominal wall consisting of skin, fat, muscle, and connective tissue. Thus the abodmen and its important contents are soft tissue structures. Palpation can therefore produce more information here than in the chest, which is limited by its bony structures.

TOPOGRAPHICAL ANATOMY

As seen from the front, the anterior abdominal wall has the approximate outline of a hexagon with the xiphoid process at the top and the symphysis pubis at the bottom. The upper edges are formed by the costal margins and the lower edges by the inguinal ligaments which extend from the iliac crests to the symphysis pubis. The sides of this imaginary hexagon are simply the right and left sides of the patient (see Figures 15.1 and 15.2). At first, it will be useful for the student to fix these points and lines by actual palpation before proceeding with the examination. It must be recalled that the abdominal contents extend up beneath the rib cage and down into the pelvis, outside this hexagon.

Due to variations in body build, the hexagon may be wide or narrow, long or short. In order to describe locations within the abdomen, the hexagon is divided into either four or nine segments. Since both systems or divisions are used, the student should be familiar with both. The simpler method is division into four quadrants made by a vertical line (the midline), from the xiphoid process to the symphysis pubis, and by a horizontal line across the umbilicus. The quadrants are simply named right upper quadrant (RUQ), left upper quadrant (LUQ), right lower quadrant (RLQ), and left lower quadrant (LLQ) (Figure 15.1).

The second system (Figure 15.2) marks off the abdominal wall by drawing vertical lines upward from the midpoint of both the right and left inguinal ligaments. Two horizontal lines are drawn — one across the lower rib margins and the other crossing the iliac crests. This produces nine areas and is a more convenient system for locating lesions or masses near the midline.

The contents of the abdomen underlying these nine areas are as follows:

Right Hypochondriac	Epigastric	Left Hypochondriac
Right lobe of liver	Pyloric end	Stomach
Gallbladder	of stomach	Spleen
Part of duodenum	Duodenum	Tail of pancreas
Hepatic flexure of	Pancreas	Splenic flexure of
colon	Aorta	colon
Part of right kidney	Portion of	Upper pole of left
Suprarenal gland	liver	kidney
		Suprarenal gland

Right Lumbar	Umbilical	Left Lumbar
Ascending colon	Omentum	Descending colon
Lower half of	Mesentery	Lower half of left
right kidney	Transverse	kidney
Part of duodenum	colon	Parts of jejunum
and jejunum	Lower part of	and ileum
	duodenum	
	Jejunum and	
	ileum	

Right Inguinal	Hypogastric	Left Inguinal
Cecum	Ileum	Sigmoid colon
Appendix	Bladder	Left ureter
Lower end of ileum	Pregnant	Left spermatic
Right ureter	uterus	cord in male
Right spermatic		Left ovary in
cord in male		female
Right ovary in female		

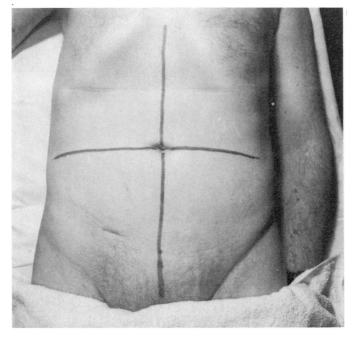

Figure 15.1 The abdomen marked into quadrants. A surgical scar is visible in the RLQ and another crosses horizontally in both upper quadrants.

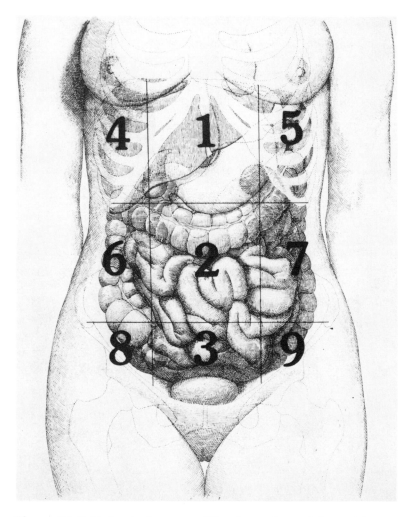

Figure 15.2 Abdominal areas: (1) epigastrium; (2) umbilical; (3) hypogastric; (4,5) right and left hypochondrium; (6,7) right and left flanks — or lumbar areas (8,9); right and left inguinal — or iliac areas. Reproduced with permission of A.H. Robins Co., Richmond, VA.

The student must review the anatomical structures present in the abdomen and their relationships before studying the physical examination. This knowledge is critical for an understanding of the techniques and results of the examination.

PHYSIOLOGY

The descent of the diaphragm on inhalation moves the liver, spleen, kidneys, stomach, and intestines downwards, producing outward motion of the upper abdominal wall. This motion is much more pronounced, on the average, in men than in women.

During the daytime, and particularly during eating, much air is swallowed. This air, mixed with ingested fluids and intestinal juices, is propelled through the stomach and intestines, producing bowel sounds which, as might be expected, sound like gurgles and bubbles. Collections of air in the gastrointestinal tract produce the hollow note on percussion called *tympany.*

As the semisolid feces are being formed in the colon, they are occasionally palpable. Urine, filling the bladder, may make it palpable and, if the full bladder is percussed, it produces a flat note.

The pregnant uterus rises out of the pelvis and, as it displaces intestine in the suprapubic area, can be appreciated as a solid mass to palpation and percussion. Late in pregnancy, the large volume of blood flow to the placental circulation may produce a bruit called the funic souffle. Fetal heart sounds may also be heard late in pregnancy.

EXAMINATION

For proper examination of the abdomen, the patient should be lying comfortably in the supine position with his head supported by a pillow. He should have a narrow towel draped across the genital area and, if the patient is a woman, the breasts also should be draped. The patient's arms should not be raised since this position tends to stretch the abdominal muscles, putting them under tension and making the abdomen harder to examine. Generally, the arms should be at the side, and if they are in the way when the flanks are examined, they may be folded across the chest.

It is ordinarily not necessary to have the patient's knees drawn up unless the patient is uncomfortable with his lower extremities flat. Should the patient desire the knees-up position, careful questioning should be done about the location of pain if one or both lower extremities are extended, as this may produce valuable diagnostic information.

The examiner should inspect the abdomen from all angles but should develop the habit of performing most of the remainder of the examination from the right side of the patient. This positioning will help to reinforce a pattern of examination. It is often convenient to sit at the bedside for detailed inspection and for auscultation.

In the evaluation of the thorax, the sequence of examination is inspection, palpation, percussion, and auscultation. Here it is advisable to vary the order and to follow inspection with *auscultation*. The reason for this is that palpation may induce tenderness if there is a painful lesion in the abdomen, and this tenderness will interfere with the motility of the bowel — sometimes producing almost no motility for a period of time. This will change the frequency and character of the bowel sounds, whereas if the examiner had listened before palpating, his findings would have been quite different.

Inspection

As for all other regions, inspection should begin with a general view of the region to detect significant variations from the normal. The examiner should keep in mind the anatomy of the area, and in his inspection should concentrate on the abdominal wall and then the abdominal contents.

It was pointed out earlier that the umbilicus is located slightly below the center of the abdomen. If it is observed to be distinctly higher than this, the examiner should be alerted to the possibility of a tumor in the suprapubic region (see diagram, Figure 15.2) or of pregnancy which causes the uterus to rise into this region. The umbilicus may be lower than normal due to tumor underlying the epigastric region, or to ascites (See Figure 15.4).

Contour

The normal abdomen should be flat and the lateral borders only slightly curved. If the abdominal wall is thin, the

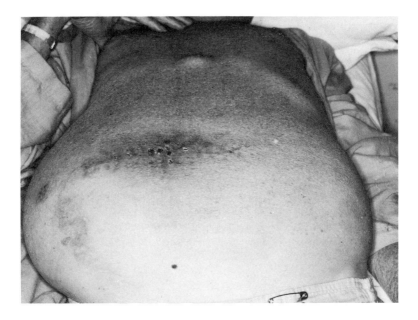

Figure 15.3 Abdominal distention. This was due to excessive fluid (ascites). The umbilicus was removed following rupture of an umbilical hernia.

abdominal contents are reduced in size and the contour will be concave rather than flat. This is described as a *scaphoid* abdomen. On the other hand, the abdominal wall may protrude forward either in a localized area or throughout its entire extent. The flanks should be inspected to see if they are not generally straight but are bulging and rounded. This is often an early finding when fluid is accumulating in the peritoneal cavity and is also commonly seen in simple obesity. Figure 15.3 shows an example of severe bulging of the flanks.

Skin

As elsewhere, the skin should be inspected for texture, color, lesions, scars, wounds, etc., which should be reported as described earlier.

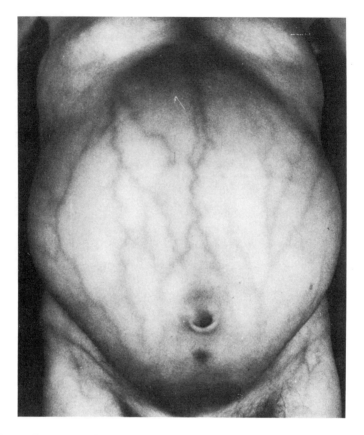

Figure 15.4 Prominent abdominal veins and abdominal distention. Photographed in infrared light. Note here that the umbilicus is displaced downward.

Discoloration

The appearance of bluish discoloration or bruises in the abdominal wall should be viewed with great suspicion, for even though they may be due to trauma, they may also represent intra-abdominal bleeding. Such discolorations may be seen in cases of extrauterine pregnancy, pancreatitis, metastatic tumors, etc.

Veins

The veins of the normal abdominal wall are usually not visible or are not prominent. A distinct increase in the number and the fullness of abdominal veins is probably abnormal and should always be reported. When prominent veins are seen (Figure 15.4), the direction of flow in them should be recorded. In the normal situation, blood flows *away* from the umbilicus, i.e., upward above the umbilicus and downward below the umbilicus.

Hernias

Inspection of the abdominal wall also reveal the presence of a hernia, which is the protrusion of tissues or an organ through an abnormal opening. There are several locations where this is prone to occur in the abdominal wall: anywhere along the midline including the umbilicus, in surgical scars, or above the inguinal ligament.

If small protrusions are noted, they may or may not be true hernias. This may be checked by having the patient strain, increasing intra-abdominal pressure. Most often, a hernia will bulge further out with such a maneuver. Palpation will also assist in confirming the bulging of a hernia when intra-abdominal pressure is increased.

Respiratory Motion

The motion of the abdominal wall should be watched through several respiratory cycles. As noted earlier, most men are "abdominal breathers" in that they utilize the diaphragm more than women. What may possibly be abnormal is the *absence* of abdominal respiratory motion, particularly in a man. This may represent the first physical finding of peritonitis which causes the patient to hold the diaphragm still to reduce abdominal pain.

Pulsation

Portions of the abdominal wall may be seen to pulsate at the same rate as the heart. This is sometimes seen in patients with thin-walled scaphoid abdomens and occasionally with distended abdomens, particularly when the distension is due to fluid (ascites).

Peristalsis

Normal peristalsis is ordinarily not visible through the abdominal wall, but in cases of intestinal obstruction, waves may be seen to ripple across the abdomen. Whenever seen, peristaltic waves should be reported, since they are almost always abnormal in the adult.

Auscultation

There is much to be gained by careful attention to abdominal sounds and this portion of the examination should not be hurried. The clinician will listen for bowel sounds, arterial bruits, venous hums, and parietal friction rubs, particularly over enlarged organs.

Bowel Sounds

The mixing and moving forward of the liquid and air in the intestines produce brief bursts of gurgling, bubbling sounds. These peristaltic sounds are of medium to high pitch (200-1000 cps) and will therefore be heard best with the diaphragm of the stethoscope, which should be pressed lightly against the abdominal wall.

Peristaltic sounds are normally variable in frequency, pitch, and loudness. On the average, sounds will occur anywhere from two to three times per minute up to 10 to 15 times per minute, depending upon the state of the digestive process at the time of examination.

The normal ranges in variability of bowel sounds must be learned by the examiner on the basis of listening to many hundreds of patients with normal intestinal function.

Examination of bowel sounds must be performed in each abdominal quadrant and for a long enough time to be certain that sounds are present in each area and are of normal quality.

The absence of bowel sounds in one area, when they are present and normal in other areas, suggests that there is no intestine underlying the quiet area — that the intestine has been displaced from that location by tumor or by fluid.

When the gut is paralyzed, as in intestinal ileus, peristaltic activity is reduced so much that sounds are produced at a very slow rate, one per minute or even less. While the

term silent abdomen is often used, total absence of peristaltic sounds for 5-10 minutes is quite rare. The examiner may
wish to be seated at the bedside for the lengthy auscultation
necessary for evaluation of a quiet abdomen.

Significantly *increased* peristalsis, with loud, rapidly
produced bowel sounds (i.e., one every 2-3 seconds) is found
in hypermotility of the gut. This condition may come from
diarrhea or from bowel irritation due to gastroenteritis or to
the presence of blood in the bowel (e.g., from bleeding duodenal ulcer).

Mechanical bowel obstruction is ordinarily associated
with periods of "rushes" of sounds. During such periods of
rushes, the sounds may be high-pitched (i.e., 1500-2000 cps),
tinkling, or splashing in quality, and are frequently simultaneous with colicky pain perceived by the patient. This combination of rushes and colicky pain is diagnostic of obstruction.
It must be understood, however, that the frequency and nature
of the abnormal sounds will vary with the degree of obstruction and the duration of the process. For example, in nearly
complete obstruction, after a period of time the bowel activity will weaken, the rushes become less frequent, and may
finally disappear — producing a true silent abdomen.

Arterial Bruits

Since these are low-pitched sounds (i.e., under 100
cps), the bell should be employed. The examiner should routinely examine several areas where bruits are most commonly heard. These include the epigastrum—a few centimeters
above the umbilicus — and the areas to the right and left of
the umbilicus. Most often, these sounds will be systolic in
timing and will be heard a fraction of a second *after* the
cardiac apical impulse or the carotid pulse is palpated. Such
bruits may be due to stenosis of the celiac artery, the renal
artery, or to arteriosclerotic narrowing of the abdominal
aorta. Renal artery stenosis may also produce a bruit lateral
to the umbilicus.

It must be recalled that some cardiac murmurs may be
transmitted quite well along the aorta, so that if the patient
has a murmur and the student hears a vascular sound over the
midline, it may be *either* a true bruit or the transmitted murmur. These are difficult to separate and the prudent student
will seek help with this problem.

Venous Hum

Another type of diagnostic sound that may be picked up is the venous hum. As the name suggests, the sound is generally less rough than an arterial bruit or murmur, is slightly higher-pitched than an arterial bruit (although the bell should still be used), and is commonly continuous through systole and diastole. Venous hums, if present, are most often found over the umbilical area, to the right of the umbilicus, or over the liver region. While some venous hums may be normal sounds produced by the vena cava, any hum should be localized carefully and reported, as it may indicate the presence of cirrhosis of the liver with portal hypertension.

Friction Rubs

These are similar in cause and quality to rubs heard over the pericardium or pleura. One should listen carefully over the liver (right upper quadrant) and over the spleen (left hypochondrium) while the patient takes several deep breaths. A rub over the liver may be indicative of a hepatoma or of cholecystitis, while a rub over the spleen may be due to inflammation or to infarction of that organ.

Percussion

As noted earlier, the stomach and intestines contain varying amounts of air so that percussion over these organs will normally produce high-pitched tympanitic sounds. While the sounds may vary somewhat from one location to another, percussion over all four quadrants should produce a predominant tympanitic note within the abdominal hexagon. Any dullness should be investigated carefully.

In some individuals, the full urinary bladder may rise above the pubis enough to produce dullness but this is ordinarily limited to 1 or 2 cm into the suprapubic area. The disappearance of that dullness after the patient voids will confirm the cause. Pregnancy also will cause suprapubic dullness, generally in the latter trimesters.

Percussion will assist in confirming the findings on palpation of an enlarged organ or mass.

The presence of a collection of fluid in the abdomen (ascites) will modify the findings on percussion also. This is described in detail later in this chapter.

Palpation

Considering the large number of organs in the abdomen and the ease with which the clinician may palpate the area, it is remarkable how little may be positively identified by this examination in the normal patient. The fingertips will sense differences in resistance but the examiner may sometimes complete a careful palpation without identifying clearly any intraabdominal organ. It may be possible to palpate a few normal structures in a patient with a thin abdominal wall: the liver edge, the abdominal aorta, the lower pole of the right kidney, the fourth and fifth lumbar vertebrae, the uterus beyond the third month of pregnancy, portions of the colon, and the full urinary bladder (Figure 15.5).

One word of caution is in order here. If the patient has identified an area of pain in his medical history, this area should be left for last in palpation. Premature palpation of a painful area may produce spasm or rigidity of the abdominal wall so that the examiner is robbed of the opportunity to evaluate the remainder of the abdomen.

There are several modes of palpation the student must learn in order to examine the abdomen thoroughly. These include ballottement, light palpation, and deep palpation.

Ballottement

A recommended technique is to begin in the lowest portion of the abdomen and to bounce the fingertips upward at 2-3 cm intervals roughly along each midinguinal line to the costal margin. If this is done lightly and rapidly, the examiner may be able to detect early *rigidity* of the abdominal muscles on one or both sides (also called guarding), which is an early sign of underlying inflammation. Or he may be able to find evidence of a mass beneath the abdominal wall. If, for example, the liver is enlarged downward to the level of the umbilicus, ballottement will provide the examiner with a definite sense of resistance as he bounces his fingers from the RLQ to the RUQ. He will also note that the sense of resistance is quite different in the RUQ from that in the LUQ.

Since ballottement should be done very lightly with the fingertips, it will rarely produce severe tenderness even in an inflamed abdomen. In a patient with a painful abdomen it may be the *only* palpation that can be accomplished, and therefore ballottement should be carefully practiced on every patient examined so that the student becomes skillful in this technique.

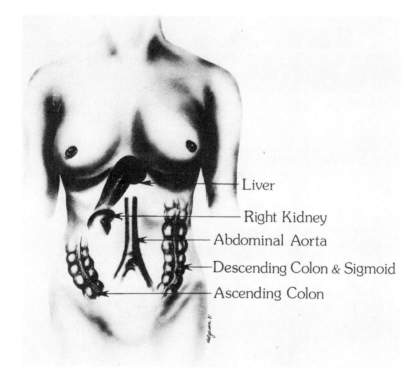

Liver

Right Kidney

Abdominal Aorta

Descending Colon & Sigmoid

Ascending Colon

Figure 15.5 Abdominal structures that may be palpable.

A more forceful type of ballottement is needed in situations where the abdomen is filled with fluid and the examiner is seeking to identify the lower edge of an enlarged organ such as the liver. As the fingers bounce upward from the lower portion of the abdomen, a distinct change of resistance will be felt as the liver is reached.

Light Palpation

Light palpation is performed by pressing the abdominal wall with the pads of the fingers lightly but firmly enough to indent the wall, but making no attempt to press deeply. All areas of the abdomen should be palpated and the sense of resistance of one side to the other should be compared. Light palpation should also be used to explore hernias identified earlier by inspection. A finger placed on a suspected hernia will pick up a thrust of the mass as the patient strains or coughs if it is, in fact, a hernia. Areas of tenderness should be felt as gently as possible to avoid muscle guarding.

Deep Palpation

When the entire abdomen has been adequately explored by light palpation, the examiner should press more firmly toward the back to identify tenderness or masses situated deep in the abdomen (Figure 15.6). It is useful to use both hands to be able to palpate deeply and not numb the fingertips (see Figure 15.1). This examination must be done *carefully* but thoroughly and the examiner must learn to distinguish between normal discomfort produced by deep pressure and true tenderness.

The student will learn, with experience, the soft and rather elastic feel of normal abdominal contents, and the sensation of more firmness over the region of the cecum and sigmoid portions of the colon, the consistency of feces within the sigmoid colon, and the movement under the fingers as he displaces gas bubbles in the transverse colon. Once again it must be emphasized that *until* the student develops his own way of sensing what is normal by repeated examinations, he will fail to sense early abnormalities.

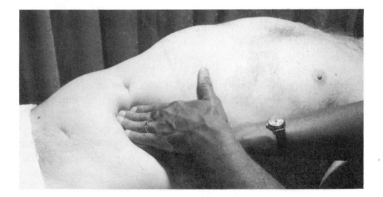

Figure 15.6 Bimanual palpation for possibly enlarged spleen.

Abdominal Pulses

In many persons, the transmitted pulsation of the aorta may be normally palpable in the epigastrium and/or the upper umbilical region. With a thin abdominal wall, the aorta itself may be palpable. It is important to distinguish a normally palpable aorta from an *aneurysm* of the aorta. There are several points that may help in this differentiation. The normal aorta is best felt in the epigastrium, while an aortic aneurysm may be located here or in the umbilical area (see Figure 15.2). Attempt to palpate by pushing two fingers deep enough to feel both sides of the structure. The normal pulsation of the aorta will not push the two fingers apart, while a pulsating aneurysm will often expand enough to move the fingers. Thirdly, an aneurysm between the fingers will have a greater diameter. The normal aorta should not be wider than 3 cm in the epigastrium, or more than 1.5 cm at the level of the iliac crests where it bifurcates into the iliac arteries. The presence of a pulsatile, expanding mass in the midline of the abdomen is nearly diagnostic of an aortic aneurysm, and should be confirmed promptly. A pulsatile mass below the level of the umbilicus is likely to be off center as it may be an aneurysm of the right or left iliac artery. Do not underestimate the value of palpation, for about 80% of all abdominal aortoiliac aneurysms are diagnosed in this way.

Although outside the borders of the abdominal hexagon, the *femoral arteries* are conveniently palpated while the patient is supine for the abdominal examination. The femoral arteries can be found in the upper portion of the thigh, just inferior to the midpoint of the inguinal ligament which forms the lower edges of the abdominal hexagon. They should be palpated simultaneously and are normally strong and equal in intensity. Absence or significant weakness of one or both pulses should be recorded, and auscultation performed for the presence of bruit.

Palpation of the inguinal area for enlarged lymph nodes is also best done at this time. One group of nodes is present along the inguinal ligament and a second group extends downward along the course of the femoral artery for a distance of 8-10 cm. Lymphadenopathy is quite common in these areas due to frequent infections of lower extremities and a search for infection in the feet, legs, and groin will often turn up the source of the lymphadenopathy.

EXAMINATION OF THE LIVER

In most adults, the liver is completely tucked up under the thoracic cage, with its top under the dome of the right diaphragm and its lower edge at or above the right costal margin. However, the edge also may normally be found several centimeters below the costal margin. If the edge has not been detected in the abdomen by ballottement or light palpation, it should be sought for near the costal margin.

This is accomplished by making use of the knowledge that the liver moves during respiration: downward as the diaphragm moves down in inspiration. A successful technique is to place the right fingertips lightly on the abdominal wall immediately below the costal margin at about the midclavicular line (Figure 15.7). Tell the patient to take a deep breath, blow it out, and take in another deep breath. As he takes in the first deep breath, hold the fingertips lightly in place; as he exhales rapidly, *push* the fingertips upward under the costal margin and *hold* them as the patient takes in his second deep breath. Now, as the diaphragm and liver descend, the liver edge taps the examiner's fingers, and both the examiner and the patient will be aware of it. This is usually not painful but the liver edge is slightly tender. The clinician should be watching the patient's face during this maneuver as the patient may wince slightly when the liver taps the examiner's fingers. If there is more liver tenderness than normal, or if the gallbladder is inflamed, the patient will suddenly stop the inspiratory movement when the examiner's fingers touch the liver edge. This "catching of breath" is highly suggestive of infection or inflammation of either or both of these organs.

This maneuver is often successful since it takes advantage of two other physiologic facts: (1) the second deep breath a person takes is usually deeper than the first, and (2) the transverse muscle fibers under the costal margin are relaxed by this breathing cycle. The location of the upper border of the liver (dome) will have been identified during examination of the thorax (see Chapter 12).

As the examiner percusses downward in the right midclavicular line, the upper border is marked by an abrupt change from lung resonance to hepatic dullness. As one continues percussion downward along the midclavicular line, there may be another abrupt change as hepatic dullness gives way to abdominal tympany at the lower border. However, this point frequently is not clearly defined, as the liver edge

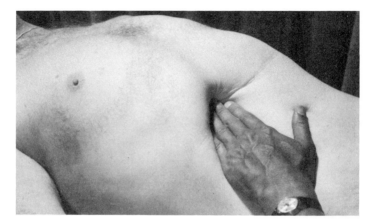

Figure 15.7 Palpation for the liver edge.

is often deeper in the abdomen than the body of the liver, giving rise to an indistinct change in percussion note.

Thus the total span of the normal liver — about 10-15 cm from dome to edge — is often best recorded by percussing the upper border and palpating the lower border in the midclavicular line.

It is critical to remember that the mere presence of a liver edge several centimeters below the costal margin does *not* define liver enlargement. In many patients the liver edge normally lies below the costal margin. Often in patients with pulmonary emphysema the diaphragms will be depressed, pushing the liver well downward into the abdominal hexagon. Only measurement of the liver span from upper to lower borders can be used as a dependable index of liver size. This measurement should routinely be taken (with the transparent ruler always in your pocket) and recorded.

Occasionally, the right lobe of the liver is congenitally elongated and may be readily palpated in the abdomen nearer the midline than the midinguinal line. If located, this long lobe (called Riedel's lobe) will move on respiration, will not be tender, but will lead to finding a liver measuring more than 15 cm from top to edge.

If there is reason to suspect liver disease — as, for example, in jaundice — blunt percussion may be of assistance in determining the presence of tenderness. This is performed

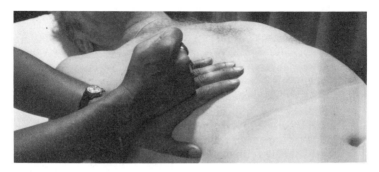

Figure 15.8 Blunt percussion for liver tenderness.

by placing one palm flat over the right lateral chest and striking the back of the hand with the ulnar side of the first (Figure 15.8). The first blow should be gentle, and if no tenderness is produced, a second harder blow can be delivered. In acute hepatitis, the liver will often hurt when jarred and the pain will persist for a few seconds. Tenderness in the area may also be due to inflammation of the gallbladder. In cases where the liver is definitely enlarged, auscultation for bruit or rub should be performed over the thoracic and abdominal portions of the liver.

EXAMINATION OF THE SPLEEN

The normal spleen is a soft, small organ located above the left costal margin centered under the tenth rib near the anterior axillary line and is, therefore, never palpable. It must enlarge to nearly *three times* normal size to be felt. Examination for the spleen should take into account the fact that this organ enlarges downward and medially. The spleen is searched for in the abdominal hexagon in the same general way as one explores for the liver, i.e., by ballottement up the left midinguinal line, then by light and deep palpation.

If the spleen is readily palpable, a distinct notch may be felt in the lower border that can confirm to the examiner that he has, indeed, felt this organ and not some other mass in the area. The spleen is a highly vascular organ, and if enlarged, should be palpated gently to avoid rupture.

When the spleen has not been located in the abdomen, it should then be sought under the costal margin. The examiner's fingers are pushed up under the left costal margin at about the midclavicular line and the patient should be asked to take deep breaths, exactly as in examination for the liver edge, described previously. Movement of the diaphragm downward to deep inspiration may push the moderately enlarged spleen onto the examiner's fingertips.

Further search may be done by bimanual examination. This is accomplished by having the patient lie on his right side, while the examiner's left hand compresses the posterior abdominal wall just below the palpable ribs. This maneuver moves the spleen anteriorly where, on deep inspiration, it may be felt by the right fingertips (Figure 15.9).

Remember that if the spleen is felt at all, it is significantly enlarged, whereas the palpable liver may or may not be enlarged.

Percussion is used also in this search. As noted earlier, the spleen is a small organ, normally centered under the tenth rib and the anterior axillary line. With the patient on his right side, as in Figure 15.9, percuss downward along the anterior axillary line starting around the level of the nipple. One will pick up lung resonance down to about the level of the ninth rib and often will detect dullness, due to the underlying spleen, for a distance of 4-6 cm before reaching an area

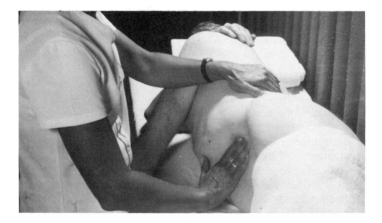

Figure 15.9 Bimanual palpation for possibly enlarged spleen.

of tympany in Traube's space, over the stomach bubble or gas-filled splenic flexure of the colon (see Figure 14.4). With significant splenomegaly, the area of dullness will extend to or below the costal margin. On deep inspiration, the area of splenic dullness may be quite pronounced and will fill much of the normally tympanitic area. At best, percussion of the spleen is difficult to perform and interpret. The student must have a considerable amount of experience to be confident of his findings with this organ.

EXAMINATION OF THE KIDNEYS

The normal sized kidneys are *not* often palpable, except in the patient with a thin or scaphoid abdomen, since these organs lie deep in the abdomen on the posterior abdominal wall. The lower pole of the right kidney is ordinarily located about 4 cm above the level of the right iliac crest at the midinguinal line. The lower pole of the left kidney is often located about 5 cm above the left iliac crest near the mid-inguinal line. Like most of the abdominal contents, the kidneys descend on deep inspiration, although they move down less than the liver or spleen.

The lower pole of the right kidney is easier to locate than the left. It should be felt for bimanually, by having the left fingers press upward in the left costovertebral angle, and pushing the right fingertips deep at the point described above (Figure 15.10), while having the patient taking deep breaths. The round lower pole may be felt as it moves downward under the left fingertips. The left kidney may be found with a similar technique, i.e., pushing upward in the left costovertebral angle with the left fingers, downward with the right fingers through the abdominal wall about 5 cm above the left iliac crest in the midinguinal line.

Because they lie so far posteriorly, ordinary percussion will not detect the presence of the kidneys. However, blunt percussion over the costovertebral angles may detect kidney tenderness due to infection (see Figure 16.3).

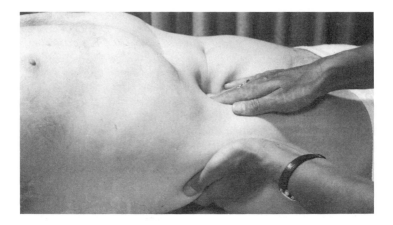

Figure 15.10 Bimanual palpation for the right kidney.

ABDOMINAL TENDERNESS

The basic aim of the clinician in examining the abdomen, where tenderness is present, is to locate the site and source of the pain as accurately as possible. This is frequently not too difficult when the patient has a localized area of pain on palpation. To locate the site of pain, whether the patient has local or generalized abdominal tenderness, one searches for the *point of maximum tenderness*. In the tender abdomen, deep palpation may produce a great deal of pain over a large area, so the examiner should try to find an area where the lightest touch produces tenderness. Gentle percussion may often pinpoint the area of maximum tenderness.

It sometimes happens that palpation in one area produces maximum pain in another area of the abdomen. Usually, this is due to transmission of the pressure by trapped gas in the intestines but, again, it is important to identify and describe the point of maximum tenderness, so the patient should be carefully questioned as to where he perceives the maximal pain when palpated.

When the peritoneum is inflamed, *rebound tenderness* may occur. This is induced by pressing over a tender area and quickly releasing the pressure. If the pain is suddenly worse when the examiner's hand is removed, rebound is said to be present and is a valuable sign of peritonitis.

Description of abdominal tenderness should include the precise location of the point of maximum tenderness, if one has been found, and the amount of pressure necessary to produce tenderness (i.e., by light palpation, moderate palpation, deep palpation, or by rebound). If the tenderness is generalized throughout the abdomen, this should be specified.

ASCITES

Small amounts of abdominal fluid may not be detectable by any methods of examination but, as fluid increases, the first sign usually is a bulging of the flanks. Bulging of the flanks is also seen in obesity, however, and it is important to distinguish between the two. Simple pinching of the flank may help, since in distention due to fluid, the examiner may sense that he has primarily skin and muscle between the fingers rather than skin, muscle, and fat. A specific test for the presence of larger amounts of abdominal fluid is the production of a *fluid wave*. This is done by placing a palm on one flank and striking the opposite flank briskly with the fingers of the other hand (Figure 15.11). If the distention is due to fluid, a distinct transmission of the blow will be felt across the abdomen. To avoid feeling vibrations transmitted across the abdominal wall itself, a third hand is needed; an assistant or the patient presses the ulnar edge of his hand deep into the midline of the abdomen.

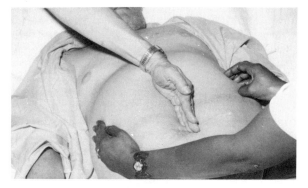

Figure 15.11 Examination for fluid wave. Note the deep compression of the distended abdomen by the assistant's hand to prevent vibrations from crossing along the abdominal wall.

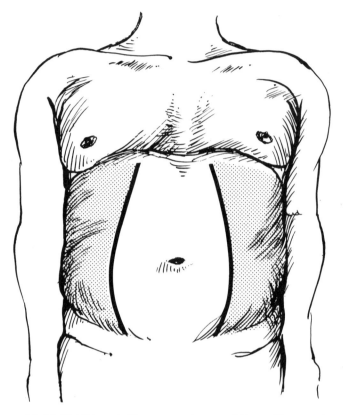

Figure 15.12 Shifting dullness, supine position. Percussion lateral to the marked lines produces dullness (shaded area) due to ascitic fluid collected in the flanks.

Another test is the examination for shifting dullness. With the patient supine, percuss the abdomen toward the flanks, marking lines where dullness begins (Figure 15.12). The patient is then asked to roll onto one side and to lie in that position for about 2–3 minutes. This will allow time for fluid to drain down from the superior flank and for air-filled intestines to float upward. Percussion of the superior portion of the abdomen will then reveal that dullness has

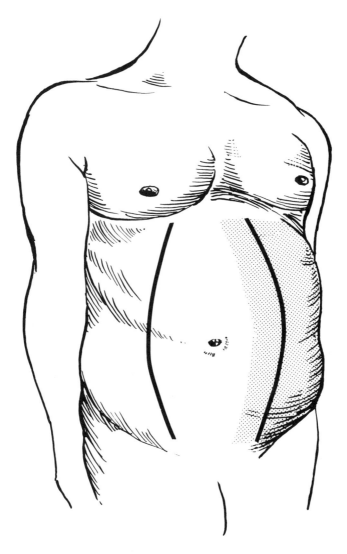

Figure 15.13 Shifting dullness, left lateral position. Dullness (shaded area) has shifted down from the superior flank. Dullness in the dependent flank now includes an area medial to the lower mark as well as lateral to it.

been replaced by tympany. Percussion of the dependent flank will show that the dull area has enlarged, being present closer to the umbilicus than it was in the supine position (Figure 15. 13). Such shifting of dullness confirms the presence of ascitic fluid as the cause of the dullness.

With severe degrees of distention due to ascites, the abdomen becomes tense and the umbilicus will be pushed outward and may even protrude above the wall. Palpation will help very little to detect anything in the abdomen causing the distention. Percussion will produce tympany, most pronounced in the umbilical and epigastric regions, with dullness elsewhere. This is due to the floating of air-filled gut toward the high point of the abdomen. Auscultation of bowel sounds will also demonstrate this central collection of intestinal gas.

RECORDING

Abdomen

Insp.:   Abdomen flat, not skin lesions, no hernia, no pulsations

Ausc.:   Normal bowel sounds q. 10 sec; no bruits

Palp.:   No tenderness or masses; spleen, kidneys not palpated, liver edge at costal margin, nontender

Perc.:   Normal abdominal tympany; liver 12 cm long

POTENTIAL NURSING DIAGNOSES

Bowel elimination, alteration in: constipation

Bowel elimination, alteration in: diarrhea

Nutrition, alteration in: less than body requirements

Nutrition, alteration in: more than body requirements

Tissue perfusion, alteration in: gastrointestinal function

PATIENT PROBLEM

Mr. A.L. is a 49-year-old male truck driver brought to primary care unit by neighbor because of abdominal distention and depression.

Problem: Abdominal Distention and Depression

S: Admits to at least 1 pt whiskey and several beers daily for past 10 yr; in past month has been fatigued, developed abdominal distention; has been attending alcohol clinic irregularly under court order because of multiple traffic violations and loss of driver's license; separated from wife, lives in rooming house, has hot plate, eats poorly.

O: *Insp:* Abdomen is distended with bulging flanks, 98 cm girth at umbilicus; numerous spider angiomata over face, neck, arms; hair sparse on chest, genitals and in axillae; dilated veins over abdominal wall with flow→umbilicus from upper quadrants; umbilicus protruding.

Ausc: Normal bowel sounds of 3-4 sec heard best in epigastric, umbilical, and suprapubic regions; sounds are distant in flanks.

Palp: Tense abdominal wall that can be indented by deep palpation to identify blunt liver edge 11 cm below right costal margin, nontender, no other masses or organs palpable; no abdominal tenderness; fluid wave present.

Perc: Dome of liver 5 cm above right costal margin; liver is 16 cm long; increased tympany in epigastric and umbilical segments, dullness over both flanks and diminished tympany is suprapubic segment; shifting dullness present.

ASSESSMENT: Appears to be series of related problems—acute malnutrition superimposed on chronic alcohol abuse, depression over loss of family and job, and development of ascites, probably secondary to cirrhosis; major problem is to relieve ascites and sort out serious socioeconomic problems leading to current debilitated state.

Nursing Diagnosis: Alterations in nutrition related to food and eating habits
and chronic alcohol abuse.
Alterations in tissue perfusion related
to ascites and abdominal distention.
Alterations in health maintenance related to socioeconomic problems.
Knowledge deficit and noncompliance
with attendance at alcohol abuse clinic.
Potential for impaired skin integrity.

PLAN:

Goals: To increase nutritional food and
fluid intake.
To maintain skin integrity during bed
rest.
To increase knowledge and compliance
with nutritional health maintenance.
To increase compliance with attendance
at alcohol abuse clinic.
To provide for a support system during
hospitalization and postdischarge.
Nursing Orders:
Diagnostic: Recommend prompt hospitalization to physician; per algo-
rithm—order SMA-12, type and x-
match 2 units blood; record urine
output.
Therapeutic: Strict bed rest in holding unit bed until hospitalization can
be arranged; orange juice 120 cc q. 1 hr;
call unit social worker to begin support
program during admission and post-
hospital stay.
Patient Education: Discussed need for
hospitalization due to probable liver
disease; explained role of social
worker and projected counseling with
staff in hospital.

IMPLEMENTATION: Provide bed rest with turning side to side q 2 hr.
Increase nutritional intake per physician prescription with frequent small feedings.
Record intake and output.
Refer to social worker for discharge planning.
Provide literature on alcohol abuse and alcohol abuse programs.
Refer to dietitian for nutritional education.

EVALUATION: Skin intact during bed rest.
Ate nutritional foods on tray and nutrition supplements.
Social worker visited.
Discussed alcohol abuse literature knowledgeably.
Requested nutritional drinks, e.g., orange juice.
Visited with AA members from the clinic.

chapter 16

The Extremities and Back

Examination Sequence

Examination of the Back

Examination of the Extremities

Recording

Spinal Screening Procedures

Potential Nursing Diagnoses

Patient Problem

The skeleton, joints, muscles, blood vessels, lymphatics, and nerves of the extremities and back do not make up a single defined system nor, strictly speaking, a region. For purposes of the physical examination, however, the extremities and the back should be looked upon as a whole and each of the component parts should be evaluated.

The skeleton consists of two parts: the central or *axial* portion and the attached or *appended* portion. The axial skeleton includes the skull, the spine, the ribs, and the sternum, while the appendicular skeleton includes the shoulder girdle and upper extremities plus the pelvic girdle and lower extremities. The functions of the axial skeleton are protection (skull and thorax) and maintenance of the upright position (spine) while the extremities provide for "fight-and-flight."

The great development of fine motion and sensation in the hand makes it unique as a tool and as a sense organ. It is a part of the legend of the Orient that the physician was limited in his examination of the harem women to inspection and palpation of the hand and wrist. Now that we are not so restricted we must not neglect the fact that careful examination of the skin, nails, joints, muscles, nerves, and pulses of the hands may detect signs of nearly 100 diseases, syndromes, or lesions! For instance, acrocyanosis, acrodermatitis, acromegaly, Addison's disease, albumin deficiency, alcoholism, amyotrophic lateral sclerosis, anemias, arteriovenous fistulae, arthritis, astereognosia, atrial fibrillation, and azotemia can begin the alphabetical list. In addition, cultural signs such as the shape and care of the nails, the wearing of rings, occupational marks and callouses, tattoos, nicotine stains, etc., may aid the practitioner in an evaluation of the patient's personality and socioeconomic status.

EXAMINATION SEQUENCE

A recommended method of examination is to perform a general inspection, then to evaluate posture, gait, and balance. Follow with an examination of the back, then upper and lower extremities, paying particular attention to range of motion of joints, strength of muscles, and competence of the vascular system. This sequence will carry the examiner's focus from the whole patient down to specific tests. Of course, here as elsewhere, the sequence and the amount of detail of the examination will be determined by the patient's history.

General

An overall view of the head and neck, back, and extremities is made here, as elsewhere, for gross asymmetry of one side as compared to the other, for deformities, for skin temperature, for skin lesions, and for the presence of swellings or masses. Because of the large number of structures present here (bones, joints, muscles, ligaments, tendons, etc.), the high incidence of trauma to the extremities, and the relative ease of examination, many swellings, masses, or deformities can be found here. One type of swelling edema, which occurs quite often in the extremities, particularly the lower extremity, deserves special mention here. Edema is the infiltration of serum into the tissues, which may occur in a localized region such as an area of trauma, or may be more generalized. By far the most common general type is dependent edema, which pits upon pressure (Figure 16.1). Since it is dependent, it will be found most often in the dorsum of the foot and the medial aspect of the ankle in patients who are not confined to bed. The dependent edema of bedridden patients will be located in the buttocks and the loose tissue over the sacrum and lower back. Distinction between pitting and nonpitting edema is an important point to establish and should always be recorded.

Dependent pitting edema has a variety of causes including right-sided congestive heart failure, renal disease, hepatic cirrhosis, lymphatic obstruction, premenstrual fluid retention, venous thrombosis, and nutritional deficiencies. All are associated with the collection of fluid under the skin being pulled by gravity to dependent areas.

Nonpitting edema, such as hypothyroid myxedema, results from soft, general thickening of the subcutaneous tissues, rather than simple fluid accumulation.

Posture

In the upright position, the patient's head should be balanced over his shoulders, his hips and his ankles. When viewed from the side, the back should have three separate curves, each of which should be present but not exaggerated (Figure 16.2): an anterior curve of the neck (cervical concavity), a posterior curve of the thorax (dorsal convexity), and an anterior curve of the low back (lumbar concavity). Viewed posteriorly, the midspinal line should be nearly perfectly straight and the shoulders should be level.

Abnormalities of posture or station may be due to skeletal deformities, muscle spasm or atrophy, joint deformities, pain anywhere in the musculoskeletal system, or to pathophysiologic needs such as the peculiar sitting position that assists the emphysematous patient in breathing (see Figure 12. 6). There are enough typical postures taken by patients with various diseases to warrant several detailed articles.

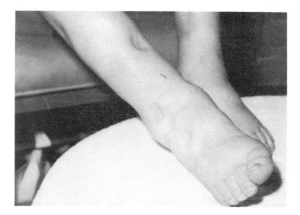

Figure 16.1 Pitting edema.

Gait and Balance

Have the patient walk away from you and then toward you. Watch for unusually short steps, and a wide-based walk, or restricted swinging of the arms, for evidence that the patient is watching the placement of his feet and, of course, for staggering or a tendency to fall (Table 16.1).

Balance is a complex function that depends upon sensation provided by the semicircular canals of the inner ear, upon position sense (proprioception), which informs the individual of the position of his body and limbs, and upon muscle coordination. These factors are examined by the *Romberg test.* Have the patient stand with feet together and eyes open to see if he maintains balance. Then have him close his eyes. Be sure that you are close to him to prevent a fall. Failure to maintain balance is called a positive Romberg sign.

EXAMINATION OF THE BACK

Inspection and palpation are done to detect and evaluate any deformities of the spine. Figure 16.2 illustrates the normal curves. An exaggerated anterior cervical or lumbar curve is called *lordosis,* while an exaggerated posterior

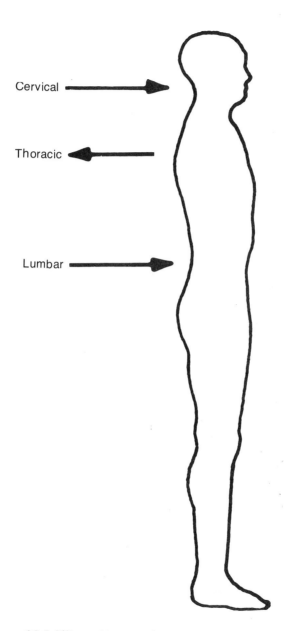

Figure 16.2 Silhouette showing proper upright posture and normal curves of the cervical, thoracic, and lumbar spines. A perpendicular line dropped from the ear canal should cross the lateral malleolus.

Table 16.1 Some Abnormalities of Gait

Type	Characteristics	Examples
Parkinsonian	Body held rigid, trunk and head bent forward; short, mincing steps, sudden uncontrolled propulsivelike movements	Parkinson's disease
Ataxic	Staggering or reeling like an alcoholic	Cerebellar disease
Slapping	Feet wide apart, legs raised high and then feet slapped on the ground; eyes fixed to floor to help guide feet for placement	Disease of posterior column of spinal cord
Spastic	Jerking, uncoordinate movements	Cerebral palsy; multiple sclerosis
Dragging	Dragging of one leg around in a semicircle	Hemiplegia
Scissors	Thighs close together due to spasticity of adductor muscles	Spastic paraplegia

dorsal curvature is called *kyphosis* (see Figure 12.8). Lateral curvature away from the midline is called *scoliosis* (see Figure 12.9). Immobility of the spine due to rheumatoid spondylitis leads to the condition known as poker spine. (At the end of this chapter there is a description of the spinal screening procedure — forward bending test for scoliosis and kyphosis.)

Palpation should be performed to determine, if possible, the cause of abnormal posture. The spine and the paraspinal muscles should be examined for tenderness, swelling, or spasm.

Range of motion (ROM) of the cervical spine has been described in Chapter 9. Active ROM of the back (thoracic and lumbar spine) can be checked by having the patient bend from standing position. The normal range is about 80° forward and about 25° to 30° backward. The trunk should flex to the right or left by around 35° from the upright position. Limitations should be noted, and the patient questioned about reasons for limitation, such as pain, stiffness, weakness, or immobility.

Blunt percussion of the back with the ulnar aspect of the fist is used in two areas, over the vertebrae from the cervical spine down to the lumbosacral joint, and over the kidney. Jarring the vertebrae may induce tenderness in the presence of inflammation or destruction of the vertebrae or intravertebral discs. Locate the lower border of the ribs where they join the spine — the costovertebral angles (CVA) — and strike each angle with the ulnar side of the fist firmly, but not hard, over the kidneys (Figure 16.3). Tenderness induced by this blunt percussion suggests kidney infection or inflammation.

EXAMINATION OF THE EXTREMITIES

Joints

Joints, of course, are designed to provide mobility, and they must be examined for this function. While the details of ROM of each joint are very complex, the examiner must develop a pattern of evaluating at least the major joints through a portion of their active ROM. Observation of the whole patient, his gait, his behavior in undressing, in moving onto and off the examination table, etc., will give the alert clinician clues as to possible limitation of motion prior to specific examination (Figure 16.4).

ROM of the upper extremities may be examined briefly by comparing the patient's motion with your own (if you have no limitation). Ask the patient to follow you in these calisthenics (moving from fingers to shoulder): open and close the hands; flex and extend the wrists; flex and extend the forearms; alternately turn the hands palm up, palm down, palm up; raise arms to the sides; touch hands overhead. This can all be done in about 10-20 seconds.

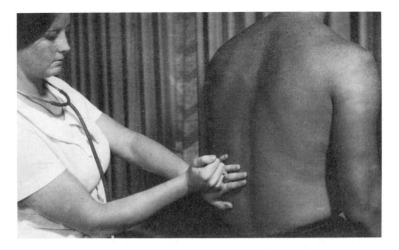

Figure 16.3 Blunt percussion of the kidney over the costo-vertebral angle.

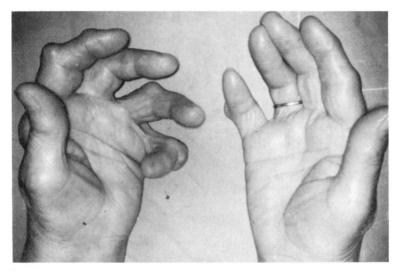

Figure 16.4 Immobile deformed joints of the fingers and hand due to severe rheumatoid arthritis.

In younger individuals, the major joints of the lower extremities can be tested as a group by simply having the patient perform a deep knee bend. It is safer in older or weak
patients to have the patient seated on the examining table
and to have the patient move individual joints separately:
flex feet up and down, bend and straighten the knees, and
raise the knees toward the chin.

Since the pattern suggested above is simply a brief
screening of joint ROM, it is to be considered adequate *only*
if there has been no history of pain or limitation of motion,
or if no limitation was detected during the examination. If
limitation has been found, closer examination by inspection
and palpation is warranted. Further tests of ROM are best
left to the physiatrist, orthopedist, physical therapist, or
other professionals specially trained in these techniques.
Many more details about expected ROM and techniques of
measurement can be found in the monograph by Hoppenfeld,
Physical Examination of the Spine and Extremities, published
by Appleton-Century-Crofts, 1976.

Musculoskeletal System

The examiner will already have had the opportunity to
notice gross deformities of the extremities or marked weakness or atrophy of muscle groups. He will have done general
inspection while the patient walked, sat down, undressed,
and moved on and off the examining table. Most easily spotted
are differences of one side from the other, although some
symmetrical deformities such as bowlegs are also readily
noticed. Even though no obvious muscle weakness is present,
a few major muscle groups of the neck, back, and extremities
should be examined against resistance.

With the patient facing forward, tell him to hold his
head still while you attempt to turn his head by moderate
pressure on first one, and then the other side of the jaw.
Unless there is gross weakness of the neck muscles, the patient should have no difficulty in holding his held still.
Press down on the patient's shoulders and ask him to raise
or shrug his shoulders. He should be able to do this easily.
Biceps and triceps are quickly tested by having the patient
hold his arm partly extended and asking him to keep that
position while you push and then pull the arm (Figure 16.5).

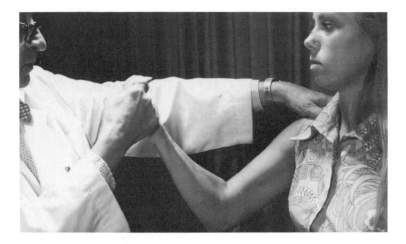

Figure 16.5 Testing strength of the biceps muscle.

Again, he should be able to resist these forces readily. Similarly, for the lower extremity, the patient should be able to resist both a pull and a push against the shin and the thigh.

Vascular System

Veins of the hand and forearm often appear dilated if the extremity is held below the level of the heart. These veins should collapse within a few seconds when the extremity is raised to about an angle of 30° above the horizontal. Failure to do so suggests increased venous pressure due to obstruction or to congestive heart failure. Veins of the lower extremities are often dilated in normal posture. Varicose veins are characterized not just by being dilated, but in being so dilated as to stand out from the underlying tissue and being tortuous (Figure 16.6). If there is any question about the presence of true varicose veins, the patient should be referred for several other examinations that can determine the competency of the venous valves.

When edema is found in the lower extremity, the examiner should be alert to the possibility of venous thrombosis since this may be a life-threatening disorder. Early venous thrombosis usually produces no symptoms, but when

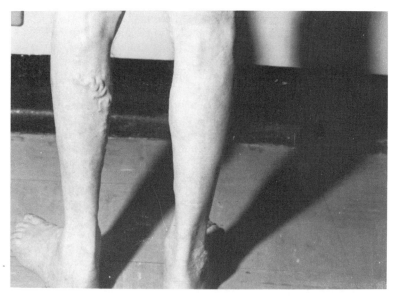

Figure 16.6 Cluster of varicose veins of the left leg. Note also the reduction of muscle bulk evident in the gastrocnemius muscles.

a vein is occluded by the thrombus there is usually pain, edema, and tenderness to palpation of the occluded portion of the vein. The extent of edema may not be readily evident, so it is advisable to use a tape measure to compare the diameter of the involved extremity to that of the other side. A good practice is to measure the diameter of the limbs at 10-cm intervals from a fixed point, such as the malleolus of the ankle, so that follow-up comparisons may be made accurately.

Examination of the radial pulse, which was performed earlier, is now repeated. Pulses are examined bilaterally simultaneously to compare their quality and the time of arrival at the examiner's fingertips. In the upper extremity, it is usually necessary to palpate only the radial pulses. If these are extremely weak or absent, the ulnar pulses should be examined, and if these two are weak or absent, the brachial arteries should then be located and examined. The brachial artery is most easily found a few centimeters below the axilla lying in the groove along the lower edge of the biceps muscle.

In the lower extremity, the femoral, dorsalis pedis, and posterior tibial arteries should be palpated routinely. The femoral arteries are readily located at about the mid-point of the inguinal ligament, i.e., midway between the anterior and superior iliac spine and the symphysis pubis, and should have been palpated with the patient supine during the abdominal examination (see Chapter 15). The dorsalis pedis artery follows a line that is drawn from the middle of the ankle into the groove between the great toe and the second toe (Figure 16.7). It is best palpated on the instep of the foot. The posterior tibial artery is slightly more difficult to locate and is best searched for with two or three fingers. Place the fingers in the groove between the Achilles tendon and the tibia just above the medial malleolus, press deeply, and move the fingers toward the tibia (Figure 16.8). These arteries are not palpable in many normal persons, so do not spend too much time searching for them.

If *neither* the dorsalis pedis nor the posterior tibial pulse can be detected on one side, the examiner should attempt to locate the popliteal artery. Although difficult to

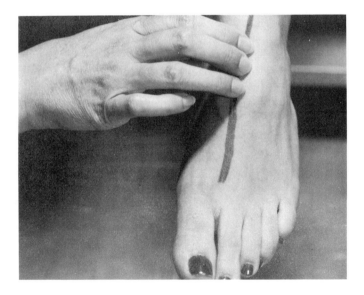

Figure 16.7 Palpation of the dorsalis pedis artery.

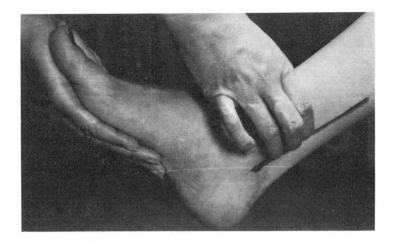

Figure 16.8 Palpation of the posterior tibial artery.

palpate, this artery often can be felt by having the patient flex the knee to relax the muscles (kneeling on a chair, if possible, is a satisfactory position). The examiner's fingertips are then pushed deep into the center of the popliteal space.

Absence of pulses in an extremity is highly suggestive of peripheral arterial disease, and the localization of obstructive phenomena may be determined generally by this type of physical examination (see Patient Problem at end of this chapter).

Hands and Feet

Although included in the examinations described above, special attention should be given to the hands[1] and feet because of their great importance to one's well-being. In addition to the hand's function in manipulating all sorts of objects

[1]The Greek word for hand is *cheir,* which is the root for words such as surgery (chirurgery), and chiropractic. The Latin word is *manus,* from which we get words such as manipulate, maneuver, and manual.

and tools, it is the prime organ of touch. This was referred to briefly in the discussion on palpation (see Chapter 6). The sensory endings in the hand and fingers are so fine that many objects can be identified by being held in the hand, with the eyes closed. The lack of ability to identify common things, such as coins, keys, pencils, or paper clips is called *astereognosis* — one of the 100 disorders diagnosable by examination of the hands listed at the beginning of this chapter.

A more common problem is arthritis of the hand. It is important to recognize *Heberden's nodes,* which are bony nodules at the distal joints of the fingers. These are due to osteoarthritis and are seen in postmenopausal women. Since they are *not* due to rheumatoid arthritis, it is useful to be able to assure the patient that she is not developing rheumatoid arthritis, the seriously deforming and crippling condition illustrated in Figure 16.4. Clubbing of the fingers has already been noted (see Figure 8.8).

Examination of the feet should include inspection and palpation and should focus on the critical function of locomotion. The feet make up only about 4% of the body surface but they serve as platforms to cushion the entire body weight in walking or running. Small and/or painful lesions therefore assume a much greater importance here than in many other regions. Problems such as blisters, corns, calluses, or bunions, which may seem to be minor problems, may interfere with walking, with serious physical and/or social consequences. Even ingrown toenails can be painful enough to cause limitation of activity which can be lethal in the aged. Mechanical defects such as pes planus (flatfoot), pes cavus (high-arched foot), or hammer toe should be sought for as well.

If there are foot problems that do lead to any difficulty in walking, these should be corrected properly and promptly. Referral to a podiatrist or other specialist is clearly indicated. The relatively simple matter of properly fitted shoes may make an enormous improvement in activity or outlook for a patient.

Lymph Nodes

Palpation of lymph nodes in the groin has been described in the previous chapter. As noted there, lymphadenopathy is frequently due to infections of the feet, legs, or genital area.

Although this is ordinarily a convenient time in the examination to perform tendon reflexes and the plantar reflex, descriptions of the technique and recording of those reflexes will be taken up in Chapter 19, Neurological and Mental Examination.

RECORDING

The normal examination may be recorded as follows:

Back: Normal curvature, no spinal tenderness, no CVA tenderness.

Extremities: No skin, hair, or nail abnormalities; full range of motion (ROM); normal gait, Romberg negative; muscle strength intact; no venous dilation; radial, femoral, dorsalis pedis, and posterior tibial pulses all palpable and equal; no lymphadenopathy.

SPINAL SCREENING PROCEDURE[2]
(Forward Bending Test for Scoliosis and Kyphosis)

The examiner should be seated.

First, have individual face the examiner. Feet should be together, knees should be straight and arms should hang loosely at sides.

Second, have individual bend at the waist 90° (toward examiner), knees straight, feet together, arms hanging with palms together and head down (Figure 16.9). In this position check for asymmetry of the thoracic and lumbar areas.

Third, have individual face away from examiner (Figure 16.10).

[2]Reprinted with the permission of the Georgia Department of Human Resources; Division of Public Health.

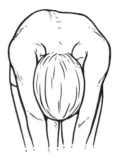

Figure 16.9

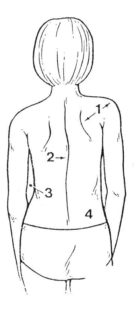

Figure 16.10

In this position check for:

1. elevated shoulder, scapula
2. curve in spinous process alignment
3. increased distance between arm and trunk
4. less prominent hip

Fourth, have individual bend forward (away from examiner) (Figure 16.11). Check for asymmetry of the thoracic and lumbar areas.

Fifth, have individual turn to the side (Figure 16.12). In this position, check for accentuated roundback.

Sixth, have individual bend forward. Check for accentuated spine hump in the thoracic area.

Note on examination (Figure 16.13):

1. Elevated shoulder, scapula
2. Curve in spinous process alignment
3. Increased distance between arm and trunk
4. Less prominent hip (iliac crest)
5. Asymmetry of thorax back (from front and back view)
6. Accentuated spine hump (from lateral view)

Presence of any one or more of these findings requires further evaluation.

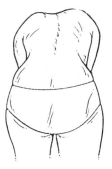

Figure 16.11

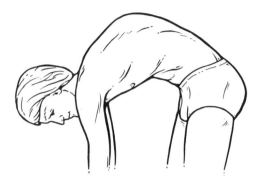

Figure 16.12

POTENTIAL NURSING DIAGNOSES

Activity, intolerance: due to generalized weakness

Mobility, impaired physical: due to musculoskeletal impairment

Self-care deficit, dressing/grooming: due to neuromuscular impairment

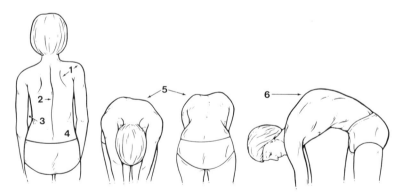

Figure 16.13

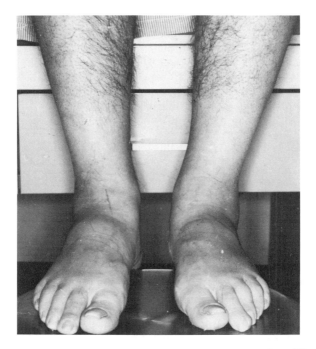

Figure 16.14 Absence of leg hair due to arterial insufficiency.
Note the sharp line of demarcation.

PATIENT PROBLEM

Mr. P. W., a 45-year-old diabetic man, presents himself
at clinic because of leg pains.

Problem: Vascular Insufficiency

S: For past 2 yr Mr. P. W. has had calf cramps that have
definitely become worse over past 2 mo. At first
these were noted only after several hours of exercise
until the present time when he can no longer walk
more than two blocks without having to stop because
of severe pains. Pain is cramping in type, involves
calves of both lower extremities, is relieved by rest
for 3-4 min. No medication ever tried for relief; is
not on a diuretic. He smokes 1 ppd.

O: No assymetry or swelling of lower extremities; legs
       are pale, feet slightly mottled; hair abruptly disap-
       pears from legs at about 15 cm above malleoli (Figure
       16.14); no hairs noted on toes. Skin below this level
       is cooler to touch than above, but is intact. Femoral
       pulses present and equal; dorsalis pedis and posterior
       tibials not palpable; popliteals not felt; no bruits heard
       along femoral arteries.

ASSESSMENT: The combination of abrupt loss of hair
                       on legs, coolness of lower portion of
                       leg, and absence of pulses of the foot is
                       consistent with reduced arterial blood
                       flow somewhere below the level of the
                       femoral arteries. Because this is
                       chronic (over 2 yr) and the patient is a
                       diabetic, this is most likely due to
                       arteriosclerosis.

                       Nursing Diagnosis: Mobility impaired:
                       related to calf "cramps" when walking.
                       Alterations in comfort related to pain
                       in both extremities.

PLAN: Goals: To minimize pain in calves when
                       walking longer than 3 minutes.
                       To increase knowledge and compliance
                       of foot hygiene and extremes of temper-
                       ature.
                       To increase fluid intake daily.
                       To stop smoking.
                       To comply with physician appointment
                       and medical regime.
                       Nursing Orders:
                       Diagnostic: Refer to vascular clinic
                         for further studies.
                       Therapeutic: None at this time.
                       Patient Education: Patient referred to
                         stop smoking clinic, advised to keep
                         feet very clean, increase fluid in-
                         take; told that blood flow to feet is
                         reduced, and that it is important to
                         continue medical workup.

IMPLEMENTATION: Make an appointment for the vascular clinic.
Review and reinforce foot hygiene.
Plan with patient a regime to change positions frequently.
Encourage increased fluid intake daily.
Avoid extremes of temperature, particularly cold.
Review with patient literature and programs to stop smoking.

EVALUATION: Consulted physician.
Participated in a "Stop Smoking" program.
Calf cramps decreasing.

The Male Genitalia and Rectal Systems

Since all malignancies of the testes can be suspected or even diagnosed on palpation, and approximately half of all rectal carcinomas are within reach of the examiner's index finger, these regions should be considered in every adult male screening health examination. Regretably, cultural and sexual problems on the part of both patients and examiners often lead to a failure to examine these areas and a report of "deferred," especially by female clinicians. This must be avoided by the development of a relaxed, yet composed, attitude on the part of the examiner who understands that disease of the genitalia and of the rectum is as important to detect as disease elsewhere. However, when there is no indication through history that problems may exist, and the patient is in the hospital or health center for specific unrelated problems, this component of the examination would not be given priority.

MALE GENITALIA

Anatomy

The skin of the penis is loose and free of hair except at the root. In the uncircumcised male it projects over the glans, forming the foreskin or prepuce. The urethral meatus is located near the center of the glans. Scrotal skin is loose and wrinkled by the dartos muscle. The scrotal sac is made up of loose skin and the thin dartos fascia and muscle. Because of the looseness of the skin and the thin sheet of dartos muscle, the scrotum is normally wrinkled. The testes are ovoid, firm organs measuring roughly 4 cm in length, about 2.5 cm in the anteroposterior diameter and about 2 cm in width. The *epididymis* is a soft, cordlike structure that can be felt from the lower testicular pole, along the posterolateral aspect up to the posterior portion of the upper pole of the testicle where it enlarges. Arising from this enlargement, called the head of the epididymis, is the *spermatic cord,* which feels harder than the epididymis and somewhat like a strand of twine. The spermatic cord enters the *inguinal canal* at the external inguinal ring and, after 3-4 cm, enters the abdominal wall at the internal inguinal ring.

EXAMINATION

General

Because of the possibilities of infection, it is a recommended practice to wear gloves in examining the genitalia. The genitalia may be most easily examined with the patient standing and the examiner seated on a low stool when possible.

Pubic Hair

The distribution of so-called male or female patterns of the pubic hair is of little clinical importance in adults since there are so many normal variations. Either absence or extreme sparseness of pubic hair, on the contrary, is usually significant and should be reported. This loss of pubic hair, along with loss or thinning of hair on the abdomen and in the axilla may be seen, for example, in advanced cirrhosis of the liver.

Penis

Because of variations in the size of the normal penis, only wide discrepancies are likely to be of significance. The penis should be inspected for edema, scars, and lesions. In the uncircumcised man, the foreskin should be retracted to expose the glans. The condition in which the prepuce is not able to be retracted is called *phimosis*. Gentle palpation for scarring or masses is carried out. Slight pressure near the tip of the glans should open the urethral meatus unless it is scarred. Observe the meatus for discharge.

Scrotum and Contents

Lesions of the scrotum are principally those of skin and should be reported as for skin elsewhere. Using the index and middle fingers of the right hand, in a scissorslike fashion, separate the two testes (Figure 17.1). This will place the right testicle in the right hand and gentle pressure by the left fingertips will allow for careful bimanual palpation of the right testicle. The testicle should be evaluated for size, consistency, and masses. Holding the right testicle in place, palpate the epididymis between the thumb and fingers of the left hand from the lower testicular pole, along the posterolateral border, to the head, and then up the spermatic cord. Common lesions of the epididymis are scarring, generalized swelling, or tumors such as *hydrocele*. The spermatic cord is also subject to these same lesions. Any tumor found should be examined by transillumination in which a small light source (penlight, flashlight) is placed behind the tumor in a darkened room to see if light passes through the tumor. Cysts generally transmit light, while solid tumors ordinarily do not.

The contents of the left scrotum are examined in the same manner, by separating the testes with the fingers of the left hand and with the right hand performing gentle palpation of the testis, epididymis, and cord.

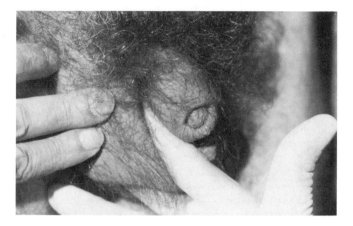

Figure 17.1 Palpation of the scrotal contents. The right testis is separated from the left by the first two fingers of the gloved right hand and bimanual palpation is thereby easily accomplished.

Cancer of the testes is the most common malignancy in men from ages 29–35. Since these tumors are readily detectable and are often curable when removed early, young men should be taught to perform self-examination on a regular basis.

Inguinal Canals

The inguinal canal, a curved 3- to 4-cm long tunnel, is the site of passage of an indirect inguinal hernia. The *right* canal is palpated most easily by the little finger or the index finger of the *right* hand, which is pushed up through the scrotum with the fingernail lying against the spermatic cord (Figure 17.2). The fingertip should not be able to enter the abdominal wall through the internal ring unless that ring is abnormally dilated. Weakness of the internal ring may signal a *potential* hernia and is tested for by holding the fingertip against the internal ring and having the patient cough or strain. Weakness or partial dilation of the ring will produce a definite tap on the fingertip as the intestinal contents are pressed downward.

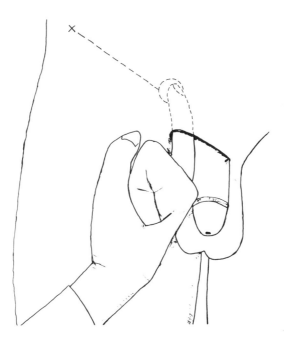

Figure 17.2 Examination for indirect inguinal hernia. The circle marks the location of the internal inguinal ring; X marks the anterior superior iliac spine.

An indirect hernia may already be present in the inguinal canal or down into the scrotum. Such a finding warrants prompt referral. The left canal is examined similarly, most conveniently with the left index or little finger.

RECTAL EXAMINATION

Anatomy

The anal canal is a muscular sphincter, 2.5-4.0 mm in length, beginning at the anus where the perianal skin joins the moist epithelium of the canal, and ending at the rectal ampulla, a dilation which marks the end of the large intestine. The prostate gland lies just *anterior* to the rectal ampulla and can be easily palpated through the thin rectal wall. It is a firm organ measuring from 3-4 cm in width and about 3 cm in length. On palpation, it seems to project less than 2 cm through the rectal wall. The normal prostate has readily palpable right and left lobes separated by a midline groove or fissure, and a median lobe, lying below the groove, which cannot be felt.

Position

The most convenient position for the routine rectal examination is for the patient to stand with his feet apart, bent forward, resting his chest on an examining table (Figure 17.3). The knee-chest position is also excellent. For the bed patient, a satisfactory position is achieved by having the patient lying on one side with the superior thigh flexed, bringing the knee as close to the chest as possible. Another position, suitable for even sicker patients, is the lithotomy position.

Inspection

The buttocks should be spread widely to visualize the entire perianal region. Skin lesions, fistulas, external skin tags (which are external hemorrhoids), or prolapsed rectal mucosa may all be seen.

Palpation

There are several techniques that are helpful in accomplishing a successful rectal examination, all of which are based upon the examiner's consideration for his patient. The more confidence and the less fear the patient has, the more likely his cooperation. First, the examiner should tell the patient that this is an uncomfortable examination, but that it should not be painful. Assure the patient that you will stop if severe pain develops. Second, do not surprise him. Tell the patient when you are about to begin palpation. Remember that the lubricant, which should be spread liberally on the gloved index finger, is at room temperature and is therefore much cooler than the anus. Tell him that he will feel the coldness. Third, and most important, *never force*

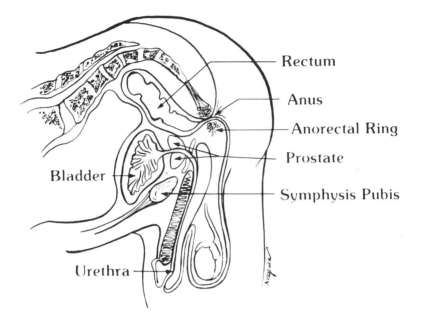

Figure 17.3 Diagram of male pelvic region with patient bent forward in routine examination position.

the examining finger through the rectal sphincter. Place the lubricated pad of the finger against the anus and hold it there with light pressure. Wait for the sphincter to relax, and the finger will almost fall into the rectum without producing pain or sphincter spasm.

As the finger slides into the rectum, curve the finger so that it remains in contact with the *anterior* rectal wall, and the patient's prostate will be directly under the pad of the examiner's finger as it enters the ampulla. Examine one lobe at a time for hard masses within the lobe, and compare one lobe to the other for size (in three dimensions), consistency, and tenderness. Identify the midline fissure. Its absence is generally evidence of enlargement of the median lobe of the prostate, the one most likely to obstruct the urethra and cause urinary retention. Carcinoma is identified as a hard mass — often described as stony hard — while benign hypertrophy of the prostate often produces a firm rubbery enlargement. In the aged male, the prostate may be atrophied, and therefore is soft and mushy or almost absent. Tenderness of one or both lobes is generally evidence of infection — acute or chronic prostatitis. Next, examine the rectal wall by rotating the finger in first one direction, then the other, so that the finger pad has swept through an entire circle across the wall to identify a tumor or internal hemorrhoids. Carcinoma of the rectum or metastatic nodules are commonly palpable here. Feces will often be present and can be identified by their ability to be indented and moved. Being too soft, the seminal vesicles are not normally palpable but, if scarred, may be felt as thickened cords lateral to the prostate.

Evaluate the anal sphincter as you withdraw your finger. Of course, if the sphincter has a painful fissure, is strictured, or is obstructed, you may not have been able to go beyond this portion of the examination. On withdrawing the finger, note the presence of weakness of the sphincter muscles by pressing in several directions within the anal canal. Provision of toilet paper or tissue for the patient should be routine at the end of the examination.

Look at the examining fingertip for fresh blood, mucus, or stool. Record the color of the feces. It is good practice (if you are properly prepared) to smear the stool on a slide or porcelain plate and to test it for the presence of occult blood by the guaiac reagent.

RECORDING

Genitalia: Normal pubic hair; penis circumsized, no lesions, no inflammation; meatus patent; no discharge; scrotum — testicles descended, symmetrical, no masses; no inguinal hernia

Rectum: No external or internal hemorrhoids, no fissures or fistulae; sphincter tone good; prostate not enlarged, no masses or tenderness; stool brown, no visible blood; guaiac negative

POENTIAL NURSING DIAGNOSES

Bowel elimination, alteration in: due to incontinence, diarrhea, constipation

Sexual dysfunction or altered sexuality patterns

Stress incontinence

Reflex incontinence

Functional incontinence

Total incontinence

Urge incontinence

Urinary retention

Self-concept, disturbance in: body image, self-esteem, role performance, personal identity

chapter **18**

The Female Genital Organs

Topographical Anatomy

Physiology

The Examination Procedure

Examination of the External Genitalia

Examination of the Internal Genitalia

Rectovaginal Examination

Recording: Normal Nullipara

Potential Nursing Diagnoses

Patient Problem

Despite an increasing openness regarding sexuality in this country, examination of sexual organs may evoke more psychologic discomfort than an examiner can anticipate. There is often anxiety and apprehension regarding exposure, as well as the possible clinical findings and their implications. It is not unusual for women, both young and old, to avoid examinations, often with serious results, because of previous unpleasant physical or emotional experiences during examination, communication from others of such discomfort, or as a result of cultural influences. Therefore, to foster relaxation, confidence, and mutual respect during this type of examination, the practitioner has a responsibility to provide a warm and

interested atmosphere rather than one which may be interpreted as clinically detached.

It has been suggested that all practitioners, male and
female, preparing to learn the procedures necessary to this
examination, role-play the part of patient, assuming the required position and experiencing the draping, exposure, and
touch. The implications are obvious.[1]

TOPOGRAPHICAL ANATOMY

The *external genitalia* (Figure 18.1), collectively termed
the pudendum or vulva, comprise the following structures:
mons pubis (veneris), a rounded puff of fatty tissue over the
symphysis pubis and covered by coarse, dark hair at puberty;
the *labia majora,* two raised, rounded, longitudinal folds of
skin, merging with the mons anteriorly and the perineal body
posteriorly; *labia minora,* small, narrow, elongated folds
between the labia majora and the vaginal introitus with surfaces that are pink, moist, and resembling vaginal mucosa;
clitoris, a slightly moist, glistening body of flesh projecting
down toward the vagina; *vestibule,* the area between the
labia minora from the clitoris to the urethral opening with
soft, hairless skin containing sweat and sebaceous glands;
Skene's glands and ducts, immediately within the urethra on
its posterolateral aspect; *Bartholin's glands and ducts,* on
either side of the lower vagina; *hymen,* circular or crescent-
shaped membrane just inside entrance to the vagina; perineal
body, including skin and underlying tissues between the vaginal entrance and the anal orifice supported by muscles; and
the *fourchette,* a low ridge formed by the labia as they con-
verge posteriorly above the perineum.

The internal genitalia (Figure 18.2) comprise the *vagina,*
a muscular, distensible canal with many folds or rugae and
lined with pink mucosa about 7–8 cm long, extending from
the external genitalia to the lower neck of the uterus; the
uterus, a pear-shaped organ about 8 cm long, consisting of
a body or fundus, a short, constricted isthmus, and a cervix
2–3 cm in diameter lying in the midline of the vagina, pointed

[1] Magee J: The pelvic examination: A view from the other
end of the table. *Annals of Internal Medicine* 1975;83:563.

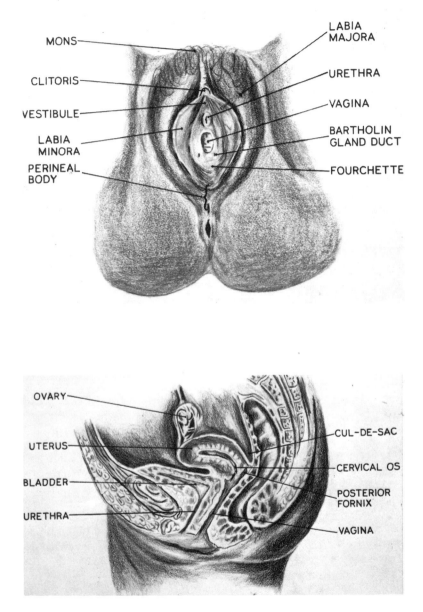

Figure 18.2 Internal genitalia.

posteriorly and covered with pink, unbroken epithelium, two almond-shaped *ovaries,* about 4 cm long, 2.5 cm wide, located adjacent to the side wall of the pelvis; and two *Fallopian tubes,* or oviducts, about 11 cm long, extending bilaterally between the folds of the broad ligament from the upper uterine fundus to an area beyond the ovary.

PHYSIOLOGY

The labia are normally close together in women who have never given birth, but then gape progressively with succeeding vaginal deliveries. They become thin with sparse hair in later years. In addition, the skin of the entire vulva becomes atrophic in the aged. White plaques referred to as leukoplakia are considered an abnormality even in postmenopausal years.

The size and development of the clitoris may be quite variable, but true enlargement usually represents some chromosomal or hormonal abnormality. Since it is analagous to the male penis, it is capable of engorgement and slight erection.

Bartholin's glands secrete into the vagina a clear, mucoid, lubricative fluid that assists the entrance of the penis during sexual intercourse. The hymen varies markedly; it may admit only a finger tip, one or two fingers, or not be present at all.

The uterus is normally tilted slightly forward and is supported by ligaments (the round ligament of the fundus, and broad ligament of the pelvis, and the uterosacral ligament from the cervix to the sacrum). The uterine body can move with considerable freedom and can change to an abnormal position (excessively vertical or excessively horizontal). The cervical opening or os varies from being small and round to being a slit in parous women. A bluish appearance of the cervix and vagina is due to increased blood supply and is usually an early indication of pregnancy (Chadwick's sign), particularly in women who have never been pregnant before.

Ovulation may be accompanied by localized abdominal pain on one side commonly referred to as *mittelschmerz* and, occasionally, by slight vaginal spotting.

Since the mucous membrane lining of the fallopian tubes is open to the peritoneum, infections from the vagina and uterus may spread into the peritoneal cavity causing inflammation (peritonitis). Amenorrhea, or failure to menstruate, is most frequently due to pregnancy but may be caused by emotional disturbances; strenuous physical training, endocrine disorders, or the presence of disease. In women who are taking the "pill," the menstrual flow may be very scant and of brief duration, while women who have an intrauterine device (IUD) in place may experience heavy bleeding of up to 8-10 days. Dysmenorrhea, or painful menstruation, relatively common in young girls, may be due to a variety of conditions which require consultation.

THE EXAMINATION PROCEDURE

Examination of the breast (see Chapter 13)

Examination of the abdomen (see Chapter 15)

Examination of the external genitalia

Cytologic smear

Examination of the internal genitalia

Rectal examination

Equipment

It will be necessary to have available:

1. Clean gloves
2. Vaginal specula
3. Sterile cotton-tipped applicators
4. Spatulas
5. Slides

---

[1] Various sizes should be available: standard Graves and larger Graves for obese multigravida patients, small Pederson for nulligravida or postmenopausal women.

Following an explanation of the necessary procedures, the patient is instructed to remove all her undergarments and is clothed only in an examination gown. It will be necessary for her to void to empty the bladder just before the examination. If cytologic examination is to be done, she should have been advised earlier to avoid douching for the previous 24 hours to maintain a normal vaginal ecosystem. Some practitioners also advise against sexual intercourse for 48 hours. Because the menstrual discharge may mask signs of discharge, lesions, or reddened mucosa, it is best to perform this examination before or after menstruation. However, in view of the dangers of unexplained bleeding and/or cancer, and despite some problems with specimens obtained during menstruation, many practitioners believe Pap smears should always be done during this examination because of the difficulty in assuring the patient's return to the office just for the Pap smear.

For the comfort of the patient, as well as for the legal protection of the male examiner, it may be advisable to have a woman in attendance during this part of the examination. Some practitioners may permit the husband or partner to stay and provide support during the examination. Among some women, either because of cultural influences or past experience, the stress of this exam may interfere with necessary muscle relaxation. When the examiner is a male the discomfort may be perceived as greater. Every effort should be made to acknowledge the patient's anxiety and suggest relaxation methods. The way the patient experiences the procedure, especially if it is her first time, can influence her entire attitude toward future pelvic examinations, as well as her concept of her sexuality and attitudes toward sexual relations. Participation in the therapeutic plan for any necessary treatments may also be affected by this experience.

EXAMINATION OF THE EXTERNAL GENITALIA

Since the mons pubis is prone to skin lesions found elsewhere on the body, look for signs of dermatitis such as lesions, reddening, or scratch marks. Edema may be a sign of vulvar varicosities or carcinomatous infiltration.

Retract the clitoral prepuce from its juncture with the clitoris and look for signs of inflammation, smegma, lesions, and adhesions. The labia majora should be separated and the area inspected for the presence of adherence, laceration, or hematoma, as well as discharge, edema, varicosities, hernia, ulcers, or tumor masses. Sebaceous cysts also develop in these structures, but although annoying, are relatively insignificant unless they become infected and present a diagnostic question.

Examine the vestibule for swelling, inflammation, and prolapsed outpouching of the urethral mucous membrane (caruncle), which is reddened and tender in infection. This area, as well as Skene ducts and Bartholin glands, is also a common site of cysts and venereal lesions, so that any discharge should be cultured for gonococcus and chlamydia.

While the lips of the labia majora are still separated, the fourchette and hymen can be inspected for old tears and scarring. The patient should be asked to strain or bear down, and the examiner alerted to any loss of urine from the urethra, or any protrusion which represents prolapse of the anterior or posterior vaginal wall or of the cervix itself.

Help the patient to relax by telling her how to relax, perhaps by concentrating on slow abdominal or chest breathing, whichever feels more comfortable.

EXAMINATION OF THE INTERNAL GENITALIA

This consists of the speculum examination and bimanual examination. Some practitioners prefer to do the bimanual examination first to locate the cervix and to facilitate proper insertion of the speculum before performing palpation. Either sequence is acceptable provided lubricating jelly is not used prior to the Pap smear.

Speculum Examination

Inspection of the cervix and the upper vagina can best be done by using a vaginal speculum (Figure 18.3). In addition, collection of vaginal and cervical scrapings for examination, culture, and cytologic study may be readily accomplished when the vaginal walls are separated. Unfortunately, thousands of women still die each year in the United States from cancer of the cervix. This is a serious tragedy when we realize that many of these women could have been cured, if their lesions had been identified early enough.

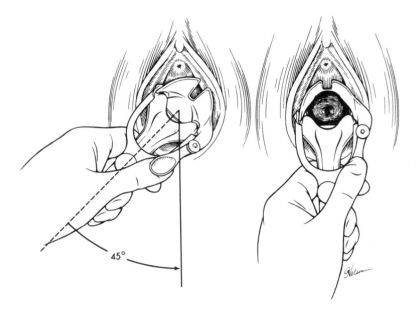

Figure 18.3 Insertion of the speculum; rotation of the speculum after insertion; inspection of the cervix. To avoid discomfort, when a very small speculum is not available, the speculum is inserted at an angle that will decrease its transverse diameter at the introitus, beyond which it can easily be rotated to the midline. The cervix is exposed by opening the blades with thumb pressure. The cervix is inspected and specimens obtained for cytologic examination (see text). From Romney, et al., 1980.

Women at risk for cervical cancer are those who have had abnormal Pap smears, have multiple sex partners, had first intercourse at an early age, or who have family history of cancer. The American Cancer Society has recommended that screening begin when a woman becomes sexually active or at age 20 (whichever occurs first), followed in 1 year by a second smear. If there are two negative smears, examination should be conducted at 3-year intervals in non-high-risk women until age 40, and annually thereafter.

Select a warmed, but not hot, speculum of the appropriate size and use water alone as a lubricant to avoid altering the results of cytology samples. Some ways to warm the speculum if warm tap water is not readily available, are: (1) heating pad on the side of the table on the low reading, (2) hold under the examining lamp. Ask the patient to breathe slowly through her mouth in an effort to relax the pelvic muscles.

Separate the labia with one hand and move two fingers inside the vagina, retracting the vaginal wall by pressing posteriorly on the fourchette. Insert the speculum by holding it closed with the other hand so that the blades are nearly vertical, the handle pointed to the side (see Figure 18.3). Direct the tip of the speculum to the posterior part of the vaginal introitus to avoid possibly painful pressure on the external urethral meatus. Rotate the speculum back to the midline so that the blades are in a transverse position and the handle points downward. Advance the speculum to full depth so the cervix can be exposed and, after opening the blades slowly, lock the speculum in its open position (Figure 18.4). It may be important to mention here that the sight of a string coming out of the os is evidence that there is an IUD in place. If a plastic tip is visualized, it would likely mean the device was partially expelled.

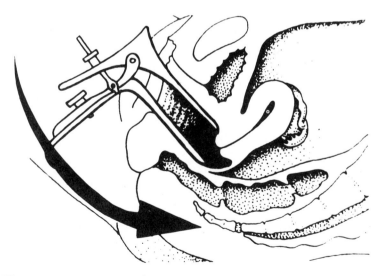

Figure 18.4 Diagram of the speculum in position with blades opened.

Once the cervix is adequately exposed, obtain specimens for Pap smear. Although there are several techniques employed, we suggest the use of cotton-tipped applicator inserted gently into the cervical os to collect the first specimen (Figure 18.5). A special spatula is used to scrape around the os (Figure 18.6), and to obtain a collection from the vaginal pool in the posterior fornix. The material should be immediately transferred to the microscopic slide, promptly fixed with alcohol and ether or sprayed with a commercially prepared fixative to avoid distorting the cells by allowing them to dry, and sent to the laboratory.

In veiw of the increasing incidence of venereal infections, especially gonorrhea and chlamydia, it is recommended that cultures also be taken routinely in young, sexually-active women during each examination even if there are no symptoms (see Appendix XI, Office Laboratory Procedures).

With the speculum still in place, the cervix should be observed for color, laceration, discharge, erosions, ulcers, and new growths.

Inspect the cervical os for size, shape, color, polyps, and beefy red appearance, as well as for bleeding spots. A marked change in position may normally occur as a result of uterine retroversion, but since any change in position may be indicative of uterine tumor, inflammation of the parametrium, or malignant infiltration, this finding should be added to the problem list and consultation requested.

The lateral walls of the vagina, visible between the blades of the speculum, should be inspected for texture, ulceration, abnormal redness or blueness, discharge, and evidence of bulging. As the speculum is unlocked and slid gently out of the vagina, the anterior and posterior walls may be inspected for cystic or solid tumors, ulcerations, and injury.

Frequently, a white vaginal discharge called leukorrhea may be found. It may occur at any age and affects almost all women at some time in their lives. Although it is not necessarily a sign of disease, but may be a manifestation of ovulation or normal desquamation of epithelial cells, leukorrhea may be a sign of a local or systemic disorder. Table 18.1 illustrates some of the typical findings in various types of vaginal discharge.

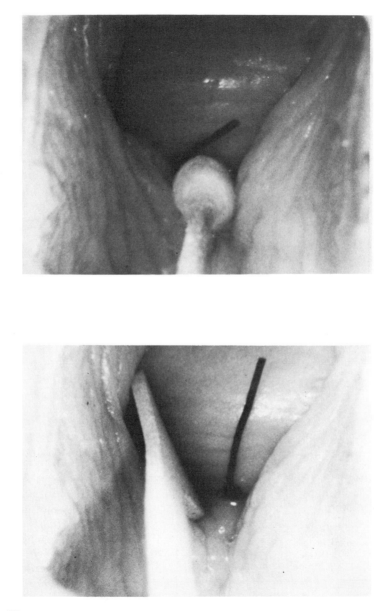

Figure 18.6 Spatula scraping the cervix for cells.

Table 18.1 Characteristics of Vaginal Discharge[a]

Color	Consistency	Amount	Odor	Probable Causes
Clear	Mucoid	+ to ++	None	Ovulation; emotional stress; increased estrogen secretion
White	Thin with curdlike flecks attached to vaginal wall	+ to ++	None to musty depending on hygiene	Vaginal mycosis, *Candida albicans*
Yellow-green	Frothy	+ to +++	Fetid	*Trichomonas vaginalis* vaginitis
Brown	Watery	+ to ++	Musty	Vaginitis; cervicitis; endometritis; neoplasm of cervix, endometrium, or tube; postradiation
Gray blood-streaked	Thin	+ to +++	Foul	Vaginal, cervical endometrial, or tubal neoplasm; Gardnerella infection

[a]Students are cautioned that these descriptions can serve only as a guide, and a great deal of variation may be expected.

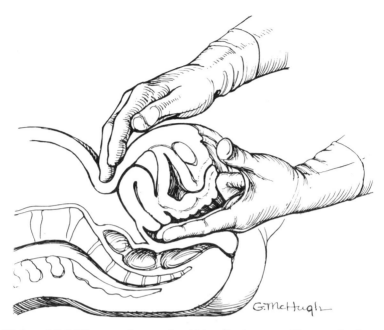

Figure 18.7 Bimanual examination, *first step:* The vaginal fingers first feel the consistency and symmetry of the cervix and its axis in relation to the axis of the vagina. They then elevate the uterus toward the abdominal wall so the total length of the uterus can be determined.

Bimanual Examination

There are two parts to this procedure: abdominal-vaginal and abdominal-rectovaginal. The examiner, again after carefully explaining the procedure, which may be slightly uncomfortable, stands before the patient who is still in dorsolithotomy position. The index and middle fingers of the examiner's gloved hand, held closely together, are lubricated and gently inserted into the vagina with slight pressure against the posterior vaginal wall (Figure 18.7). The hand is then turned so that the back surface is parallel to the floor and the finger pads facing the anterior vaginal wall, in an attempt to avoid pressure on the sensitive urethra. Notation should be made of any firmness, induration, tenderness, tumors, or cystic masses in the vaginal wall, as well as the amount of relaxation present. Estimation of vaginal muscle tone is done by having the patient bear down to evaluate the pubococcygeus muscle. Patients can be taught the importance of Kegel exercises at this time and encouraged to do them regularly. The examiner should be alerted to bulging of the posterior vaginal wall into the introitus, which is indicative of a rectocele, or bulging of the anterior wall, which occurs with cystocele.

Consideration should then be given to the consistency, tenderness on mobility, or fixation of the cervix. Normally the cervix feels like a button with a rounded face and a central depression; its consistency is similar to the tip of the nose. Feel for nodules and old lacerations.

Press downward with the abdominal hand while the pelvic structures are swept up against it with the vaginal fingers, and attempt to feel the uterus between the examining fingers and the abdominal hand (Figures 18.8 and 18.9). With the vaginal hand palm up, separate the two fingers laterally so that one finger is on either side of the cervix, and attempt to outline the uterus. The five important characteristics requiring attention include: *size, mobility, position, consistency,* and *contour.* Irregularity in surface such as in myomata usually can be easily identified. The cul-de-sac area should be examined for bulging, tenderness, and masses. Remember to explain your movements and the sensations she will have to your patient.

To locate the ovary, place the vaginal fingers on one side of the cervix and push up and back. Place the abdominal fingers just medial to the anterior superior iliac spine and, by pushing downward so their tips approach the vaginal fingers, you should be able to locate an ovary. (The right-handed practitioner may have to reglove and change hands to feel for the left-sided organs with the left hand. See Figures 18.10 and 18.11.)

Fallopian tubes can rarely be palpated unless enlarged, inflamed, badly scarred from old pelvic inflammatory disease (PID), or immobilized by adhesion, or endometrial implants.

The ovary may not always be felt in the normal or postmenopausal woman. If the ovary is located, it should be evaluated for size, shape, and mobility. It is important to remember that it is sensitive to pressure, so gentleness is imperative. The presence of unusual tenderness, enlargement over 5 cm, a fixed position from which it cannot be moved, or evidence of any irregularity in shape is noted.

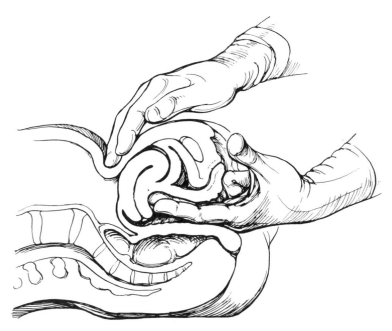

Figure 18.8 Bimanual examination, *second step:* The vaginal fingers are moved into the anterior fornix to permit palpation of the uterine corpus. If the abdominal wall is thin and well relaxed, it is possible by this maneuver to define even minor irregularities in contour or consistency of the uterus. *Third step:* with the vaginal fingers still in the anterior fornix and with the aid of the abdominal hand, the uterus is moved gently toward the retroverted position and then from side to side to determine its mobility and the presence or absence of pain on movement of the uterus.

RECTOVAGINAL EXAMINATION

This is another important part of the examination that can help identify the presence of serious inflammation, tumor of the pelvis, or undiagnosed fistulas secondary to birthing trauma. After changing gloves, gently insert the index finger into the vagina and the second finger into the rectum (Figure 18.12). The presence of any inflammatory reaction, extensive malignant tumor, or granulomatous masses of the

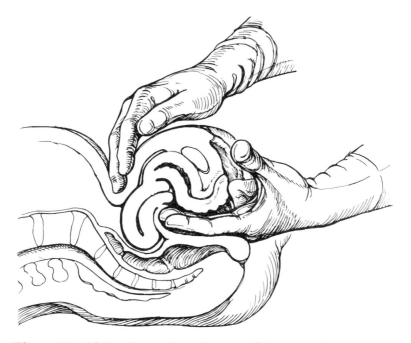

Figure 18.9 If the fingertips of abdominal and vaginal hands come together in carrying out step 2, one concludes that the uterus is retroverted; the vaginal fingers are then moved to the posterior fornix to outline the symmetry, consistency, and mobility of the retroverted corpus.

pelvic cellular tissue may be palpated in this manner. A guaiac test for occult blood might also be done as described in Chapter 17. (See Appendix XI, Office Laboratory Procedures.)

Once the examination has been completed, the patient's vulva should be cleansed of examining lubricant, her legs removed from the stirrups, and she can be assisted from the table.

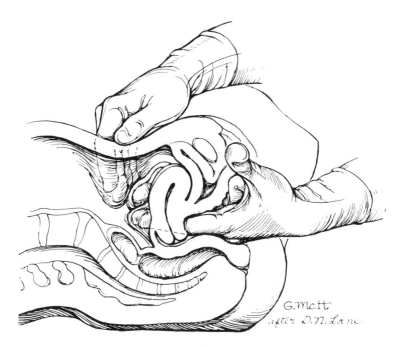

Figure 18.10 Bimanual examination, step 4: To outline the adnexa the vaginal fingers are moved to the left fornix, and one attempts to bring the abdominal and vaginal fingers together at a point presumed to be superior to the tube and ovary.

RECORDING: NORMAL NULLIPARA

Genitalia

External: Normal pubic hair, no labial swellings or lesions; normal clitoris; introitus admits two fingers; no urethral redness, swelling, or discharge; Skene's and Bartholin's not inflamed; perineum intact, no scars

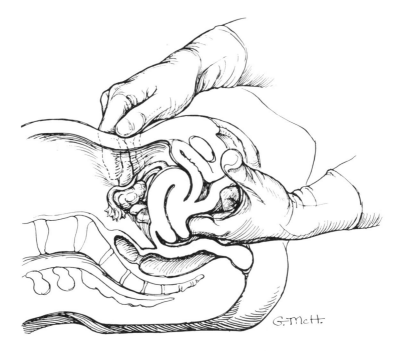

Figure 18.11 Bimanual examination, step 5: When the fingers of abdominal and vaginal hands are quite close together (it is desirable, but not always possible, to approximate these fingers), they are then moved gently toward the examiner so the adnexa slip between the fingers, and can so be outlined.

Internal: Vagina: No bulging or masses, mucosa intact and pink.

Uterus: Anterior, average size, regular shape, mobile, normal consistency.

Adnexa: Tubes not palpated, ovaries not enlarged, slight tenderness.

Cul-de-sac: No bulging, tenderness, or masses.

Discharge: Clear, mucoid, 1+, no odor.

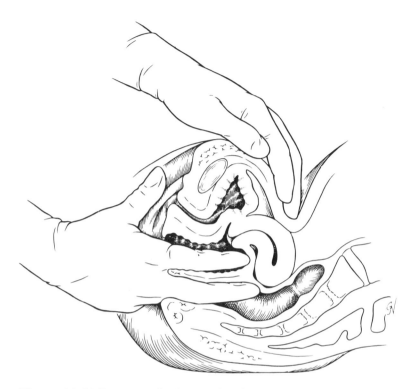

Figure 18.12 Rectovaginal examination. The retroverted or retroflexed corpus uleri can best be identified as shown. (From Romney et al., 1980, with permission.)

Pap: To lab.

Rectum: No external or internal hemorrhoids, no fissures or fistulae; sphincter tone good; no masses or tenderness; stool brown, no visible blood; guaiac negative.

POTENTIAL NURSING DIAGNOSES

Anxiety

Knowledge deficit

Rape trauma syndrome or posttrauma response

Self-concept, disturbance in: body image, self-esteem, role performance

Sexual dysfunction or altered sexuality patterns

Urinary elimination, alteration in patterns (see page 327)

PATIENT PROBLEM

Mrs. S. D. is a 22-year-old, well-developed, white, married female, with CC "vaginal itch, burning on urination and vaginal discharge of 1-wk duration."

Problem: Pruritis, Dysuria, Vaginal Discharge

S: Treated with erythromycin 4 wk ago for RUL pneumonia. Was well until 7 days ago when she first noticed increased vaginal discharge with severe itch and burning on urination. Has taken low dose pill for birth control past 2 yr, no untoward effects. Doesn't remember name of pill. Menses of 28 days x 3 days, no dysmenorrhea, no clots or spotting, uses 4 tampons q.d.; no dyspareunia; urine neg. for sugar in hospital; history diabetes maternal grandmother.

O: Vestibule and urethra red and irritated.

Vagina: Reddened mucosa, white curds clinging to wall.

Uterus, cervix and adnexa: Within normal limits.

Discharge: Thin, watery 2+, no odor.

Pap: Done — to lab.

Urine: Neg. sugar.

KOH prep: No trichimonads seen, cells typical of *Candida albicans.*

ASSESSMENT: In view of recent Rx with erythromycin, increased susceptibility due to birth control pills, typical monilia cells seen on KOH prep, suggest *Candida albicans* vaginitis.

Nursing Diagnosis: Comfort, alteration in: due to "vaginal itch and burning on urination." Alteration in health maintenance related to vaginal discharge.

PLAN: Goals: To verbalize understanding of need to continue medical regime until discharge clears. To minimize discomfort of burning on urination and vaginal itch. Nursing Orders: Diagnostic: 2-hr pc blood sugar. Therapeutic: Nystatin (Mycostatin) suppositories b.i.d. 1 wk; encourage increase in fluid intake. Patient Education: Advise to avoid sexual intercourse, use of tampons and douching 2 wk; use cotton panties changed regularly; if not cleared, return for consultation; advised against use of perfumed type douching, occasional vinegar OK; take showers instead of baths.

IMPLEMENTATION: Instruct in the appropriate application of vaginal suppositories and medical regime. Discuss importance of hand washing and feminine hygiene. Encourage increase in fluid intake. Encourage frequent pericare and use after voiding.

EVALUATION: Verbalized understanding of medical regime and importance of compliance until vaginal discharge clears.

The Neurologic and Mental Examination

In performing the history and physical examination described to this point, the clinician has already included almost all of the elements of a screening mental and neurologic examination. The purpose of this chapter is to arrange these elements into an organized whole, to describe several additional tests that should be performed for a more complete evaluation, and to recommend a format for reporting this examination.

GENERAL EXAMINATION

The essential portions of this evaluation can be divided into the examination of *cerebral function,* the *cranial nerves,* the functioning of the *cerebellum* and *motor* and *sensory* systems, and the *reflexes.* The examination summarized here is an adequate screening examination and is *not* a full, detailed evaluation of all psychiatric or neurologic functions, which must be left to the specialist.

CEREBRAL FUNCTION (Mental Status)

The mental status of the patient is a critical portion of any evaluation and is properly recorded here. The entire medical interview, with appropriate questions, plus careful observation of the patient during the history-taking and the physical examination should provide the clinician with a sound estimate of the patient's mental status.

In earlier chapters, several sections indicated specific ways to elicit information about the emotional and mental condition of the patient. These include nonverbal communications, the third ear (Chapter 3), review of systems, family history, personal and socio-cultural history, activities of daily living, habits, sleep, sexual history, and interpersonal relationships (Chapter 5). In Chapter 28, special tools developed to assess the level of emotional distress, anxiety, and depression are described.

Although there is some degree of overlapping in any classification, the mental functions may conveniently be placed in groups as follows: (1) state (or level) of consciousness, (2) affect (or mood), (3) behavior, (4) intellect, and (5) speech.

State of Consciousness

State of consciousness refers to the actual wakefulness of the individual: his level of responsiveness. This varies from full alertness to lethargy to stupor to coma. Lethargy and general psychomotor retardation can be present in depression as well as organic disease. (See Chapter 28.) The student must also be aware of the fact that the state of consciousness may be changeable over short periods of time. This lability is a most important phenomenon to note — and to report promptly.

Affect

Affect refers to the emotional tone — the mood — of the person. The affect encompasses anger, anxiety, elation, euphoria, depression, dullness, or unvarying sameness of mood — a "flat affect."

The examiner should note and record the patient's dominant mood exhibited during each visit. It is also vital to note moods that seem inappropriate to the patient's actual life situation.

Behavior

Behavior refers to physical clues including general appearance, dress, and motor activity. The general appearance will, most often, relate to the affect. Thus, a person who is depressed may slump in a chair, answer questions very briefly, and move about slowly. On the contrary, an elated or euphoric individual will be alert, lively, generally appropriately dressed, talkative, and animated.

Nonverbal communication is a distinct form of behavior that is most often closely related to the person's emotional tone. Personal appearance also has a tendency to mirror affect. The man who has not shaved for a couple of days, or the woman with no makeup at all may be telling the world how they feel. Rumpled clothing or inappropriate dress may also be clues to affect. Inability to maintain eye contact or attentiveness to the examiner may be a sign of mental illness.

Intellect

This category includes a large number of cerebral functions, of which only a few ordinarily need to be tested.

Orientation

The normal, intact individual is fully aware of time, place, person, and situation. He knows the approximate minute, hour, day, and date; he knows his name and those of his family or friends; he knows where he is; and is aware of why he is in this place at this time.

Memory

There seem to be at least three "memory banks" in the cerebral cortex: one for events of the distant past, one for events of the recent past, and the third for immediate recall. The standard medical history will have tested abundantly memory of the distant past ("Childhood diseases?", "Military service?", "Previous surgery?"). The recent past will have been explored with questions about current diet, home address, present illness, etc.

Recognition

The subject should be able to recognize familiar objects such as a coin, pencil, chair, or picture. He should also be able to recognize common words by giving simple definitions of a car or a door, for example. He should be able to state how a pair of words are alike, such as a shoe and a stocking or a dog and a cat.

These require some verbal ability plus simple reasoning.

Other

These include intelligence, mathematical ability, judgment, general knowledge, ability to perform abstraction, etc. These cerebral functions are rarely, if ever, tested in a *screening* evaluation.

Speech

Speech is a complex act that includes both language formation and actual articulation. The involved structures are the cerebrum, the cerebellum, the cranial nerves, the mouth, palate, tongue, larynx, and the respiratory system. It was suggested earlier that evaluation of speech should be recorded in the general survey (Chapter 7) and it should also be included in this summary of cerebral functions.

The report for a person with normal findings might be summarized as follows:

Mental status: Alert and responsive; thought process, memory, orientation intact. Appropriate behavior and speech.

Lack of ability to perform these basic cerebral functions may
be a reflection of a disturbed thought process. Also, the
presence of delusions, hallucinations, or bizarre expressions
are indicative of impaired intellect. Once again, if the routine history and physical examination have turned up evidence
of mental impairment, the task of the general clinician is to
refer the patient to an appropriate practitioner.

CRANIAL NERVES

General

The function of each of the cranial nerves will have
been tested in the physical examination of the head and neck;
therefore, the technique for examination of each will not be
repeated here. The functions of the cranial nerve or group
of nerves will be listed so that abnormalities can be related
to the appropriate nerve.
The sense of taste (cranial nerves VII and IX) need not
be routinely tested and is not included in the listing below.
For cranial nerve VIII only the cochlear branch function is
listed. The vestibular branch is concerned with balance but,
routinely, this nerve function is not tested. Gait and balance
are reported under the examination of the cerebellum in this
summary. Similarly, nystagmus, which, if present, will have
been identified and recorded during examination of the extraocular movements, should also be reported as a lesion of
cranial nerves III, IV, and VI here, although, in fact, it may
be due to a lesion elsewhere.

Specific Nerves

  .I. Olfactory: smell
  II. Optic: visual acuity, visual fields, color vision
 III. Oculomotor ⎫   extraocular movement (EMO),
 IV. Trochlear ⎬   nystagmus, elevation of upper
 VI. Abducens ⎭   lids, pupils
  V. Trigeminal: sensations of forehead, cornea, face and
     jaw; closure of jaw
 VII. Facial: movement of facial muscles, closure of eyes
VIII. Acoustic: hearing, Weber test

IX. Glossopharyngeal ⎫ phonation, position of the uvula,
 X. Vagus   ⎭ swallowing, gag reflex
XI. Accessory: movement of head, shrugging of shoulders
XII. Hypoglossal: protrusion of tongue, tremor of tongue

CEREBELLAR FUNCTION

The cerebellum serves as the higher center for balance and muscle coordination. These functions should be tested separately. Only a few of the many possible tests are listed below, but these are adequate to identify possible cerebellar disorders. If either muscle weakness or impaired position sense (proprioception) is present, the above tests may be misleading. This is particularly true for weakness or impaired proprioception in the lower extremities.

Balance Tests

1. *Gait:* Characteristic of a cerebellar disorder is a staggering, ataxic gait similar to that seen with alcohol intoxication. If the abnormality of gait is not due to an obvious physical abnormality, such as paralysis of a lower extremity or muscle wasting, this abnormality should be reported here.
2. *Romberg:* This is a test for defective position sense leading to ataxia and has been described during the examination of extremities (see Chapter 15). Have the patient stand with his feet together and eyes open. If he does not begin to fall, have the patient close his eyes. With an impairment of station or posture, the patient may begin to fall — be prepared to catch him! Such a response would be recorded as a positive Romberg test.

Coordination Tests

1. *Finger-to-nose:* Have the patient extend his arms fully to the sides and ask him to touch his nose rapidly, first with one fingertip and then the other. If this can be performed easily, have the patient repeat this with the eyes closed. An abnormal response would consist of "past-pointing" in which the fingertip will be brought beyond the nose, missing the target widely (Figure 19.1).

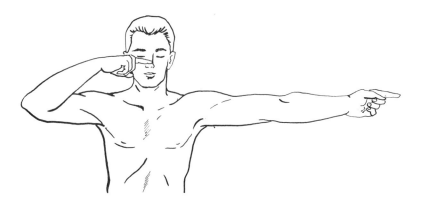

Figure 19.1 Finger to nose coordination. The movements should be smooth and rapid with little or no head or body movement.

2. *Heel-to-shin:* With the patient lying on the examining table, have him place one heel rapidly down the shin to the ankle. Ask him to repeat this using the other heel. Failure to do this smoothly and accurately will suggest a cerebellar disorder.
3. *Alternating motion:* The normal individual should be able to coordinate alternating motions such as *rapid* pronation and supination of the hands or tapping the floor with his toes. These activities will be slow and inaccurate with cerebellar dysfunction.
4. *Heel-to-toe:* This simple maneuver may bring out minor degrees of unsteadiness not gross enough to affect gait or to produce a positive Romberg.

TENDON REFLEXES

The routine physical examination should include testing the biceps, triceps, patellar, and Achilles reflexes. These reflexes are tested by striking the tendon and watching for contraction of the stretched muscle. It is not necessary for the muscle to contract forcefully enough to move the limb, but simply to contract. The reflexes may be difficult or impossible to elicit when the patient is tense and holding himself rigid, so relaxation is imperative for proper testing.

Distracting the patient is often necessary. Reflexes on corresponding sides are compared with each other and against an arbitrary scale:

    0   = Reflex absent
    +   = Reflex hypoactive
    ++   = Normal reflex
    +++ = Hyperactive reflex
    ++++ = Hyperactive reflex with clonus

There is a wide range of normal and it is more important to compare reflexes from one side of the patient to the other than to fit an arbitrary scale.

The biceps reflex is obtained by supporting the patient's arm, placing the thumb firmly on the patient's biceps tendon (Figure 19.2), and striking the thumbnail briskly with the reflex hammer. Watch the biceps muscle for contraction.

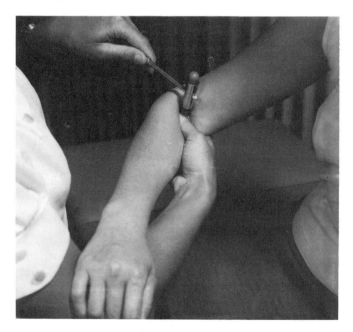

Figure 19.2 Testing the biceps reflex. Note the way in which the examiner supports the patient's arm to afford relaxation.

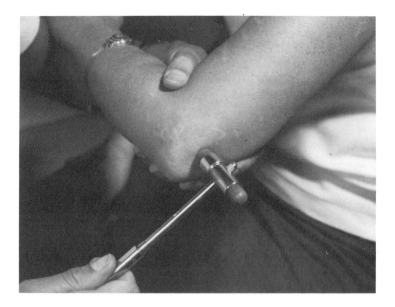

Figure 19.3 Testing the triceps reflex. Again, the examiner is seen supporting the patient's arm.

Similarly, the patient's arm is supported to relax the muscles, and the triceps tendon is struck with the hammer just above the olecranon process (Figure 19.3).

The patellar reflex is most easily obtained with the patient seated on the examining table with the legs dangling free. Tension may be relieved by having the patient swing his legs loosely for a moment before testing. The patellar tendon is struck just below the patella, and the quadriceps muscle group should be observed for contraction (Figure 19.4).

With the patient seated on the table, the Achilles reflex is obtained by having the foot *lightly* supported by the examiner's free hand while the tendon is struck with the hammer. Sometimes, slight jiggling of the patient's foot before tapping the tendon will assist in obtaining relaxation (Figure 19.4).

When the patient is to be examined in bed, some variation of these positions is necessary but the principles to be followed are the same: get the patient and the limb as

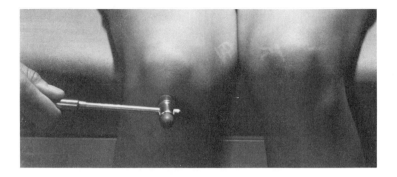

Figure 19.4 The patellar reflex.

relaxed as possible and then strike the tendon briskly and with equal strength for all reflexes.

Plantar Reflex

Using a hard, blunt object such as a key, applicator stick, or the handle of a tuning fork, stroke the foot firmly. Start near the heel, stroke up the lateral surface of the sole and across the ball of the foot (Figure 19.5). An *abnormal* response (the Babinski sign) consists of dorsiflexion of the great toe and spreading of the other toes. This would be reported as *Babinski present.* Any other response is to be considered a normal plantar reflex.

MOTOR SYSTEM

Muscle Atrophy

In the examination of the neck as well as in the upper and lower extremities, the clinician should observe and palpate for atrophy of muscles and significant asymmetry of one muscle group from adjacent groups or the corresponding group on the opposite side. Such atrophy should be recorded here to give a picture of the motor system as a whole in one place.

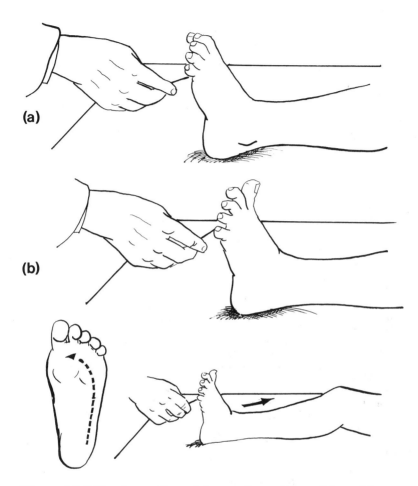

Figure 19.5 Plantar reflex: (a) negative; (b) positive. The line drawn on the foot is the course of the instrument along the lateral aspect of the sole starting at the heel to elicit a plantar reflex.

Muscle Strength

This testing was also performed in examination of the extremities (Chapter 16) and, if abnormal, should be recorded here, also.

Involuntary Body Movements

A variety of involuntary movements may occur in either alert or comatose patients. These should be recorded here, although they may have been noted earlier in the region where observed (Table 19.1).

SENSORY SYSTEM

General

As for other portions of the detailed neurologic examination, there are many sensory modalities capable of being tested. Routinely, *light touch, superficial pain,* and *vibratory sense perception* are tested in a few locations. Start the examination by testing opposite, corresponding parts of the body, going from distal to proximal regions, asking the pateint to compare the sensation on one side to that on the other. *Slight* differences ordinarily are not significant. This examination should be done with the patient's eyes closed, although he should be told what is to be done and what responses are expected of him.

If a definite difference is reported by the patient between opposite sides, the abnormal area should be carefully outlined. Thus, if the patient notes diminished pain to pinprick on the right forearm, testing should be done to determine at which level the abnormality is first noted, how low on the forearm it extends, and how far it extends on the flexor and extensor surfaces. A useful method for reporting the extent of such an area of abnormal sensation is to draw a diagram.

Light Touch

Using a wisp of cotton, touch, in order, the forehead, cheeks, hands, forearms, arms, chest, feet, legs, and thighs. The abnormality will usually be in perception of diminished touch sensation.

Table 19.1 Characteristics of Involuntary Movements

Fibrillations	Spontaneous fine contractions of individual muscle fibers that accompany peripheral denervation, visible, if at all, only in tongue
Fasciculations	Delicate, spontaneous, simultaneous contractions of a bundle of muscle fibers that are innervated by a single peripheral axon; contractions are visible through the skin, variable and slow in frequency, and associated with motor neuron or motor nerve root disease
Tics	Sudden, large amplitude, irregular muscle movements that most often involve face, tongue or trunk movements; often producing bizarre grimacing or abrupt twisting, they may appear to be behaviorally related
Tremor	Fine, rapid (10-12/sec) tremors can affect peri-orbicular or peripheral muscles with fatigue, anxiety, thyrotoxicosis, or alcohol abuse; coarse tremor accompanies extrapyramidal or cerebellar dysfunction
Motor Seizures	Can be several types: *Myoclonus* includes sudden unexpected abrupt contractions of a single muscle or group of muscles involving limbs more than trunk and usually producing flexion *Focal motor seizures* can affect face, hand-arm or, less often, foot-leg; movements are semibehavioral or repetitive myoclonic *Generalized motor seizures* can be clonic or tonic, sometimes both in sequence, and produce gross powerful, symmetrical muscle contractions of extremities and trunk

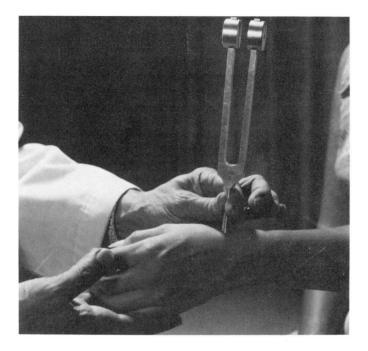

Figure 19.6 Testing vibratory sense at the wrist.

Superficial Pain

Using a sharp pin, prick lightly on the above areas. Either decreased or increased sensation may be noted.

Vibratory Sense

Strike the tuning fork (C256) before touching each location to obtain roughly the same intensity of vibration. Place the base of the fork on the area to be tested, pressing firmly against the underlying bone (Figure 19.6). Test the fingers, wrists, elbows, shoulders, toes, ankles, shins, and knees. Hold the fork on the part and note the patient's ability to feel when the fork stops vibrating. An abnormality is either stating that vibration has stopped while the fork is still vibrating briskly, or feeling no vibrations at all.

RECORDING

Cerebral Function: Alert and responsive, thought process, memory, and orientation intact. Appropriate appearance, behavior and speech.

Cranial Nerves:

I. Identifies alcohol

II. Vision 20/20 OD, 20/20 OS; color intact; fields normal by gross confrontation; fundi normal

III. IV. VI. EOM intact; no ptosis; no nystagmus; PERRLA

V. Sensory intact, jaw closure normal

VII. Facial muscles symmetrical, no weakness

VIII. Hearing intact, Weber test normal

IX. Swallowing and gag reflex intact; uvula rises in mid-
X. line on phonation

XI. Head movement and shrug of shoulders normal

XII. Tongue protrudes in midline, no tremor

Cerebellar function: finger to nose, heel to shin coordination intact; gait normal, Romberg negative

Motor system: no atrophy, weakness, or tremors

Sensory: intact to light touch, pinprick, and vibration

Reflexes: these are best reported either in chart form, or by use of a stick figure (Figure 19.7).

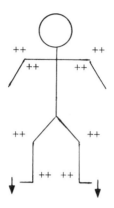

Figure 19.7 Recording of normal deep tenson reflexes.

POTENTIAL NURSING DIAGNOSES

Anxiety

Communication, impaired verbal

Grieving, dysfunctional

Sensory-perceptual alteration

Thought processes, alteration in

chapter 20

The Sequence of a Complete Physical Examination

Suggested Sequence

For purposes of clarity of teaching, the physical examination of each region or organ has been described as if each were a separate entity. Chapter 12 described inspection, palpation, percussion, and auscultation of the thorax and lungs from anterior, lateral, and posterior positions. Chapter 14 then described inspection, palpation, percussion, and auscultation of the heart, anteriorly. To actually perform a complete examination of a patient in this manner would require a repetition of examination of the same body region, resulting in much movement of the patient and the examiner, as well as a significant loss of valuable time for both. These repetitions must be eliminated by the development of a pattern of examination of the whole patient that will not miss any portion of the examination and will minimize wasted time. There is no single "right" order of examination that is used by all practitioners, or even by the same practitioner for all patients. The examination of a bedridden patient, of an ambulatory patient in the office or clinic, or of a seriously ill, feeble, or uncooperative patient will be varied according to circumstances. Additionally, if the patient presents a specific disturbing abnormality (e.g., abdominal pain, mass in the neck), this part may be examined first to reassure the patient that his major problem will receive priority, and not be relegated to the routine sequence of the examination. As mentioned earlier nurses will examine the patient selectively based upon the presenting complaints, acuteness of the situation, risk factors, goals of the interaction, and institutional policies. It is strongly recommended, however, that the student develop a pattern for the complete basic physical examination and stay with this routine until it becomes a habit pattern. In this way, he will not skip around from one place to another wondering what to do next, and he will be less likely to miss a portion of the examination.

SUGGESTED SEQUENCE

The following is a suggested sequence for the routine examination of a fully cooperative ambulatory patient and is presented simply as one of several possible logical models.

1. Observe body movement and general status on entry
2. Interview for current problem, health history, and initial mental status assessment
3. Record vital signs, test vision with Snellen chart
4. Body as a whole
   Inspect gait, balance, body build
5. Head and neck
   Inspect and *palpate* head, eyes, ears, nose, mouth, pharynx and neck
   Auscultate cranium, carotids, and thyroid, if indicated
6. Anterior thorax
   Inspect anterior and lateral chest wall
   Palpate shoulders, supra- and infraclavicular spaces, axillae, breasts, ribs and sternum, precordium
   Percuss lungs (anterior and lateral chest), heart
   Auscultate lungs (anterior and lateral chest), heart
7. Posterior thorax
   Inspect neck and back
   Palpate lungs
   Percuss lungs, diaphragm, costovertebral angles, spine
   Auscultate lungs
8. Abdomen
   Inspect anterior abdomen and flanks
   Auscultate bowel sounds and bruits
   Palpate abdomen, flanks, and femoral arteries
   Percuss abdomen and flanks

9. Extremities (examine upper, then lower extremities)
   Inspect
   Palpate joints, muscles, and arteries
   Percuss tendon reflexes
   Test touch, pinprick, vibratory senses, and plantar reflex
10. Genitalia
    Inspect and *palpate*
11. Rectal
    Inspect and *palpate*

It should be reemphasized that this sequence is a suggested model and that it is useful in developing a pattern of routine examination for the clinician. More detailed examinations of a region, part, or organ will be added when abnormalities are detected. On the other hand, no complete examination can be called thorough that does not include all of these elements of the workup, no matter what the order of examination.

Part Four

COMPLETING
THE DATA BASE

chapter 21

Nutritional Assessment

Dietary History

Physical Examination

Laboratory Evaluation

Additional Assessment

Potential Nursing Diagnoses

Patient Problem

Food is life; everyone must eat and what we eat influences our growth and, to some degree, our state of health. Because of the influence of food on our well-being, there is an enormous amount of folklore pertaining to the benefits of various food substances. While there are bona fide experts in the field of nutrition, there is also an extensive population of self-styled "experts," both professional and nonprofessional. Food has been a constant source of argument from the discussions about certain fruit in the Garden of Eden to the role of Nutrasweet in national diets, going on today.

Many people have faith in the role of certain foods, vitamins, or herbs in preventing, ameliorating, or curing various conditions or diseases. Certainly it is proved that chronic thiamin (vitamin B_1) deficiency leads to beriberi. It is also clear that it is necessary to remove phenylalanine from the diet of patients with phenylketonuria (PKU). Not so clear, however, are the benefits of massive doses of vitamin C in the treatment of cancer, the liberal allowance of martinis in weight-reduction programs, or the use of black-strap molasses and cider vinegar in the treatment of arthritis. Eating, like sleeping, is a physiologic necessity, requiring time, effort, preparation, and choices. Unlike sleeping, eating is a public activity and can be used to express social, religious, economic, or political beliefs. The eating of pork is prohibited to Jews and Muslims. The eating of the meat of cattle is rejected by the Hindu for religious reasons, while the vegetarian may be making a social statement by refusing meat. Fasting in public or in prison can be a powerful political weapon, whereas the gourmet uses food and drink to express an attitude and a socioeconomic position. Against this background, it is evident that the clinician must continuously increase his knowledge of nutrition. It is also evident that a careful nutritional assessment may provide valuable clues to the patient's general health and to some of his psychosocial dynamics.

This chapter is concerned with the general principles and techniques of nutritional assessment. It also deals with the nutritional status of the adult. Considerations of special pertinence during pregnancy, in the newborn, the infant, the child, the adolescent, and the elderly will be found in the "life cycle" chapters that follow.

DIETARY HISTORY

The dietary history may be incorporated as a portion of the history of present illness, the past history, or the personal and social history. The time for actually taking this element of history and the place for recording it will depend on the clinician's impression of the relative importance of the patient's nutritional status relative to his major problem. For example, in patients who present with gastroenteritis, gross obesity, anorexia, or chronic alcoholism, the dietary history may be considered to be a part of the HPI. In such cases, it may be desirable for the examiner to seek assistance from, or referral to a dietitian, nutritionist, or gastroenterologist, depending upon the problem and the availability of these specialized professionals.

While the clinician need not have the detailed knowledge of food required by a dietitian, a certain amount of information is useful. He should have a reasonable idea of the caloric content of various foods, and some idea about the components of a balanced diet. A well-rounded diet, generally, is one that consists of foods from each of these four major groups:

1. Protein-rich: meat, fish, poultry, beans, eggs, hard cheese
2. Milk: whole milk, buttermilk, skim milk, butter, ice cream, cottage cheese
3. Fruits and vegetables: citrus fruits, leafy and yellow vegetables
4. Grains: bread, cereal, pasta

A brief overview of a patient's diet may be obtained by the technique of 24-hour food recall. Here, the patient is asked to list all the foods and beverages consumed during the previous 24-hour period. If the previous day was not typical, the individual may be able to provide a 24-hour food recall for a typical day's food intake. (An example is provided in Appendix IV: Sample Case Report.) Another method is the use of the nutrition scan devised by Christakis.[1] The patient is asked to list the frequency of use of foods that are pertinent to specific nutritional problems:

1. How many times a week do you have the following for breakfast in usual portions?
   a. Citrus fruit (oranges, grapefruit, whole or juice)
   b. Whole grain cereals, hot or cold
   c. Eggs (plain, or with bacon, ham, sausage)
   d. Pancakes, waffles
   e. Coffee, milk (whole, 2% or skim)
2. Of the 14 lunches and dinners you eat a week, how many consist of
   a. Beef, lamb, pork or organ meats (liver, heart, kidneys)
   b. Poultry (chicken, turkey, or duck)
   c. Fish, shellfish
3. How many times a week do you eat or drink
   a. Bread, rolls
   b. Vegetables of all types
   c. Cheese
   d. Legumes (peas, beans, chick peas)

[1]Christakis G: How to make a nutritional diagnoses without really trying. A. Adult nutritional diagnosis. *J Fla Med Assoc* 1979, 66:349-356.

e. Pasta (spaghetti, noodles)
f. Fruit
g. Butter
h. Margarine
i. Vegetable oil/salad dressings
j. Ice cream
k. Alcoholic beverages (beer, wine, hard liquor)
l. Snacks (pretzels, potato chips, chocolate, etc.)
m. Cookies
n. Nuts
o. Raisins
p. Soft drinks
4. How much water do you drink daily?

Such a listing will give the dietitian or nutritionist an *estimate* of:

1. The adequacy of the overall diet
2. The relative proportions of saturated versus unsaturated fats
3. Adequacy of dietary protein
4. Cholesterol intake
5. Dietary fiber intake
6. Excessive snacking or alcohol intake

Along with information on the type and quantities of specific food items consumed, some questions about general eating habits should be included. Information should be obtained on how often meals are skipped, when and where meals are taken, food intolerances or allergies, weight changes, constipation or diarrhea, *pica* (i.e., eating of substances not usually considered as foods, such as clay, chalk, laundry starch), and any self-imposed restrictions on calories or specific food items.
Either of these methods for obtaining a brief review of dietary history should uncover enough personality or nutritional clues to enable the clinician to move on to another area or to pursue the subject further. The finding of unusual factors such as tension at meal times, use of "health" foods, megavitamin dosing, meals "on-the-run," excessive use of salt or sugar, absence of vegetables or citrus fruits, or a totally vegetarian diet, may suggest some further exploration of the dietary history.

PHYSICAL EXAMINATION

It will become obvious that the general physical examination described in Chapters 6-20 will cover all of the elements of the examination needed for nutritional assessment. The items associated with malnutrition are collected here for purposes of illustrating their relationship to nutritional diagnosis.

One of the most obvious physical signs will be the general state of nutrition of the patient. This is simply evaluated in terms of malnutrition or obesity at the extremes. In any event, weighing the patient is a very important element of the physical examination and one too often neglected. Table 21.1 gives guidelines for desirable weights for adults. These tables are labelled *guidelines* or *suggested desirable weights*, whereas many older tables carried the title of Ideal Weights. The ideal weight tables had the clear meaning that persons above or below the printed value were at higher risk for illness or death than those within the "ideal" range. Today, experts are still arguing the accuracy of such a statement. Unless the clinician has had considerable experience in nutrition or dietetics, it would be prudent to refer a patient whose weight is outside the guidelines for further guidance by a dietitian or specially trained physician. Table 21.2 lists *some* of the major clinical signs of nutritional deficiencies. Although many of these signs may be due to nonnutritional causes, their presence should alert the examiner to the possibility of malnutrition in his patient.

LABORATORY EVALUATION

While the full evaluation of the patient by clinical laboratory studies is beyond the scope of this text, a few general comments are in order. Common clues of malnutrition include the presence of anemia, small or large red blood cells (increased or decreased mean corpuscular volume [MCV]), reduced serum iron, low serum albumin, low blood urea nitrogen, reduced blood sugar, high serum levels of cholesterol, or high serum triglycerides.

Table 21.1 Guidelines for Body Weight

	Metric				
	Men Wt (kg)[a]			Women Wt (kg)[a]	
Ht (M)[a]	Av.	Accept. wt		Av.	Accept. wt
1.45				46.0	42 to 53
1.48				46.5	42 to 54
1.50				47.0	43 to 55
1.52				48.5	44 to 57
1.54				49.5	44 to 58
1.56				50.4	45 to 58
1.58	55.8	51 to 64		51.3	46 to 59
1.60	57.6	52 to 65		52.6	48 to 61
1.62	58.6	53 to 66		54.0	49 to 62
1.64	59.6	54 to 67		55.4	50 to 64
1.66	60.6	55 to 69		56.8	51 to 65
1.68	61.7	56 to 71		58.1	52 to 66
1.70	63.5	58 to 73		60.0	53 to 67
1.72	65.0	59 to 74		61.3	55 to 69
1.74	66.5	60 to 75		62.6	56 to 70
1.76	68.0	62 to 77		64.0	58 to 72
1.78	69.4	64 to 79		65.3	59 to 74
1.80	71.0	65 to 80			
1.82	72.6	66 to 82			
1.84	74.2	67 to 84			
1.86	75.8	69 to 86			
1.88	77.6	71 to 88			
1.90	79.3	73 to 90			
1.92	81.0	75 to 93			

		Nonmetric		
	Men Wt (lb)[a]		Women Wt (lb)[a]	
Ht (ft, in.)[a]	Av.	Accept. wt	Av.	Accept. wt
4 10			102	92 to 119
4 11			104	94 to 122
5 0			107	96 to 125
5 1			110	99 to 128
5 2	123	112 to 141	113	102 to 131
5 3	127	115 to 144	116	105 to 134
5 4	130	118 to 148	120	108 to 138
5 5	133	121 to 152	123	111 to 142
5 6	136	124 to 156	128	114 to 146
5 7	140	128 to 161	132	118 to 150
5 8	145	132 to 166	136	122 to 154
5 9	149	136 to 170	140	126 to 158
5 10	153	140 to 174	144	130 to 163
5 11	158	144 to 179	148	134 to 168
6 0	162	148 to 184	152	138 to 173
6 1	166	152 to 189		
6 2	171	156 to 194		
6 3	176	160 to 199		
6 4	181	164 to 204		

Source: Bray GA (ed): *Obesity in America.* Washington, DC, DHEW Pub No (NIH) 79–359, 1979.

[a]Height without shoes; weight without clothes.

Table 21.2 Clinical Signs Suggesting Malnutrition

Body Systems	Signs
Hair	Becomes dull, dry, brittle, wirelike, thin, straight, reddish in blacks, bleached out in bands in whites ("flag sign"), easily and painlessly plucked
Face	Diffuse depigmentation, malar and supraorbital pigmentation, lumpiness or flakiness of skin of nose and mouth, moon face, enlarged parotid glands, nasolabial seborrhea
Eyes	Pale conjunctivae, conjunctival injection, Bitot's spots, angular palpebritis, conjunctival xerosis, corneal xerosis, kerotomalacia, corneal opacities and scars, circumcorneal injection
Lips	Cheilosis, angular stomatitis, angular scars
Tongue	Swollen, glossy, scarlet and raw tongue (glossitis), magenta tongue, atrophic filiform papillae, hyperemic and hypertrophic filiform papillae, fissures
Gums	Spongy, bleed easily, recession of gums
Neck	Thyroid enlargement (goiter)
Skin	Xerosis, dyspigmentation, follicular hyperkeratosis, pellagrous dermatosis, flaky paint dermatosis, scrotal or vulval dermatosis, petechiae or ecchymoses, excessive bruising, lack or excess of subcutaneous fat, xanthomas, edema

Body Systems	Signs
Nails	Brittle, ridged, flattened, spoon-shaped, thin
Muscular and skeletal systems	Muscle wasting, protuberant abdomen, epiphyseal enlargement, beading of ribs (rachitic rosary), knock-knees, bowlegs, deformities of thorax, winged scapula, musculoskeletal hemorrhages
Cardiovascular system	Tachycardia (heart rate above 100), enlarged heart, abnormal rhythm, elevated blood pressure
Gastrointestinal system	Hepatomegaly, ascites, splenomegaly
Nervous system	Mental irritability and confusion, listlessness and apathy, paresthesia, loss of position and vibratory sense, weakness and tenderness of muscles (may result in inability to walk), decrease or loss of ankle and knee reflexes, tremor

Source: Christakis G (ed): Nutritional assessment in health programs. *Am J Public Health* 1973;63:Suppl Nov.

ADDITIONAL ASSESSMENT

In the workup of a patient who has, or is likely to have, a nutritional problem, a dietitian or physician might add to the basic assessment presented above. Additional history might include an inventory of food likes and dislikes, a 3-day or 7-day food recall, or a comparison of actual food intake to the National Academy of Sciences Recommended Daily Dietary Allowances (RDA).

In a specialized examination, measurement of the skin-fold thickness over the triceps muscle, measurement of mid-arm circumference, and calculation of midarm muscle circumference are all useful indices of body fat and muscle mass. Additional laboratory examination, such as actual blood levels of certain vitamins and blood enzyme studies, are also available to the specialist.

Although it is true that there is a low prevalence of serious malnutrition (except for obesity) in many of the "developed countries," the nutritional assessment should become a routine part of patient evaluation. It may identify symptoms and signs of actual nutritional disorders and may reveal the presence of conditions that place the patient at higher risk for such entities as coronary heart disease, diabetes, or renal disease. Additionally, the presence of even minor nutritional disorders may add to the disability of a patient suffering from other unrelated problems. While all patients will not need referral to a dietitian or nutritionist, it is expected that all professionals will recognize their limitations and will learn through experience when referral is indicated.

POTENTIAL NURSING DIAGNOSES

Nutrition, alteration in: less than body requirements

Nutrition, alteration in: more than body requirements

Nutrition, alteration in: potential for more than body requirements

Health maintenance, alteration in

Self-care deficit: feeding

Tissue perfusion, alteration in: gastrointestinal

Oral mucous membrane, alteration in

Fluid volume deficit, actual

Fluid volume, alteration in: excess

Fluid volume deficit, potential

PATIENT PROBLEM

Problem: Generally Not Feeling Well — Fatigue, Weakness, Tiredness, and Loss of Appetite

S: Complains of fatigue, weakness, tiredness and loss of appetite over the past month. Says he has lost 10 lb over the past 2 mo. Often feels sad and lonely due to the death of his wife 6 mo ago.

O: 67-year-old white male; widower for 6 mo.; lives alone.
Wt.: 130 lb (desirable body wt. = 145 lb); ht.: 5'8".
Triceps skinfold: 94% of standard.
Mid arm circumference: 93% of standard.
Mid arm muscle circumference: 93% of standard.
Lab data:
  Urine: pH = 6, protein = 0, glucose = 0, acetone = 0.
  Blood: Hb = 10 g/100 ml, Hct = 36%; total protein
  = 6 g/100 ml; serum albumin = 3.2 g/100 ml; cholesterol = 175 mg/100 ml.
Dietary data: 24-hr food recall indicates a typical dietary intake of 1600 calories, 44 g of protein and a lack of adequate amounts of iron-containing foods in the diet.

ASSESSMENT: Iron deficiency anemia.

Nursing Diagnosis: Nutrition, alteration in: Less than body requirements.
Grieving, dysfunctional: Due to loss of wife.

PLAN: Goals: To regain weight loss.
To establish social contact in community.

Nursing Orders:
Diagnostic: Therapeutic trial of iron salts per protocol, then return to clinic to repeat laboratory analysis of hemoglobin and hematocrit.
Therapeutic: 50 mg ferrous sulfate, fumarate, or gluconate daily; daily multivitamin and multimineral supplement; daily diet: at least 2500 calories, at least 56 g of protein (i.e., 100% of the RDA) and foods high in iron (per MD orders).
Patient Education: Referral to social service for psycho-social assessment and counseling; refer patient to a nutritionist or dietitian to be instructed on his diet and the principles of good nutrition; referral to a community feeding program for the elderly.

IMPLEMENTATION: Appointment made for home visit by nutritionist and social worker; schedule for community lunch program offered; part-time homemaker recruited by social service; one-month supply of vitamin and mineral supplements provided by hospital pharmacist under Medicare.

EVALUATION: Patient returns in one month—has gained 5 pounds; attending community lunch and recreation program for senior citizens at church.

chapter 22

The Laboratory Examination

Types of Laboratory Tests and Special Procedures

Purposes and Categories of Diagnostic Tests

Interferences in Laboratory Test Results

Errors and Pitfalls

Laboratory Screening Schedule for Asymptomatic Adults

Office Laboratory Procedures

Although this textbook is concerned primarily with health history and physical examination, a brief overview of the laboratory examination is in order. Laboratory data represent the third element of the data base, and for the full evaluation of the patient, these findings will take their place along with findings from the history and physical examination. For the most part in the past, the physician or dentist alone assumed responsibility for ordering laboratory studies; however, professional nurses have always been concerned with monitoring results of laboratory studies, preparing patients appropriately, and collecting and routing specimens. In certain settings, such as emergency rooms, when physicians were not immediately available they ordered diagnostic tests according to established protocols. Today in many health care settings, nurse clinicians, physician associates, and other primary health care providers share responsibility with physicians for ordering laboratory tests to initiate a thorough data base for early problem identification and management.

There are literally thousands of bits of information that can be determined by laboratories in modern medical centers and dozens to hundreds in smaller offices and clinics. Every year more and more bedside and or office systems are becoming available for immediate analysis of body fluids.

The proper selection of appropriate laboratory tests requires knowledge of biochemical, physiologic, and pathologic processes associated with various disease entities. The task of the clinician is to add to the data base the laboratory findings likely to be of assistance in defining the patient's problems more clearly and in managing them with consideration for the economics of his decisions. In the past, claims have been made that the laboratory has been overused and abused as a result of a suit-conscious public and governmental audit regulations. Since health care costs represent a significant part of every dollar spent in this country, it is essential that the practitioner be aware of "utilization guidelines" and order no tests unnecessarily.

Hospital laboratories usually account for 15-20% of all hospital revenue. The clinician should be aware of the cost of laboratory work. Although these figures will probably be higher on the day this book is published than at this writing, it is interesting to note that a laboratory workup in a clinic for a student with a sore throat could cost as much as $59.00 (CBC with differential, $22.00, throat culture, $21.00, Monospot slide test, $16.00).

The clinician also must keep in mind what specific variable is to be measured when multiple tests may be part of a series done on one specimen, as well as the importance of time relationship. In monitoring the blood count of a patient receiving potentially toxic drugs, the order "daily CBC" may be written where it should be "daily WBC" and possibly weekly "hemoglobin" with the option of studying further any deviations indicated as a result of the single test.

TYPES OF LABORATORY TESTS AND
SPECIAL PROCEDURES

Chemical studies: blood, urine, feces, spinal fluid, and other body fluids such as gastric juice, saliva, and joint fluid

Microbiological studies: bacteria, fungi, viruses, and other organisms

Microscopic examinations: urine, blood, spinal fluid, sputum, cells from Papanicolaou smears of the uterus, cervix, vagina, bronchi, esophagus, and other organs, tissues and cells from biopsy material, etc.

X-ray studies, CAT scan: bone and soft tissue

Biophysical technique: electrocardiography, electroencephalography, electrophoresis, electromyography, echoencephalography, thermography, etc.

Isotope studies: scanning of the thyroid gland, brain, or lung, uptake of radioactive materials, distribution of radioactive substance in body fluids or tissues, etc.

Instrumentation: bronchoscopy, esophagoscopy, gastroscopy, sigmoidoscopy, etc.

Physiologic testing: pulmonary function tests, cardiac catheterization, intestinal absorption studies, renal function tests, Lupus Erythematosis (LE) cell preparations, skin sensitivity tests, blood typing, complement fixation tests, Ripid Plasma Reagin (RPR) tests, etc.

This listing is neither intended to be complete nor overwhelming, but is designed to illustrate the tremendous assistance available from the laboratory and the complexity of making intelligent selections from these resources.

PURPOSES AND CATEGORIES OF DIAGNOSTIC TESTS

Individual diagnostic tests may have multiple purposes. When no definite symptoms are present the purpose of a test may be to screen and uncover pathology early, especially in an individual or population "at risk." Some tests are very specific for a particular condition, while others give generalized information. For example, the Gamma Glutamy/Transpeptide (GGT) enzyme test (unlike other liver tests) has been shown to be capable of detecting abnormalities in the liver while they are still reversible. This can improve the early identification of people who are drinking too much or who are hidden alcoholics, despite the individual's reluctance to acknowledge excessive drinking.

Screening

PKU is a common screening test performed on newborns, and all black children should be screened for sickle cell trait. Other diagnostic procedures, such as chest x-ray, ECG, Papanicolaou smear, skin tests for pulmonary infections (PPD, or Tine, etc.), and serological test for syphilis (RPR), are commonly utilized as screening examinations for specific high risk populations. AIDS virus screening is still controversial.

There are several tests and procedures which by experience are so useful in detecting early evidence of disease that they are referred to as routine laboratory tests. These vary from one medical center to another and depend upon the data previously collected for the patient and the presenting complaint or reason for seeking assistance. In some hospitals every patient admitted has a CBC and urinalysis regardless of previous test results done in the physician's office or of the admitting diagnosis. Tests done for a healthy adult during complete examination, such as CBC, urinalysis, ECG, and chest x-ray, are referred to as screening tests for this event, but have other purposes when specific disease conditions are suspected.

Another type of screening examination, called multiphasic screening, has become popular with the development of automated laboratory equipment which can produce 6, 12, 18, or more tests on a single blood sample. Because the system is automated, the cost is little more than that for a single test. When used, the information obtained is more than the clinician would ordinarily order initially, but the principle is the same as for the routine laboratory tests, i.e., it identifies conditions that might otherwise go undetected. It is important that the practitioner become aware of the individual laboratory tests included in a panel of tests and the expected range of normal values according to the laboratory selected. Normal values are often identified directly on the ordering form, but the practitioner may wish to refer to Appendix X for a Table of Normal Values for a selected group of common tests.

Qualitative or Confirmatory

Following the completion of a history and physical examination, the clinician may have developed several clues to the presence of disease. These clues are then followed up by the selection of tests or procedures that will confirm or deny the presence of such disease entities or will identify the type of disease process. Presented with a patient in whom the history and physical examination suggest the presence of gallbladder disease, the clinician may, for example, order a gallbladder series.

Quantitation

Where the presence of disease is evident, laboratory tests may be useful in determining how severe or how extensive the process is. Examples of this are determination of the blood urea nitrogen (BUN) in patients with known renal disease, the determination of blood indices in anemic patients, the measurement of bilirubin in jaundiced patients, and thyroid function tests in a patient with obvious hyperthyroidism.

Management

As the clinician will follow changes in symptoms or physical signs during the course of his patient's illness, so will he use serial laboratory tests to detect improvement — or failure of improvement — as the patient undergoes treatment. He will follow changes in plasma ketone bodies in a patient with acute diabetic coma, repeated chest x-rays to follow the healing of a tuberculous lung lesion, serial electrocardiograms in the course of an acute myocardial infarction, urinary albumin in a patient with nephrotic syndrome, and white blood cells in a patient receiving chloramphenicol.

INTERFERENCES IN LABORATORY TEST RESULTS

Several different factors which the clinician should be aware of may interfere with laboratory testing. For example, certain drugs and foods alter test results. Failure to obtain a history of a recent intravenous pyelogram will lead to an un-explained high level of protein-bound iodine in a patient's plasma. The fasting state for blood sugar requires that the patient not eat for at least 8 hours and preferably 12. Diuretics will alter blood electrolyte concentrations.

ERRORS AND PITFALLS

It is sometimes assumed that laboratory procedures are very accurate and less subject to error than the history-taking or the physical examination. However, since laboratory procedures are ordered, performed, reported, and interpreted by human beings, they too, are subject to human error. In addition, a certain calculated error is incorporated into many laboratory results by the establishment of "normal" values. As there are persons whose normal blood pressures are lower than average or whose normal pulse rate is higher than average, so there are people whose normal blood sugar level is outside the range established for the "normal" person. The laboratory normal values are often established by a gaussian distribution curve and may be expected to include 95% of a given population, not 100%.

Actual inaccuracies in the results of laboratory tests may arise from diverse human errors such as collecting the specimen from the wrong patient, using unsterile equipment for collection of material for culture, or delay in examination of a specimen with fragile materials, such as red blood cells in urine. Errors will occur because of selection of the wrong test, the wrong timing, or lack of knowledge of the limitation of the test itself. An example of this type of error is the use of the fasting blood sugar to detect diabetes: about 30% of diabetic patients will have normal fasting blood sugars. Since the electrocardiogram does not detect all acute or old myocardial infarctions, wrong conclusions may be drawn from the report of a normal ECG.

These errors and pitfalls can occur; therefore, it is incumbent upon the clinician to be careful in his selection of tests and to use judgment in the addition of laboratory results into the data base. Skill, knowledge, and experience are necessary when the clinician is faced with a laboratory result that is unexpected. He must be prepared to question either his own clinical judgment or the laboratory result and must decide on a course of action to try to resolve conflicts between the clinical findings and the laboratory results.

LABORATORY SCREENING SCHEDULE
FOR ASYMPTOMATIC ADULTS

There are very few fixed and agreed upon patterns of laboratory tests that should be done "routinely" on episodic or on annual health examinations. Most offices, clinics, and hospital departments make up their own lists. It should be obvious, however, that the lists will vary depending upon the risk factors identified in the individual patient, the incidence of hidden diseases, and the difficulty of the laboratory test to be used. For example, almost all lists made up for women in the childbearing years will include some measure to check for the anemia commonly present due to loss of iron through the menstrual blood. The following is to be considered a sample routine screening list and not an absolute and necessary pattern for adults *not* known to be at high risk.

Blood Pressure

Since this is a readily obtained test for a common disorder (with a high incidence in blacks), and one that is readily treated with good results, it should be present in most "routines."

Hematocrit

Recommended, as noted above, for all adult women prior to menopause.

Urinalysis

A useful routine to identify unsuspected diabetes or kidney disease (see Appendix X).

Breast Examination

The American Cancer Society recommends self-examination monthly for women over age 20, examination by a practitioner every 3 years from age 20-40, and annually after age 40.

Papanicolaou Smear (Cervix)

The American Cancer Society recommends that screening begin when a woman becomes sexually active or at age 20 (whichever occurs first), followed in 1 year by a second smear. If there are two negative smears, examination should be conducted at 3-year intervals in non-high-risk women until age 40, and annually thereafter.

Intestinal Cancer Screening

Stool testing for occult blood is inexpensive, noninvasive, and fairly acceptable to patients; however, it is nonspecific for cancer. The false-positive rate is minimal, but false-negatives may be over 20%. The American Cancer Society guidelines are for annual testing of stools for occult blood on men and women over 50 years of age, utilizing three to six slides per patient. The American Cancer Society recommends sigmoidoscopy every 3-5 years in persons over 50 years of age, following 2 negative examinations 1 year apart.

Chest X-Ray

The subject is under careful review at present, and many practitioners do not perform routine chest x-rays on asymptomatic patients who have no increased risk factors. Smokers, coal miners, and others exposed to dusty environments do have increased risks, and should be examined on a regular basis.

Mammography

Current opinion is also changing, so a reasonable recommendation is for a baseline mammogram for all women over 35 years of age, and further mammograms for those without increased risk factors or the discovery of a breast mass only upon physician's recommendation. (See Table 13.1, Breast Cancer Risk Factors.)

Cholesterol Level

The basic findings of the famous Framingham Study show that the higher a person's serum cholesterol, the more at risk he is for a myocardial infarction. New studies have demonstrated that lowering serum cholesterol is beneficial in preventing heart attacks. For estimating this risk factor, a baseline cholesterol is considered useful by most practitioners today.

Tonometry

In view of the fact that over 2% of the American population over age 40 are at risk for glaucoma, that glaucoma is responsible for thousands of cases of blindness, and that it is a readily treatable condition, ocular tonometry fits the criteria stated earlier of an easy-to-do, cost-effective routine test. This yearly test should be recommended for all persons over the age of 35.

Electrocardiogram

Because of the very high incidence of coronary artery occlusion among American men, it seems prudent to have a baseline cardiogram on all men over the age of 35, and all postmenopausal women. While women seem to be protected before menopause, that protection may not exist if she is a diabetic or a smoker. Therefore, all diabetic women over 35 probably should also have a baseline tracing.

OFFICE LABORATORY PROCEDURES

Examination of urine for glucose, acetone, and proteinuria has been possible for years using reagent tablets or dipsticks. New developments in laboratory technology have now produced complex analytic systems that are simple to operate, relatively reliable, and inexpensive. These systems allow the practitioner to perform test analysis in an office laboratory and can provide timely information useful for diagnostic and clinical management decisions. Systems are available for urine and blood cell analysis, determination of the sedimentation rate, coagulation testing, biochemical analysis, bacteriologic and virologic testing, analysis for fecal occult blood, allergy profiles, and others.

The advantage in providing immediate analysis is clear, not just for the clinician but for the patient as well. The outpatient does not have to make a special trip to the laboratory and the specimen does not get lost or delayed if it has been collected by the practitioner.

Part Five

THE LIFE CYCLE

chapter 23

Prenatal Assessment

Health History

Physical Examination

Laboratory Tests

Potential Nursing Diagnoses

In this text we have presented a general guide for collection of information relating to history and physical examination that can be applied in almost all situations. There are occasions, however, when, to guarantee the thoroughness of the data base appropriate to that situation, additional information will be required. During pregnancy, for example, it becomes important to know not only about the health history of the mother and her family, but to include information about the father, as well. We know that certain genetic conditions transmitted from the father or his family may place the fetus in a high-risk category.

Specific signs and symptoms accompany the physiologic changes occurring in the mother's body as a result of the pregnancy. However, signs and symptoms that may indicate real or potential problems must be recognized early and reported appropriately so that proper therapeutic measures may be instituted rapidly. It is well-accepted knowledge that the sharp drop in maternal and infant mortality occurring in the twentieth century is directly related to the quality of prenatal care received.

In attempting to provide, in this text, a guide for prenatal assessment and yet avoid redundancy, we have preferred to include only that information that would serve as a supplement to the general guide. During the interview it is most important that the woman's response to the reality of the pregnancy and its implications be evaluated. Many women need time and guidance to help work through their feelings about pregnancy. It is important to stress that the emotional response of each pregnant woman to her pregnancy is unique. Many personal and interpersonal factors influence acceptance or rejection of the reality of pregnancy. Feelings of helplessness, fear of nonsupport from spouse, partner or family, and/or anxiety related to economic implications may lead to self-concept disturbance, ineffective coping, and potential for alteration in parenting.

The ability to elicit and identify emotional problems relating to impending motherhood is a special skill worthy of development in those who deal with expectant parents. Therefore, the guidelines presented earlier for development of a mutually beneficial relationship should be remembered during the initial encounter for prenatal evaluation and for subsequent continuing visits. The practitioner must demonstrate the ability to be concerned, supportive, and nonjudgmental, even in the most unusual situations. This will undoubtedly affect the woman's willingness to continue and cooperate with the health supervision so vital to the well-being of the mother and the fetus.

HEALTH HISTORY

The health history should be as complete as one collected for any other patient, with attention given to factors that place the mother and fetus at risk.

Chief Complaint. In most cases this will be simply, "My period is 3 weeks late — I think I'm pregnant," or "I used a home pregnancy test, and it was positive."

History of Present Illness. An introductory statement identifying the age, marital status, gravida, and parity is usually preliminary to specific information, which includes the date of the *first day of the last menstrual period* (LMP) and presumptive symptoms of pregnancy experienced by the patient such as nausea and vomiting, fatigue, constipation, tingling of breasts, and increasing urinary frequency. Bleeding and cramping since the last normal menstrual period are noted. Include any statements that pertain to how the patient and her partner feel about the possibility of pregnancy, planned or unplanned, and whether due to contraceptive failure.

Past History

Medical Conditions. Include questions about diabetes, hypertension, rheumatic fever, tuberculosis, urinary diseases, venereal disease, phlebitis, pulmonary embolus, epilepsy, as well as specific infections or environmental hazards that may have a bearing upon the health status of the mother and/or fetus. A history of hematologic disorders as well as any known allergies should be included. If anemia is present, question the patient to determine if the type has genetic implications.

Surgical Procedures. Include those operations that may affect or involve the reproductive system. Information gathered should include a summary of the events of hospitalization, types of intervention required, anesthesia, and any related problems or complications. Include information about back problems or surgery that might interfere with regional anesthesia. Information about whether the patient has ever been examined vaginally is important to note.

Immunizations. An up-to-date record of immunizations should be noted, especially immunization to rubella.

Medications and Drugs. Include all over-the-counter drugs, including aspirin and decongestants, and physician prescribed medications. Women with a history of drug addiction should be carefully evaluated. The use of infertility drugs for contraception and the date of discontinuation of oral contraceptives must be noted. List allergies to medications and specific reactions to them. Be alert to herbs and teas used by some members of certain cultures.

Previous Pregnancies. A record of previous pregnancies, including significant history about the mother, father, and baby, is necessary.

Obstetrical History for Each Previous Pregnancy

Age at time of delivery

Date of delivery

Where delivered, e.g., hospital (name), home, birthing center

Weeks of gestation

Weight gain during pregnancy

Antepartal complications, e.g., toxemia, bleeding, premature labor

Length of labor; type of delivery — forceps, spontaneous, or cesarean

Presentation, e.g., vertex, breech

Anesthesia, analgesia, or oxytocic drugs administered

Premature rupture of membranes

Episiotomy, bleeding, infection, or blood transfusions

Puerperal problems, e.g., infection, bleeding thrombophlebitis

RhoGAM administered

Significant health problems

Genetic conditions or anomalies in family

Abortions, spontaneous or induced

Breast or bottle feeding

Paternal History for Each Previous Pregnancy

Blood type

Significant health problems

Genetic conditions or anomalies in his family

Infant History for Each Previous Pregnancy

Sex

Birthweight, large or small for gestational age, dead or alive

Weeks of gestation

General condition at birth, congenital anomalies or neonatal complications, e.g., jaundice, respiratory

Apgar score (if information available)

Multiple births

Present status, living and well, emotional and physical development

Current History

Review of Systems

The usual review of systems should be obtained with special attention to the following areas.

Breasts. Changes, such as tingling and fullness, color of areola; increase in size of areola, nipple, and breast, and secretion from nipples, should be noted. Self-examination of the breasts should be done monthly.

Reproductive System. Include age at menarche, regularity of cycle, number of days and amount of flow, clots, intermenstrual bleeding, dysmenorrhea, premenstrual problems, frequency of coitus and postcoital pain or bleeding, methods of contraception used, douching, history of infertility, date and findings of last Pap smear, and information about vaginal discharge, such as odor, consistency, associated pain, and itching. Determine trimester of pregnancy by EDC (estimated date of confinement), presence of Braxton-Hicks contractions, quickening, or lightening.

Family History

The family history should be as complete as that mentioned in Chapter 5, but certainly should include the history of any genetic conditions or congenital anomalies, as well as multiple births. Extended family relationships and locations are important to ascertain.

Activities of Daily Living

Occupation of the patient and responsibilities in the areas of child care and household management should be evaluated. Recreation, hobbies, personal hygiene, elimination, clothing, and personal habits, such as smoking and drinking, all should be included.

Diet History

Because the quality of life for the unborn child is closely related to prenatal nutrition, it is essential to assess the patient's diet carefully. Methods employed should include a 24-hour recall, a common foods and food categories checklist, and questions about food purchasing (who does, what bought, and for how many). The responses then can be cross-matched. The nutrients that need specific calculation and instruction are calories, protein, iron, folic acid, calcium, and vitamin C. There must be adequate calories as well as protein to assure a positive nitrogen balance so that protein will be used for tissue growth and not energy requirements.

Patients at *high risk nutritionally* may need higher than the normally recommended 300 additional calories and 30 additional grams of protein per day. High-risk conditions include adolescence, underweight at time of conception (greater than 5%); undernutrition, defined as a deficit in daily protein intake as assessed by the methods described, and nutritional stress. Nutritional stress is defined as the existence of one or more of the following: uncontrolled vomiting, pregnancy spacing less than 1 year, poor obstetrical outcomes in the history, failure to gain 10 lb by 20-weeks gestation, and serious emotional problems or upsets.

Fads, cravings, and cultural food preferences also should be identified. Pica, the ingestion of nonnutritive substances such as laundry starch, clay, ice, or plaster, frequently occur during pregnancy. Fast-foods, common in the diets of teenagers and many Americans, must be assessed carefully to identify deficiencies.

Cultural practices must be assessed; for example, a practice common to the Hispanic culture is that of the hot and cold theory of disease. An example in foods is the avoidance of cold foods (also called acid or drying foods) such as fruits and leafy vegetables during menstrual flows, including 40 days postpartum. The yin and yang in the Chinese tradition relates to food taboos during pregnancy including a number of foods high in vitamin C content, as well as certain meats and fish. A lactose deficiency present in many adult blacks and Orientals will affect the established practice of prescribing milk and milk products for these pregnant patients. Vegetarian diets vary in what nutrients are included and the basis for adherence may be religious or cultural.

The major task for the clinician is to establish the woman's nutritional status as early as possible during pregnancy, consulting with a dietitian or nutritionist when necessary since there are many special problems and rapidly changing concepts of the diet in pregnancy. Modern recommendations, for example, are for a weight gain of 25–30 lbs, or more, during pregnancy. Sodium-rich foods such as cheeses, meats, fish and milk should not be avoided, but salt should be cautiously added to food during cooking and at the table. Diuretics should be avoided. The emphasis during pregnancy nowadays is not so much on weight reduction, even in obese patients, but is on *what* and *when* the pregnant woman should eat, rather than what she should *not* eat. These standards are different from those given only a few years ago.

Personal-Social History

Gather data about adequacy of housing, ability to maintain a family unit, financial need in regard to prenatal care and hospitalization; assess ability of parenting, race/ethnicity, religion, education, as factors that will influence the relationship between patient and practitioner.

Psychologic History

This assessment must be made based on the particular trimester of pregnancy. There is a wide variety of behavior among individual patients, but common to most are shifts in mood, an openness to sharing feelings, fears of the unknown about self and infant, feelings of dependence, and demanding behaviors. During each trimester the relationship with the baby's father should be assessed. In the *first trimester,* note whether acceptance of the pregnancy has become a reality. Is there ambivalence, disappointment, rejection, anxiety, depression, unhappiness, concern over weight gain, or need for loving without sex? *Second trimester* assessment should include comments on whether there is a radiant affect, quickening, reevaluation of the relationship between the patient and her own mother, a need for attention and love, socializing with other pregnant mothers or caring of other's newborns. Is the focus of concern the pregnancy and childbearing preparation? During the *third trimester,* is there an impatience for the baby's arrival; are names chosen; classes attended; equipment and clothing bought; nursery prepared; fears for own life, baby's life, abnormalities, labor and delivery, recognizing labor and prematurity? What is content of dreams? Has grief work begun in anticipation of separation of fetus from her body, sometimes recognized by depression and introversion? Does she feel awkward, ugly, sloppy, uninterested in sex due to size of abdomen?

Patient Profile

The same guidelines mentioned earlier in the text should be followed with exploration of the meaning of this pregnancy to the parents and evaluation of risk factors.

PHYSICAL EXAMINATION

The physical examination, in addition to identifying the existence of any medical problems, will serve to reinforce the history in establishing the existence of pregnancy. It should include a general examination as outlined in this text with special attention given in later months to palpation and auscultation of the abdomen for size and position of the fetus. Vaginal examination will provide additional data to support the diagnosis, as well as the capacity of the birth canal. At this time, estimation of pelvic measurements may also be accomplished.

It may be of value for the student to review the normal changes that occur as a result of pregnancy and those which the examiner can expect to identify during the examination.

Physical Measurements

Measurements should include: temperature, pulse, respiration, blood pressure, height, and weight.

General Inspection and Skin

In general, the woman who is relatively healthy, well-developed, and well-nourished will not be adversely affected by pregnancy. Occasionally, there will be a loss of weight and dehydration early in the first trimester due to nausea and vomiting. If nausea becomes severe and persists, it may represent a serious problem that requires consultation for specific diagnostic treatment.

During pregnancy there is a general heightening of skin pigmentation so that the following become classic signs: chloasma (mask of pregnancy) (see Figure 26.1), linea nigra (darkening of vertical line from umbilicus to symphysis pubis), and striae gravidarum (silvery or reddish streaks on the abdomen and thighs due to stretching of tissue). In addition, there is an increased tendency to spider angiomas, which are not especially significant during pregnancy. Exposure to the sun may increase freckling during this period. Most of the signs disappear soon after delivery.

Head and Neck

It is most important to recognize that a generalized headache and blurred vision in the pregnant woman may be a sign of hypertension. These signs accompany a rise in both systolic and diastolic pressures. Edema of the face and eyelids should also be noted. Ask about contact lenses, which sometimes do not fit correctly due to eye contour changes.

Palpation of the thyroid gland, which occasionally may become enlarged during this period, should be carefully conducted in several positions.

Eye examination should include fundoscopy to detect retinal aberrations. The nose, throat, and teeth should be checked. Otoscopy should be performed and the anterior cervical, posterior cervical, and supra clavicular nodes should be palpated.

The Breast

The breast becomes generally enlarged during pregnancy but should still remain symmetrical in development. Tingling and tenderness similar to that experienced premenstrually is an early sign of pregnancy. The primary areola about the nipple becomes elevated, edematous, and pigmented during the second month of pregnancy. It becomes soft and velvety to the touch and elevated above the level of the surrounding skin. Colostrum may be expressed from the nipple by the end of the third month, while the nipples themselves become larger and more sensitive. The secondary areola appears at the fifth month of pregnancy and is characterized by a series of washed-out spots surrounding the primary areola due to the presence of nonpigmented sebaceous follicles. This sign is of diagnostic value in the woman who has never been pregnant.

Heart and Lungs

Pregnancy may impose a risk for a woman who has a history of rheumatic heart disease. The naturally occurring increase in circulating blood volume places an increased burden on an already damaged heart. As the fetus grows, the pressure on the diaphragm with subsequent limitation of the ability of the lungs to expand may create an additional problem of dyspnea and orthopnea.

The existence of hypertension prior to or occurring during pregnancy also creates problems for the expectant woman; a rising blood pressure in the second half of the pregnancy should be considered a possible sign of impending hypertensive disorder (toxemia). The finding of blood pressure above 135/85 (140/90 is abnormal) should always be considered a danger signal and medical consultation should be sought.

The Abdomen

Enlargementof the abdomen is apparent after the third month when the uterus rises by its increased growth out of the true pelvis. This enlargement is steady and progressive until the last month of gestation. Early in pregnancy it is more

pronounced in multigravidas than in primigravidas because
the abdominal walls may have lost part of their tonicity and
may be flaccid so that they afford little support to the uterus,
which then sags forward and downward. The fundal height is
approximately at the pubis by the third month, the umbilicus
by the sixth month, and the lower part of the sternum by 8.5
months. During the last two weeks of gestation in primiparas
the fetus usually starts descending. This descent, known as
lightening, leads to easier breathing and to more frequent
voiding due to the shift of the uterus away from the diaphragm
and toward the bladder. Multigravidas may not experience
this until the onset of labor. Explore with the patient any
scars on the abdomen; often new information not elicited in
the review of systems will come to light.

The linea nigra, which may be observed from the end
of the second month, although marked in brunettes, may be
absent in blondes. The pigmentation may remain after the
pregnancy has terminated. In brunettes, a dark circle appears about the umbilicus, and pigmented patches are ob-
servable over other parts of the abdomen. The umbilicus
itself should be observed for signs of hernia.

The abdominal signs of pregnancy on palpation are progressive increases in the size of the pregnant uterus. The
fundus at the end of the third month is palpated in the plane
of the pelvic brim, but is felt higher as each month passes.
The pregnant uterus presents certain definite characteristics
in shape. After the first two months, the uterus is egg-shaped,
smooth, symmetrical, and soft. The fetal parts are detectable as early as the fifth month.

By placing the hand on the fundus, the examiner may
detect painless intermittent uterine contractions as early as
the fourth month. These contractions, known as the Braxton-
Hicks sign, occur periodically throughout pregnancy, thereby
preparing the uterus for labor.

Fetal movements first detected by the patient, known
as *quickening,* occur between 16 and 20 weeks. Fetal movements detected by an experienced examiner may be considered a positive indication of pregnancy. They may be elicited
by suddenly placing the hand upon the woman's abdomen, but
are seldom elicited before the fifth month. During the fourth
and fifth months the fetus is small in relation to the amount
of amniotic fluid present, and a sudden tap on the uterus
makes the fetus rise and rebound to its original position and

tap the finger of the examiner. This is referred to as *ballot-tement,* which was described earlier in the chapter on examination of the abdomen.

The auscultation of fetal heart sounds is a positive indication of pregnancy. They are first heard by the eighteenth or twentieth week, using a fetoscope. With the Doppler method, they are heard between the tenth and fourteenth week, and with ultrasound the fetal heart has been seen beating at 7-weeks gestation. Varying from 120-140 beats per minute, they are double sounds, closely resembling the tick of a watch under a pillow. The rate should be compared with the maternal pulse. In the early months, the heart should be sought just over the symphysis pubis, but later it varies according to position and presentation of the fetus. In vertex presentations, fetal heart sounds are heard the loudest midway between the umbilicus and the anterosuperior spine of the ilium. In LOA and LOP positions, sounds are generally heard best in the left lower quadrant. In ROP, the heart sounds are loudest in the flank toward the anterosuperior spine. Breech presentations are heard loudest at the level of the umbilicus. Later in pregnancy, other sounds auscultated include the funic souffle, uterine or placenta souffle, and sounds due to movement of the fetus, as well as the gurgling of gas in the mother's abdomen. The *funic or fetal souffle* is a sharp, whistling sound synchronous with the fetal pulse, which is heard in about 15% of cases. It is inconsistent in appearance due to the rush of blood through the umbilical arteries when they are subject to torsion, tension, or pressure, such as when the cord is around the baby's neck. The *uterine souffle* is a soft, blowing sound, synchronous with the maternal pulse and usually is heard distinctly upon auscultation in the lower portion of the uterus, because of the passage of blood through the dilated uterine vessels. It is not only characteristic of pregnancy, but may be present in any condition where the blood supply to the internal genitalia is increased markedly, i.e., with large uterine tumors or enlarged ovaries.

Abdominal palpation for the determination of fetal position can be accomplished by four *Leopold maneuvers* once the uterus rises out of the pelvis. To perform this procedure, ask the patient to void, then position her flat on her back with her knees flexed. The examiner should make sure the hands are warm before the examination to avoid contraction of the patient's abdominal muscles. In the first maneuver, the practitioner faces the patient and places both hands flat on the upper abdomen to ascertain which part of the fetus is at the fundus of the uterus. Generally, the mass felt will be either the head or the buttocks. The practitioner determines which part of the fetus is felt by the consistency, shape, and mobility of the mass. The head is harder than the buttocks; the head is round and hard and the transverse groove of the neck may be felt, whereas the breech has no groove and feels more angular. The head moves independently of the trunk while the buttocks move with the trunk. Malpresentation prior to 36-weeks gestation is no cause for concern, as there is room in the uterus for frequent changes of position.

The second maneuver attempts to locate the back of the fetus in relation to the right and left sides of the woman. Facing the patient, the practitioner places the palmar surfaces of both hands on either side of the abdomen with deep but gentle pressure. The hand on the right side of the abdomen remains fixed to steady the uterus while the left fingers are used to slowly palpate the fetal outline. To palpate the opposite side, the functions of the right and left hand are reversed. During the procedure the examiner will note that on one side of the abdomen the back is felt as a fairly firm, straight plane, while the other side has numerous nodulations indicating the knees, elbows, and small parts of the fetus.

In the third maneuver, the practitioner attempts to find the head at the pelvic inlet and determine its mobility. Using one hand, the examiner gently grasps the lower portion of the abdomen above the symphysis pubis, using a thumb and fingers. If the presenting part is not engaged, a movable mass will be felt.

The fourth maneuver determines if the fetal head is flexed, confirms the location of the back, and aids in the determination of how far the head has descended. It is performed by facing toward the feet of the patient and using the fingers of both hands to palpate the lower abdomen around the Poupart ligament.

Pelvic Signs

There are changes in the appearance and character of the vagina and uterus that occur quite early in pregnancy and assist in the diagnosis. The purple color of the cervix and vagina, referred to as the *Chadwick sign,* is due to the marked congestion of pregnancy. This sign may be observed in the cervix from the first month after conception, but since it may remain in the vagina from previous pregnancies, it is not a specific diagnostic factor except in primigravidas.

Goodel's sign is a softening of the cervix. This sign can usually be determined in the primipara by vaginal examination as early as the sixth week. It begins at the lower border of the cervix and feels like a thin, velvety layer covering a firm body. As gestation progresses, the softening extends upward from below until it involves the entire cervix by the end of the eighth month. It is described as giving a sensation to the finger similar to that produced by palpating the lip.

In addition, there are changes in the shape, size, and consistency of the uterus itself. These changes, detected by bimanual examination at about the second month of gestation, are enlargement of the body of the uterus and change in shape to one which is irregular and globular and feels soft and elastic. *Hegar's sign,* in which the examiner can feel the softening of the lower uterine segment, appears at approximately the second month of gestation.

Internal ballottement of passive fetal movement is accomplished by placing two fingers in the vagina against the anterior uterine wall above the cervix, while the other hand steadies the fundus. With the two fingers, toss the fetus upward in the amniotic sac; feel it fall back against the fingers. This ballottement indicates the presence of movable solid content and is usually detectable during the fifth and sixth months.

Pelvic examination should be done routinely during the bimanual at the first visit; but because the pelvic examination may be anxiety-producing for many women, pelvic measurement assessment (clinical pelvimetry) may be delayed until 36-weeks gestation when ligament softening renders the examination less uncomfortable. This delay also allows the patient to come to feel more comfortable with and trusting in the clinician-patient relationship.

X-ray pelvimetry is used less often, but is delayed until labor to protect the growing fetus from the possibility of teratogenic effects. In some cases, a long protracted labor may be the first evidence of cephalopelvic disproportion (CPD), leading to the decision to perform a cesarean delivery.

Since the ability of the pregnant woman to deliver her infant vaginally with minimal difficulty is affected by the capacity of her pelvis, it may be necessary to carry out an additional component of the examination measurement. Estimation of pelvic measurements to determine the existence and extent of pelvic contraction before the onset of labor requires special techniques we believe are not germane to the objectives of this text. The student is, therefore, referred to obstetric texts for specific descriptions of the techniques employed.

Examination of the Lower Extremities

Important information regarding the cardiovascular system may be learned. Significant varicosities can be an indication of future problems, thus health teaching regarding elastic stockings should be planned early. Edema should also be assessed, with suggestions for decreasing it by use of the left lateral recumbent position at least once a day.

LABORATORY TESTS

Pregnancy tests that are based on the detection of human chorionic gonadotropin (HCG) secreted into maternal urine and serum are the tests of choice. These include the following: immunologic tests, which are accurate one to two weeks after a missed menstrual period; the radioimmunoassay test, which is accurate six days from conception; and home pregnancy tests, which are accurate two weeks or more after a missed menstrual period.

Laboratory work usually done at the first prenatal visit includes hemoglobin and hematocrit, urinalysis for protein, glucose, and microscopic examination, pap smear, RPR for syphilis, blood type, Rh factor, indirect Coombs if Rh negative, rubella titer, sickle cell prep and Tay-Sachs test for patients at risk, and tuberculin test (unless previously positive). At each subsequent visit the urine test for glucose and protein is repeated. Hematocrit and RPR are repeated at 34- or 36-weeks gestation. The Coombs test on Rh-negative patients is checked at least four times at appropriated intervals, and other tests are ordered as indicated by other findings.

Consideration is now given to administering Rho Gam (Rho immune globulin) to any woman who is Rh negative, or Coombs negative, at 28-weeks gestation to 72 hours following delivery, since Rh sensitization is possible during pregnancy. RhoGAM should also be administered after abortions, ectopic pregnancies, and during amniocentesis, as well as after term and premature delivery.

Carbohydrate metabolism is affected by the changes of pregnancy. Levels of fasting blood sugar are lower and the secretion of insulin is increased. Subclinical diabetes mellitus may be detected during the prenatal assessment.

Antenatal Tests for Fetal Maturity

When the fetus is suspected of being at risk, any or all of the following measures may be incorporated into the physical assessment. Amniocentesis with amniotic fluid analysis is the most accurate determinant of gestational age. Identifiable changes indicating fetal maturity are:

1. The presence of phosphatidylglycerol (PG) and phosphatidylinositol (PI)
2. Lecithin/sphingomyelin (L/S) ratio of 1:2 or greater
3. Creatinine levels reaching 2 mg/100 ml
4. The absence of bilirubin in the amniotic fluid
5. Fat cells totaling 20% of cells examined

Risks and discomforts involved in amniocentesis make ultrasonography a much safer and more practical procedure. Ultrasound poses no known risks to mother or fetus and is highly accurate in determining gestational age. With the use of ultrasonic (high-frequency) sound waves, echo signals are produced as the sound waves rebound off the fetus. As these echo signals are displayed on a screen, the size of the head and fetal and placental positions can be determined. A biparietal measurement of 9 cm, or more, usually indicates fetal maturity. A series of sonograms, usually beginning at 20-weeks gestation, establishes the growth of the biparietal diameter and is a more accurate diagnostic tool than a single measurement.

Other tests of fetal maturity include the urinary estriol test. Estriol is produced by the placenta and is excreted primarily in the maternal urine in increasing amounts to 12 mg/24 hr or greater as pregnancy progresses. A 24-hour urine collection is essential for the accuracy of this test. Plasm estriols are equally valid and the ease of collection is a factor that must be considered. The oxytocin challenge test (OCT), or stress test, also can be useful in determining fetal status before delivery. Uterine contractions and fetal heart rate are monitored during the administration of dilute oxytocic drugs. During this simulation of labor, the fetal heart rate is studied and the ability of the fetus to withstand labor is evaluated. A nonstress test (NST) evaluates the fetal heart rate in relation to fetal movement. The use of oxytocin is thus avoided. If the test is nonreactive, an oxytocin challenge test probably will be the next step in assessment.

Roentgenologic studies during pregnancy have essentially been replaced by these antenatal tests for fetal maturity. Respiratory distress syndrome (RDS) can now be avoided following cesarean section due to more accurate determination of lung maturity with the L/S ratio before scheduling the surgery. Determining gestational age is also useful in the presence of maternal disease when timing of a termination of pregnancy is crucial to mother and fetus.

POTENTIAL NURSING DIAGNOSES

Coping, ineffective individual due to unanticipated pregnancy

Parenting, potential alteration in: due to lack of support from partner

Self-concept, disturbance in: due to feelings of helplessness

Impaired adjustment

chapter 24

Assessment of the Newborn

History: Risk Factors

Examination

Potential Nursing Diagnoses

The earlier chapters in this assessment guide have focused almost exclusively on the adult patient. Most of the information previously presented is transferable to the evaluation of the infant and child. However, the idea that the neonate and the child are but small adults is an erroneous concept. It is important to recognize that physiologic, anatomic, and developmental considerations make physical examination somewhat different. Some variations in examining techniques, in approach to the patient, and in interpretations of findings are necessary. Birth events, patterns of growth, and the accomplishments of developmental milestones are assessed in the health status of infants and children. This chapter deals with examination of the newborn and the methods used to assess and maintain wellness. Chapter 25 expands the assessment to include the infant and child. It is important to assess all the functional health patterns in the newborn as well as across the life cycle.

When examining the newborn, you are primarily concerned with congenital deformities and metabolic disturbances. During the developing years, attention will be given to signs of infection, nutritional-metabolic patterns, malignancy, and degenerative conditions, as well as impairment of physiologic functioning as a result of trauma. Throughout the

developing period, the clinician will be evaluating nonphysi-
cal accomplishments: thought processes, family coping, and
development of self-concepts. All of these develop concur-
rently, and continuously interact and influence each other.
There are specific techniques to use, specific observations
to make, and specific questions to ask. The examiner must
know what he is looking for. Serendipity is not an asset in
the examination.

   We would like to point out that when you are examining
the infant or the child, you are also dealing with the mother, or
perhaps both parents. Careful explanation of each aspect of
the examination and findings to the parents who are standing
by is a wise course to follow. It serves to reassure them of
competence and thoroughness in your procedures, affords an
opportunity for questions to be answered, and helps to establish a relationship that may be extremely valuable if referral
or consultation for identified problems becomes necessary.
Every new parent is primarily concerned with the question,
"Is my child normal?" and when illness is evident, "What is
the problem?"

HISTORY: RISK FACTORS

   Before examination of the newborn, it is important to
review the health history of the parents and siblings in terms
of known alterations in health patterns with hereditary characteristics that may influence the infant, such as diabetes
and sickle cell anemia. The existence of genetically transmitted anomalies in the family also will give cues to observations that must be made. Does the mother smoke, use alcohol,
drugs, or appear malnourished? In addition, it is important
to obtain information about the pregnancy and delivery. Was
there exposure to infections, such as German measles, or
teratogenic agents, such as x-ray or drugs, early in the pregnancy? What were the results of Rh typing and serology?
Was there an elevation of the mother's blood pressure, indicating preeclampsia or bleeding due to placenta previa with
possible fetal anoxia? Was there premature rupture of membranes, foul smelling fluid, or stained membranes? Was there
use of analgesics and anesthetics throughout a long and difficult labor? Were forceps required or cesarean section performed because of cephalopelvic disproportion? Any of these risk

factors might indicate potential problems with the infant and emphasize the necessity for close observation in the neo-natal period. It is also a time when verbal and nonverbal cues to alterations or potential alterations in parenting are revealed.

EXAMINATION

The neonate is examined several times: immediately after birth, in the nursery, and once again before hospital discharge. This is usually when the effects of maternal anal-gesia and anesthesia have passed and some adjustment to the new environment has occurred. The neonate is observed con-stantly by hospital staff while quiet, active, and while feeding.

General

Cry, color, posture, size, heart rate, respirations, body proportions, nutritional status, and movements of the head and extremities are evaluated.

The Apgar score at one minute and then at five minutes will give the examiner a beginning clue to the infant's general status (Table 24.1).

Obvious malformation, such as anencephaly, missing limbs, and omphalocele, will be recorded here, and then described in detail under the system involved. The weight and length of the infant, as well as the head circumference, should be noted and then compared against norms in order to be useful.

The newborn's temperature is taken first by rectum to determine rectal patency, but may be taken later by axilla or groin. It is not unusual to find a temperature of 34.5–36°C (94–97°F). Normal skin temperature range is 36.2°C (97.1–98.6°F). Lower readings may occur as a result of birth trauma or a low environmental temperature. Elevated temperatures may mean dehydration after the third day, brain damage, or infection.

Table 24.1 Apgar Score[a]

	Score		
Criterion	2	1	0
Heart rate	100–140	100	0
Breathing and cry	Immediate and strong	Slow and weak	Apnea
Reflex irritability	Good	Fair	No response
		OR	
	Cough, sneeze or cry to bulb suctioning	Slight grimace to suctioning	No response
Muscle tone	Well flexed	Some flexation	Flaccid
Color	Pink	Body pink, extremities blue	Blue/pale

[a]A score of 8–10 is excellent, 4–7 guarded, and 0–3 critical.

Behavioral and Gestational Age Assessment

The low-birth-weight infant is one who weighs under 2500 g, and who may be preterm and/or small for gestational age (SGA). Preterm infants are those of less than 38 weeks of gestational age; full-term is between 38 and 42 weeks; post-term gestational age is more than 42 weeks. However, infants may be small, average, or large in size for their gestational age. Small-for-dates or SGA may be caused by intrauterine malnutrition, congenital infection, or chromosomal abnormalities.

Assessment of gestational age provides data related to true prematurity. Prematurity is now based strictly upon the amount of time the infant has spent in the womb, not by birth weight. The behavior and needs of the small for gestational age baby are different from the true premature. A scoring system for gestational age in the newborn infant based on ten neurologic and eleven "external" criteria has been developed by Dubowitz et al. (see Appendix VI), and validated to differentiate the short gestation from the small for date infant. A number of clinical parameters have been used, i.e., neurologic signs such as postures and primitive reflexes, and a series of superficial or external characteristics, e.g., edema, skin texture, color, opacity, lanugo, and plantar creases. The higher the score, the greater the gestational age.

The Brazelton Neonatal Behavioral Assessment Scale is a well-established tool developed to evaluate the behavioral capacity of newborns. This evaluation requires skill in techniques learned through a special training program and through much experience with newborns. Assessment includes evaluation of six major areas of behavior: habituation, orientation, motor maturity variation, self-quieting ability, and social behavior. Significant information related to the newborn's individual responses to his environment may be learned.

A variety of tools has been developed to assess the maternal-infant interaction. The practitioner working with mothers and newborns should review the criteria identified with regard for cultural variations to formalize the assessment process and identify potential alterations in parenting early.

Guides for perinatal assessment of the newborn have been developed to identify risk factors by maternal components and neonatal components. One example can be found in Appendix V Maternal-Child Health Care Index.

Most examiners find it helpful to proceed as in the adult, with the physical evaluation from head to toe, in order to establish a systematic approach and ensure a thorough assessment. However, with infants, it may be a wise decision to auscultate the heart and the lungs first, for once the baby begins to cry as a result of turning and lifting, listening with the stethoscope becomes more difficult.

Body Systems

Skin

The skin of the newborn should be observed as in the adult for color, hydration, texture, hemorrhages, tumors, and other alterations in skin integrity.

Cyanosis, frequently present on the hands and feet, is referred to as *acrocyanosis,* and is due to sluggish capillary blood flow and cool surface temperature, but may be quite normal during the first 4 hours or even throughout the neonatal period. It will most likely diminish gradually, first from the hands and then from the feet, but if cyanosis remains beyond that time, a pathologic cause may exist. *Circumoral cyanosis* in the neonate is definitely a danger signal. Since cyanosis is also influenced by the infant's crying, this phenomenon should be specifically recorded, if present.

In evaluation of pallor in the newborn, accompanying cardiac signs must be identified. For example, bradycardia usually accompanies the pallor of anoxia, while tachycardia usually accompanies anemia.

Although an erythematous flush over the body may be normal for 24 hours, a prolonged beefy red color over the entire body may indicate significant polycythemia, or possible hypoglycemia. Vasomotor responses to temperature changes leading to mottling or marmoration, especially over the trunk and extremities, are not unusual. The *harlequin sign,* when half the body is red and the other half pale, is usually temporary and not pathologic.

Jaundice is usually a normal physiologic finding after 48 hours of age, but its occurrence before this time is most often pathologic. It should be carefully looked for in the skin, sclera, mucous membrane, and nail beds of the newborn. For the most part, jaundice appearing within the first 48 hours may signify hemolytic disease or infection, while jaundice that appears afterwards would more likely be physiologic in nature. Persistent jaundice may be due to breast feeding or possibly biliary obstruction.

Scratches, petechiae, and ecchymosis as a result of birth trauma are not unusual, particularly when forceps have been used; however, since they may also be indicative of infection or hemorrhagic diseases, they must be noted. A blue to blue-black flat lesion that may resemble an ecchymosis is called a *mongolian spot.* It can occur anywhere, but usually appears over the back or buttocks and is of no clinical significance (Figure 24.1).

Telangiectases are quite common on the base of the neck, base of the nose, and the center of the forehead, as well as on the eyelids, where they are known as nevi flammeus. Pigmented nevi and hemangiomas are birthmarks found any time during the first year of life, but the disfiguring permanent port-wine stain shows itself at birth.

Although local edema may be seen temporarily on the presenting part as well as on the genitalia of both sexes, generalized edema is characteristically seen in premature infants, infants of diabetic mothers, and infants with severe Rh incompatibility. Lymphedema of hands and feet may be a presenting sign of Turner's syndrome.

Additional normal characteristics of the newborn's skin include desquamation and milia, which are pinpoint white spots not surrounded by erythema, usually over the bridge of the nose, chin, or cheeks, and erythema toxicum, a pink papular rash appearing on the trunk and face 24-48 hours after birth.

Head

Examination of the skull of the neonate is different because there are open sutures and anterior and posterior fontanelles. The fontanelles must be evaluated for their size and tension. The anterior fontanelle measures 4-6 cm in its largest diameter at birth and normally closes between 5-18 months (Figure 24.2). The posterior fontanelle is 1-2 cm at birth and usually closes by 2 months (Figure 24.3). Pulsations reflect the peripheral pulse. Bulging fontanelles are an indication of increased intracranial pressure, most commonly caused by hydrocephalus, meningitis, or intracranial hemorrhage. Depressed fontanelles are most commonly seen in dehydration and inanition. It will be necessary to measure the head circumference to have a base from which to observe skull growth which, in turn, indicates the development of the brain. At birth, the normal range of head circumference is 32-37.5 cm for boys and 32-36 cm for girls (Figure 24.4). We expect to find that the head circumference is 0.5 or more greater than the chest or abdomen. Tables are available indicating the norms for head circumference at various ages. (See Appendix VIII.)

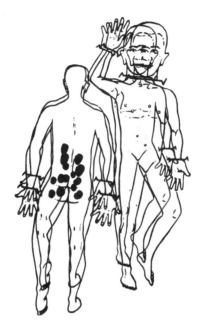

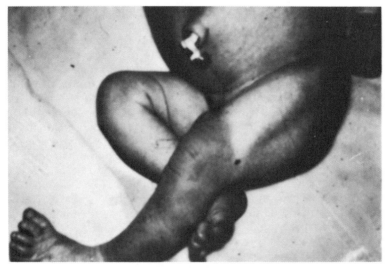

Figure 24.1 Mongolian spot.

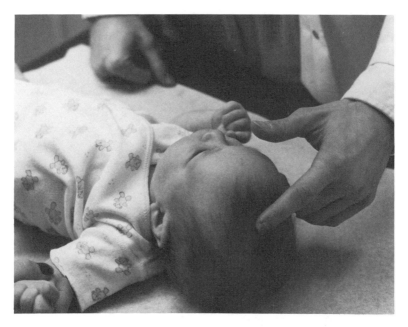

Figure 24.2 Anterior fontanelle.

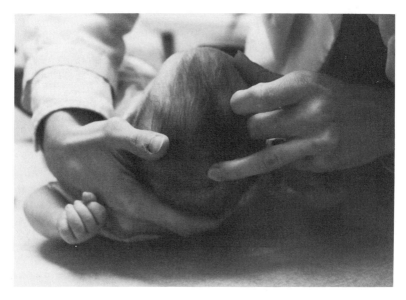

Figure 24.3 Posterior fontanelle.

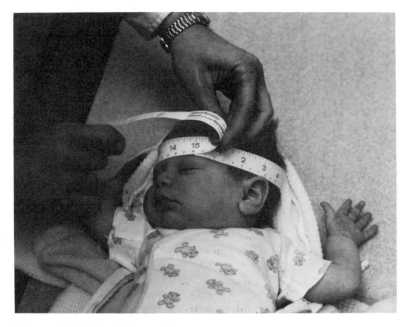

Figure 24.4 Head circumference.

It is not unusual to observe asymmetry of the head because of intrauterine molding, or to find masses such as
cephalohematomas or caput succedaneum. *Cephalohematoma*
is a soft and fluctuant, well-defined mass confined within
the edges of the bone margin, not crossing the suture lines.
Caput succedaneum is characterized by a soft, but ill-defined
enlargement crossing suture lines, not fluctuant, and pitting
on pressure. Although representing birth trauma, neither of
these is cause for alarm in the absence of neurologic signs.
    Palpation of the newborn's head for craniotabes can
best be accomplished by pressing the scalp firmly just behind
and above the ears in the temporoparietal or parieto-occipital
area. A crackling sound (crepitation) represents a softening
of the outer table of the skull found in premature infants,
some normal infants under six months of age, and a variety
of conditions such as hydrocephalus, syphilis, and osteogene-
sis imperfecta (Figure 24.5).

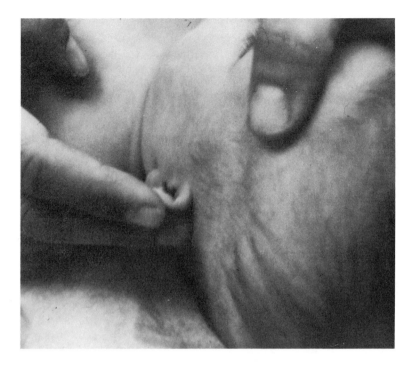

Figure 24.5 Palpation of the head for craniotabes.

Look at hair whorls, as they are a sign of underlying brain growth. Is there a parietal hair whorl (crown)? Two or more whorls may indicate that brain growth was interrupted.

Face

In general, the face is inspected for symmetry and paralysis. The distribution of facial hair is noted, especially in the premature baby. A small-sized chin referred to as *micrognathia* has importance because the infant can experience breathing difficulties due to the tongue falling backward and obstructing the nasopharynx.

Ears

The height or positioning of the ears in the neonatal skull is important to evaluate because there is a strong association between low-set ears and renal malformation or other chromosomal aberrations such as Down's syndrome. Be careful, as you examine the newborn's ears, to visualize the tympanic membrane. The largest speculum possible for the size of the canal should be used, but not passed deeply into it (Figure 24.6). Pull the pinna downward in infants. The light reflex may be diffuse and not cone shaped. If he fails to respond within a few days of birth with an eyelid twitch or a complete Moro reflex to the snapping of fingers or a loud noise, sensory perceptual alterations such as deafness may be identified in the neonate. (The reflex is described in the chapter on neurologic examination.) Note helix formation, preauricular skin tags and/or pits with ears.

Eyes

The eyes of the neonate should be examined for structure and function; however, since only peripheral vision is present during the first few weeks, eye movements normally are uncoordinated. Since the newborn's eyes usually are held tightly closed at rest, lift him upright and turn him slowly to observe sclera, pupils, and extraocular movements. Discharges may be evident soon after birth, primarily due to chemical irritation at first, ophthalmia neonatorum (gonorrhea) within the first week, and chlamydial infection later. This latter organism also is responsible for causing protracted afebrile pneumonias in the first months of life.

An upsweep of the eyes, represented by a lateral upward slope with an inner epicanthal fold, may suggest chromosomal abnormality. Also note downslants and hypertelorism — wide spacing of the eyes. This can be determined by measuring the inner and outer canthal distances and comparing with known normals.

The newborn's eyes frequently demonstrate a searching nystagmus and intermittent strabismus, but these conditions should disappear. Ptosis of the eyelids is always a cause for concern. Drooping eyelids reduce the amount of light the retina receives and stunts its development. The assessment of vision is based on the presence of visual reflexes, direct and consensual pupillary constriction in response to light,

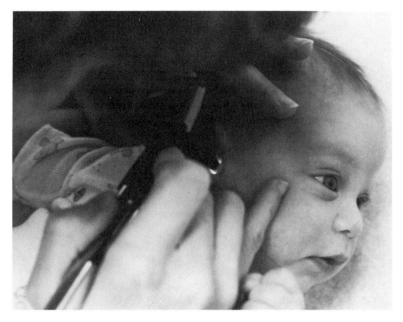

Figure 24.6 Examination of the ear.

blinking in response to bright light and an object quickly moved toward the eyes, as well as nystagmus produced by rapid movement of vertical black lines across the visual fields.

Conjunctival or scleral hemorrhages are commonly found in the newborn and are rarely significant.

Although absence of the pupillary reflex is not uncommon during the first three weeks of life, unilateral constrictions or dilation or continued absence of the reflex may represent pathology. It may be difficult to examine the fundus of the newborn because a strong orbicularis muscle keeps the eyelid closed and retraction is almost impossible. Examination will be facilitated in a slightly darkened room. Use of a cotton-tip applicator placed adjacent to each row of lashes or an infant lid retractor may be necessary to observe for the red reflex and fundal landmarks with the ophthalmoscope.

Nose

Patency of the nose may be tested immediately after birth with the attempt to insert a tiny suction catheter. A nonpatent nasal passageway, represented by ineffective breathing patterns, may be associated with choanal atresia. Although sneezing of mucus is common, thick bloody discharge suggests congenital syphilis. Flaring of the nostrils is a positive finding that indicates respiratory distress.

Mouth

The mouth should be inspected for cleft lip and cleft palate, as well as for the presence of tumors and cysts. The sucking, rooting, and gag reflexes should be tested. A nipple pressed to the side of the mouth should elicit a turning and sucking response by the newborn. After a day or two, absence of these reflexes may indicate brain damage. The presence of flat, white curds clinging to the mucous membranes of the newborn's mouth may represent *thrush,* a fungus infection that is a serious threat to the nutritional status of the infant because he is unable to suck without pain. Although spitting up and occasional vomiting are common in the newborn infant, persistent and projectile vomiting may indicate serious intestinal obstruction or neurologic problems.

The pharynx can best be examined while the baby cries (Figure 24.7). Avoid inserting the tongue blade, as it may create a strong reflex elevation of the tongue and block the view. A shrill or high-pitched cry may be indicative of a central nervous system disorder. There should be very little saliva. Large amounts present in the newborn may indicate tracheoesophageal fistula. Tonsillar tissue should not be present at birth.

Neck

The neck is observed by placing one hand behind the upper back and allowing the head to fall gently into extension. The finding of a mass or deviated trachea may indicate any one of a variety of problems such as torticollis, fractured clavicle, congenital goiters of the thyroid, or cystic hygromas.

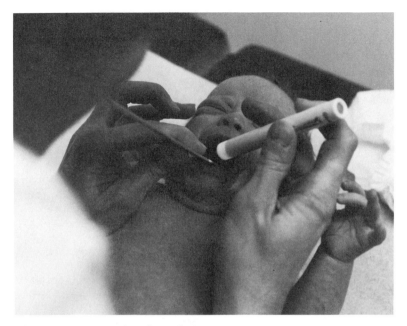

Figure 24.7 Examination of the pharynx.

The neck should be turned from side to side to elicit the normally found *tonic neck reflex*. When the head is turned in one direction, with the infant on his back, the arm and leg on that side extend while the opposite arm and leg flex. This is the *fencer position*. Absence of this reflex, which normally continues for 2-3 months, or prolonged maintenance to 4-5 months, may indicate central nervous system damage.

Chest

The chest and abdomen of the newborn should be examined as a unit for their symmetry or fullness. Asymmetry may be due to a variety of pulmonary conditions as well as the presence of a diaphragmatic hernia with the intestine lodged on one side of the chest. Unequal excursion of the chest during respiration can point to atelectasis of a lung or a spontaneous pneumothorax, as in the adult. The AP diameter is usually equal to the transverse diameter at birth.

Enlargement of the breast, usually due to maternal hormones, may be seen in both sexes. Secretion of small amounts of milk from the newborn's nipple is rarely significant unless there is redness around the nipple. When this is apparent on only one side, a breast abscess is suspected. Extra nipples may be found. Wide-set nipples may be an indication of genetic disorder, e.g., Turner's syndrome.

Lungs

Respiration in the newborn is chiefly abdominal, and from 30-60/min, irregular in rate and depth. Weak, grossly slow or very rapid rates, and grunting are clues to pathologic situations, but rales are normally heard in the newborn for the first few days. The breath sounds of the infant are bronchovesicular, relatively louder than those of the adult, and may vary according to position. Breathing is usually alternatingly shallow and slow, then rapid and deep. The sound may be diminished on the side of the chest opposite the direction in which the head is turned. Intercostal, subcostal, and suprasternal retraction indicate labored breathing found in respiratory distress syndromes. Apnea may be found for short periods in normal newborns. Apnea also may be a presenting sign for metabolic disease so ineffective breathing patterns following feedings should be carefully evaluated.

Heart

Upon palpation, the apex of the newborn's heart may be found lateral to the midclavicular line and in the third or fourth interspace because it lies more horizontally than in the adult. The heart rate is regular but varies from 100-180 at birth. It soon regulates itself at 120-140 beats per minute. The first heart sound (S_1) is usually louder than the second heart sound (S_2) in infants at the apex. In the newborn, because of changing hemodynamics during the neonatal state, murmurs may become obvious only after the first several days, so that the need for repeated examinations becomes evident. It is often difficult to identify slight murmurs in infants because of their crying during the examination, so that it may become important to use a pacifier to quiet the baby (Figure 24.8). Murmurs are usually heard at the left sternal border in the third or fourth interspace or over the base of the heart, rather than at the apex. The most significant factor related to the differentiation between innocent

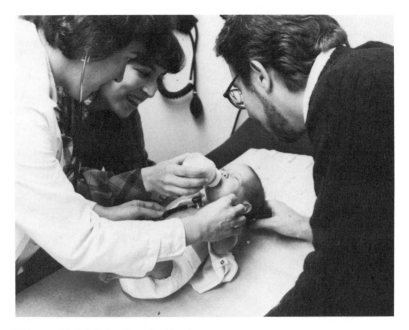

Figure 24.8 Listening to the heart.

and organic murmurs is the finding of other significant signs
of decreased cardiac output, e.g., abnormal pulses, color, and
respiration.

In the aortic area a thrill that radiates to the right side
of the neck may indicate aortic stenosis, while in the pulmonic area a thrill radiating to the left side of the neck may indicate pulmonary stenosis.

Abdomen

Examine the neonate's umbilical cord for the presence
of two umbilical arteries and one vein. A single umbilical
artery may be associated with other anomalies, especially of
the heart and kidney. In the newborn, the abdomen is pro-
tuberant because of poorly developed musculature. It should
be examined for distention, scaphoid abdomen (depression due
to dehydration or large diaphragmatic hernia), weakness or
absence of abdominal muscles, dilated veins, and visible peristaltic activity. Although the infant is an abdominal breather,

excessive excursion may indicate pulmonary disease. A common finding is *diastasis recti,* a linear protrusion noted in the midline due to underdeveloped musculature, which is more common in Down's syndrome, but may be seen in many preterm babies.

Palpation of the abdomen for masses is especially important in the newborn, but ausculatation for bowel sounds should be done before palpation because palpation may stimulate crying. Metallic tinkling every 10-30 seconds can be heard normally. Usually the spleen tip may be palpable under the left costal margin, and a liver edge can be felt 2-3 cm below the right costal margin. When examining the newborn, it is wise to begin the palpation in the lower quadrants and move upward so as not to miss these organs. Hold the legs flexed at the knees and hips with the left hand and palpate with the right (Figure 24.9).

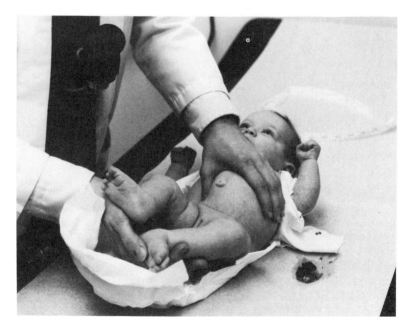

Figure 24.9 Palpation of the abdomen.

To palpate the kidneys, the infant should be raised at a 45° angle with one hand supporting the occiput and neck and flexing the knees for relaxation, while the other hand palpates for the lower half of the right and the tip of the left kidney, which normally can be felt in the newborn. Flank masses are usually of renal or adrenal origin, such as congenital hydronephrosis and Wilm's tumor.

The bladder may be percussed or palpated 1-4 cm above the symphysis or at the level of the umbilicus. A markedly distended bladder may be difficult to palpate, so percussion is also necessary. Distention may indicate congenital urethral obstruction or other impairment of urinary elimination.

Genitalia

There are a variety of malformations that may affect the genitalia. Some are chromosomal in origin, while others may be due to the ingestion of hormonal drugs during the first trimester. An unusually large clitoris is found in *pseudohermaphroditism,* but since it may be a small penis, the urethral meatus should be identified. In the male, *hypospadias,* in which the urethral meatus is not on the glans, is common. Occasionally, there is an opening in the glans, but a secondary opening on the ventral surface of the penis is also present. The foreskin should be partially retracted, allowing inspection of the urethral meatus for patency and position. The testes should be palpated in the scrotum, which may appear enlarged, especially after breech delivery. The observation that one or both of the testes have not descended is significant. Although this is usually accomplished during the eighth lunar month of fetal development, it may take several months after birth or even years to occur and may require medical or surgical intervention. Look for hydroceles and hernias, which are common findings in male infants.

In the female, a vaginal vault must be seen. The hymenal ring generally is protruding through the introitus and the labia are engorged due to the effect of maternal hormones. Fusion of the labia indicates a serious anomaly whereas simple adhesion may be due to inflammation. A slight bloody discharge may be quite normal in female infants for as long as a month and a thick white discharge also may be normally present.

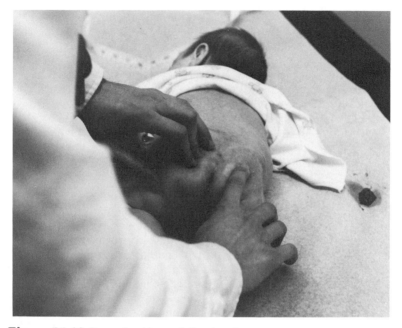

Figure 24.10 Examination of the back.

Rectal temperatures should be taken judiciously, since an imperforate anus may exist. It is imperative that consultation for rectal examination be made immediately in any suspicious case. If substantial amounts of normal meconium stool have been passed and there is no abdominal distention, there is no need to question the patency of the rectum. Small amounts of meconium may be extruded via sinus tracts connecting the blind rectal pouch to the perianal skin.

Back and Extremities

The newborn should be placed on the abdomen and the spine inspected and palpated for spina bifida, pilonidal sinus, and curvatures of the spine such as scoliosis (Figure 24.10). Tufts of hair over the spine and sacral areas may mask spina bifida occulta. The observation of symmetrical bilateral muscle movement of the hips and knees as the infant assumes intrauterine position will give clues to possible problems. The extremities of the infant are noted and fingers counted.

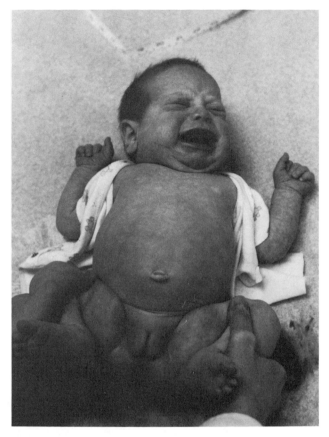

Figure 24.11 Examination for hip dislocation.

Polydactyly (extra) and syndactyly (fused fingers) are noted. Normally his elbows, hips, and knees do not extend completely. The infant's hips must be examined for dislocation by rotating the thighs with the knees flexed. Usually they may be abducted and externally rotated so that the knees touch the table top. Unilateral subluxation will result in limited abduction on the affected side. Flexion, external rotation, and abduction of his hip can reveal limitation of motion or cause a "pop" or sharp click of dislocation. Although soft clicks are common in the hips and knees, any suspicious findings such as an uneven buttock and nonsymmetrical thigh crease posteriorly should warrant referral for hip x-ray of the infant (Figures 24.11, 24.12, and 24.13).

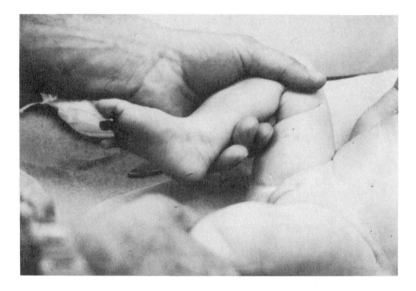

Figure 24.12 Note position and action of examiner's hand as he checks for dislocation clicks.

The feet of the newborn may appear to be deformed since they retain their intrauterine position. In examining the newborn's feet for anomalies, first scratch the outside, then the inside of the lower border of the foot, which should make his foot assume a right angle with his leg. If he has a clubfoot or metatarsus varus, it will not respond appropriately, or may possibly respond only with forceful stretching. True deformities do not allow manipulation to even the neutral position. Minor abnormalities may be evident, such as bowing of the tibia. This is generally self-correcting. Metatarsus abductus, which is a fixed angulation between the forefoot and the hindfoot, generally requires orthopedic care. Signs

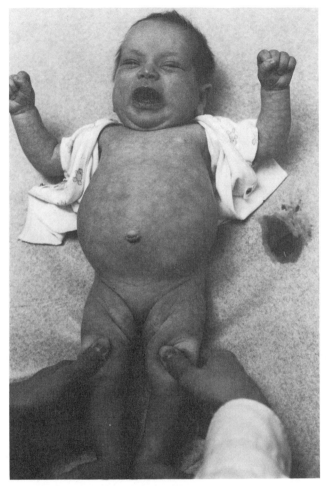

Figure 24.13 Thigh creases.

of congenital anomalies and chromosomal defects such as Down's syndrome include hyperextension of the phalanges and wrists, short, spadelike hands, simian crease (continuous crease across the palm), and a divergent great toe with a deep line on the sole between the first and second toes.

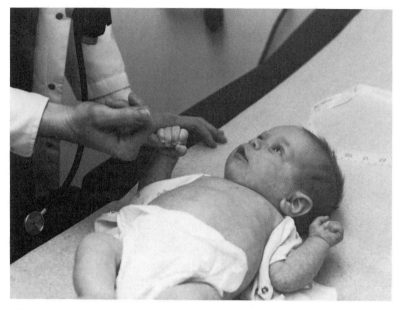

Figure 24.14 Grasp reflex.

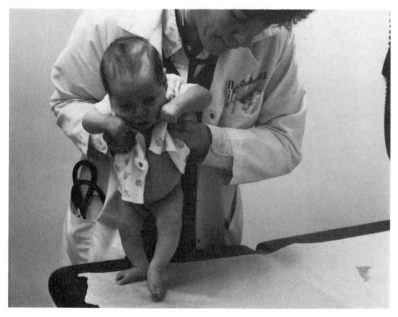

Figure 24.15 Walking reflex.

Neurologic

Throughout the examination we have been evaluating the neurologic function, much of which was included in *Behavioral and Gestational Assessment,* earlier in this chapter, observing positioning, examining muscle tone and reflex patterns, and listening to the cry. The normal lusty cry of the newborn can readily be distinguished from the weak, catlike cry referred to as cri-du-chat of a neurologic disorder. Since the nervous system is not completely developed, findings in the neonatal period will not coincide with those of the older infant or child.

A variety of responses that are present at birth, or appear shortly thereafter, including the grasp reflex (Figure 24.14), will remain for only a short time or persist for a year or two. Several of these are mentioned here. The normal, waking newborn infant will engage in reflex stepping movements if placed in an appropriate position, as shown in Figure 24.15. To elicit the Moro reflex (Figure 24.16a and b), which should be present at birth, support the infant under the sacrum and buttocks with one hand, and the occiput and back with the other while allowing the head to fall slightly back. The neonate should react by extending his arms, then flexing them with his hands clenched, and drawing his knees and hips up. This reflex should be present until about 3-5 months of age; its absence at birth or persistence after five months is indicative of severe central nervous system damage. In addition, if you observe him during his response for symmetry of movement of the arms and legs, you may observe signs of asymmetry due to fractured humerus, brachial nerve palsy, or recently fractured clavicle in the upper extremities; spinal cord injury, dislocated hip, and myelomeningocele, identified by irregular reflex of one leg, in the lower extremities. Other examples are tonic neck reflex, which also disappears after 4-5 months, as well as the sucking and rooting reflexes. The Babinski reflex is normal in the infant, but should not be present past the age of two (Figure 24.17 a and b).

Neonatal reflexes that persist for an abnormally long time may indicate a potential for cognitive impairment or impaired physical mobility.

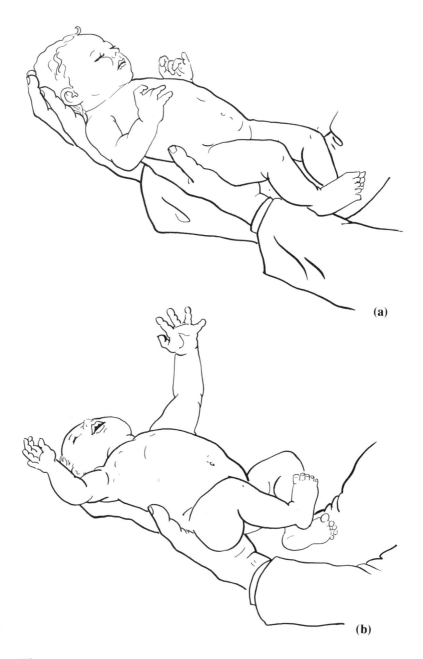

(a)

(b)

Figure 24.16 Moro reflex.

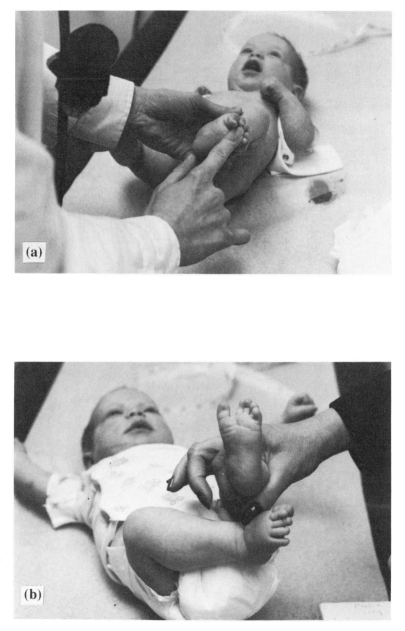

Figure 24.17 Babinski positive or present.

POTENTIAL NURSING DIAGNOSES

Parenting, alteration in: actual or potential

Sensory-perceptual alteration

Airway clearance, ineffective

Breathing pattern, ineffective

Gas exchange, impaired

Ineffective thermoregulation

Alteration in skin integrity

chapter 25

Assessment of the Infant and Child

History

Child Abuse and Sexual Abuse of Children

Approach to Examination of the Child

Examination

Development

Potential Nursing Diagnoses

Patient Problem

A regular schedule of examinations during the first year and continuing annually throughout childhood and adolescence sets a pattern for comprehensive health supervision that results in the early detection of health problems. For the most part, normal ranges of physiologic development and behavioral abilities have been well-defined and are used as a comparison for the development and behavior observed in the child being evaluated.

The *Recommendations for Preventive Health Care of Children and Youths* represents a guide for the care of well children who receive "competent parenting," who have not demonstrated any significant health problems, and who are growing and developing satisfactorily (Table 25.1). Additional visits or procedures may be recommended when there are actual or potential alterations in parenting such as:

Table 25.1 Recommendations for Preventive Health Care of Children and Youths

AGE[2]	2-4 Wks.	2-3 Mos.	4-5 Mos.	6-7 Mos.	9-10 Mos.	12-15 Mos.	16-19 Mos.	23-25 Mos.	35-37 Mos.	5-6 Yrs.	8-9 Yrs.	11-12 Yrs.	13-15 Yrs.	16-21 Yrs.
HISTORY														
Initial					At first visit									
Interval					At each visit									
MEASUREMENTS														
Height & Weight					At each visit									
Head Circumference	✓	✓	✓		✓		✓		✓					
Blood Pressure										✓	✓	✓	✓	✓
SENSORY SCREENING														
Sight[3]	✓	✓	✓		✓					OR	✓	✓	✓	✓
Hearing[4]					✓					OR				
DEVELOPMENTAL APPRAISAL[5]					At each visit									
PHYSICAL EXAM					At each visit									
PROCEDURES[6]														
Immunization		✓	✓	✓		✓	✓			✓	✓		✓	
Tuberculin Test[7]						✓				✓		✓		
Hematocrit or Hgb.						✓				OR		✓		
Urinalysis[8]										✓				✓
Urine Culture (girls only)[9]										✓				
DISCUSSION & COUNSELING[10]					At each visit									
DENTAL SCREENING[11]					At each visit									
INIT. DENTIST'S EXAM[12]									✓					

1. Applicable in context of accompanying explanatory text and footnote references.
2. If a child comes under care for the first time at any point on the Schedule, or if any items are not accomplished at the suggested age, the Schedule should be brought up-to-date at the earliest possible time.
3. *Manual on Standards of Child Health Care*, 2nd Edition. Page 8 for details.
4. Ibid. Page 9, 127-130.
5. Ibid. Page 23-32, 120-126, 132-134, 140-144. Developmental appraisal is an integral part of each visit. Employ a standardized format at any time there is suspicion of developmental delay.
6. Ibid, page 131. *Report of the Committee on Infectious Diseases*, (Red Book) 17th Edition, 1973.
7. May be indicated yearly in certain areas and population.
8. At least 5-test dipstick.
9. Taken in morning, see Kunin, C.M., *Detection, Prevention and Management of Urinary Tract Infection*, Lea & Febiger, Philadelphia, 1972, Pages 60-69, for suggested methods.
10. *Manual on Standards of Child Health Care*, 2nd Edition, Pages 13-21. Discussion and counseling of child by the physician is of increasing importance at age 11 years and thereafter.
11. Ibid., Pages 11-13. Appendix 1, I. 135. Physician should inspect teeth and check on dental hygiene throughout childhood.
12. Subsequent exams as prescribed by dentist.

Key: ✓ to be performed.

Source: Committee on Standards of Child Care, American Academy of Pediatrics: *Standards of Health Care*, ed 3. Evanston, IL, 1977.

For firstborn or adopted children, or those not with natural parents;

For parents with a particular need for education and guidance;

For children of a disadvantaged social or economic environment;

For children who present with signs or symptoms of possible abuse, or

In the presence or possibility of perinatal disorders (such as congenital defects or familial disease); and

For acquired illness or previously identified disease or problems.

HISTORY

The general guidelines for taking a thorough health history are adapted as necessary for the age of the child and the conditions surrounding the visit. Whenever possible, permit an older child to tell as much of his own story first.

It will be necessary during an initial visit to gather data significant to the child's previous health. No matter what the age of the child, no assessment can be complete if the examiner is not aware of the antenatal, natal, and neonatal history. Significant factors relating to the health of the mother during pregnancy, parents' medical problems, infections during pregnancy, vomiting, toxemia, and bleeding complications are all pertinent. The examiner should know about the birth process: gestation, birth weight, duration of labor, type of delivery, sedation and anesthesia, and state of infant at birth. In addition, significant events occurring during the neonatal period, such as jaundice, cyanosis, convulsions, and feeding difficulties, should be reviewed. The parents' perceptions of the perinatal period may reveal an alteration in parenting.

The accomplishment of developmental milestones and nutrition must be evaluated carefully, for this may uncover the earliest clues to the presence of disease or nutritional deficiency. When did he first roll over, sit alone, walk, talk, and attain bladder and bowel control? How did he compare to his siblings? What of growth events and adjustments to school? Breast or bottle feeding, type of formula, solid foods, eating habits, and allergies are relevant factors in the health history, depending upon the age of the child.

Proper nutrition is most critical during periods of rapid growth, so although serious malnutrition may be uncommon in the United States, the clinician should do a careful nutritional assessment on all children. The growth tables in Appendix VIII are useful in following growth patterns.

Pertinent elements of the dietary history are similar to those of the adult, once the child is eating solid foods. The 24-hour dietary recall is a quick method of obtaining information about the intake of foods in the four major groups: proteins, dairy foods, fruits and vegetables, and grains. Inquiry about dietary intake should always include questions about the frequency and amount of the use of candy, soft drinks, syrup, and jam.

Parents should be asked directly if they have any concern about the child's development, about his health status generally, and specifically about his hearing or other sensory-perceptual alterations. Be aware of religious-cultural patterns related to children, but recognize that beliefs and values will vary among individuals within families and groups.

A review of all immunizations received, including response, should be clearly established and recorded.

No history of the child is complete without reference to personality factors, such as relationship with siblings, other children, adjustments, and achievements in school. The child's habits should be reviewed (eating, sleeping, exercise, urinary, and bowel), and any evidence of disturbance should be clarified (e.g., excessive bedwetting, breath-holding, temper tantrums).

The relationship between parents and child can be observed throughout the interview and the examination and is of invaluable assistance in identifying potential or existing alterations in parenting that require guidance, referral, and perhaps reporting to child protective services or law enforcement agencies.

CHILD ABUSE AND SEXUAL ABUSE
OF CHILDREN

In recent years we have become more aware of the incidence of child abuse and sexual abuse of children, and even small infants, from within the family and outside the home.

Every clinician who works with children should be alert to the physical and behavioral signs of abuse and keep them in mind throughout the examination (Tables 25.2 and 25.3). Use of the problem-oriented record helps to assure that no data is lost. The health record should be carefully maintained throughout the duration of the relationship between health professional and the family and made available whenever referral or consultaton is necessary. Sample of a Child Health Data Base is included in Appendix IX.

APPROACH TO EXAMINATION
OF THE CHILD

Establishing rapport with the child is particularly important. The clinician will need to develop the skill in approach to children that is similar in objective to that cited earlier when relating to adults. Since each child is unique in his behavior and response to strangers, depending upon his age, relationship with parents and emotional health, it is often difficult to anticipate the response he will make to introductions and procedures necessary during the physical evaluation. When he is ill, it is even harder to accept interference from the stranger examining him, who may remove him from the secure arms of his parent. Talking with the parent first to allow a young child to "eyeball" the examiner before he is approached may facilitate comfort. Understanding the developmental level is absolutely necessary to communicate effectively with the child. Much of the examination may be done while the child is sitting on his parent's lap or held over the shoulders. When the child sits on the high examining table, he is approached by the examiner at eye level, which may initiate an atmosphere of mutual respect. A friendly, kind, gentle, patient examiner with a soft voice will certainly have a better chance to accomplish his mission than one who rushes and quickly resorts to force and restraint (Figure 25.1).

Every attempt should be made to develop a trusting relationship by explaining what is being done, whether or not the child is old enough to understand every word. Even if the child is not old enough to fully understand what you are explaining, the words may be soothing and reassuring, if only to his mother standing nearby. Speak in language that is appropriate, but not demeaning to the child or parent (Figure 25.2).

Table 25.2 Behavioral Indicators of Child Sexual Abuse

1. Overly compliant behavior.

2. Acting-out, aggressive behavior

3. Pseudomature behavior

4. Hints about sexual activity

5. Persistent and inappropriate sexual play with peers or toys or with themselves, or sexually aggressive behavior with others

6. Detailed and age-inappropriate understanding of sexual behavior (especially by young children)

7. Arriving early at school and leaving late with few, if any, absences

8. Poor peer relationships or inability to make friends

9. Lack of trust, particularly with significant others

10. Nonparticipation in school and social activities

11. Inability to concentrate in school

12. Sudden drop in school performance

13. Extraordinary fears of males (in cases of male perpetrator and female victim)

14. Seductive behavior with males (in cases of male perpetrator and female victim)

15. Running away from home

16. Sleep disturbances

17. Regressive behavior

18. Withdrawal

19. Clinical depression

20. Suicidal feelings

Source: Sgroi SM, Porter FS, Blick LC: *Validation of Child Sexual Abuse,* in Sgroi SM (ed). Boston, DC Heath, 1982, pp 39–79, with permission.

Table 25.3 Physical Indicators of Child Sexual Abuse

---

1. Trauma to the genital or rectal area (soft tissue injury or lacerations to the urethral, vaginal, or rectal opening

2. Pain or discomfort on urination

3. Unusual frequency of urination

4. Blood in the urine

5. Inability to pass urine

6. Pain on defecation

7. Rectal bleeding

8. Blood stains on underwear

9. Difficulty in walking or sitting still

10. Avoidance of strenuous play activities

11. Foreign body in the newborn, vagina or rectum

12. Abnormal dilatation of the urethra, vagina or rectum openings

13. Sperm in the vagina

14. Trauma to breasts, buttocks, lower abdomen, or thighs

15. Presence of sexually transmitted disease, i.e., painful blisterlike lesions of genital or rectal area (Yeast, trichomonas or mixed bacterial infections of the vagina in young children do not necessarily indicate sexual abuse)

16. Pregnancy

Source: Sgroi SM, Porter FS, Blick LC: *Validation of Child Sexual Abuse*, in Sgroi SM (ed). Boston, DC Heath, 1982, pp 39–79, with permission.

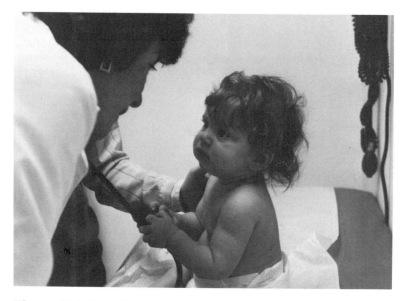

Figure 25.1 Establishing rapport (eye contact) with the child.

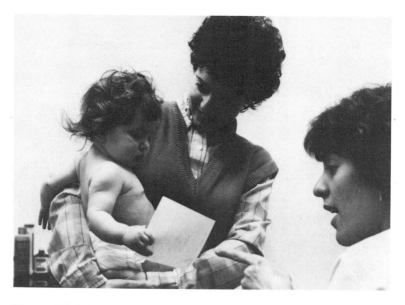

Figure 25.2 Communicating with the child.

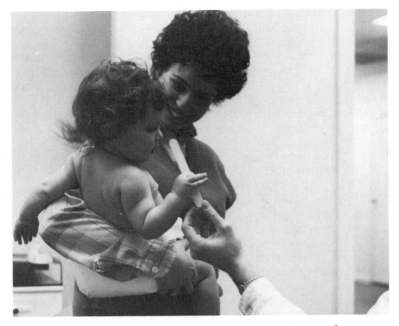

Figure 25.3 Play activities for developmental screening.

Often developmental screening involves play activities
(Figure 25.3). Doing this first with the child promotes comfort and familiarity and trust in the examiner. Assessment
procedures that require restraint or discomfort should be
integrated into the examination after confidence has been
established. Activities that restore comfort and security
should follow such procedures so as to leave the child with
positive feelings about the examination.

Although there may be differences of opinion on whether
it is appropriate or wise to give the child advance notice of
a potentially painful procedure, we find that most children,
regardless of the age, prefer to be told the truth. Do not tell
him it will not hurt if, in fact, it might.

The practitioner with imagination may dispel many of
the fears a child may have of the variety of instruments used,
by developing techniques of storytelling and games; but, of
course, the ability to use these effectively or the assurance
that the child will respond appropriately cannot be universally guaranteed. Engage the child's cooperation in helping with

the examination as is developmentally appropriate. For example, "Will you hold my hammer while I listen to your chest?"
There may be times when no amount of creativity or playing
will work, and some gentle restraint will be necessary. Some
feel that parents should not be the restrainer (if restraint is
required), but should be present in a supportive role. If the
need is explained in terms of safety and prevention of pain,
a greater degree of cooperation may be elicited and may
minimize any long-term negative effect.

EXAMINATION

The examiner should always wash his hands in warm
water before touching the child. Undress the infant slowly
to avoid drafts and chills. When appropriate, have the child
himself, or his parent, do the undressing. Never assume that
an infant is too young to roll off the table or a toddler reliable enough not to try to jump off. Watch that no sharp objects are left within the child's reach. The examination
sequence may need alteration to deal with a restless child
or prevent a painful or frightening task from stimulating
a response in the child that will make continuation difficult.
Some examiners prefer to reverse the order of adult examination and work from toes to head, while others begin with
auscultation of the chest. This is usually painless and mysti-
fying to the child and, if accompanied by an opportunity to
hear his own heart (providing the age is suitable), it can be
a fascinating experience that may make him more cooperative throughout the remainder of the procedure. In any event,
you may have a few minutes of quiet before he responds with
hysterical crying, making auscultation almost impossible.
It is wise to leave the examination of the ears, nose, and
mouth to the end, for these may more likely initiate negative
responses.

It also may be necessary to skip some minor parts of the
examination that consistently have been negative in findings
during previous examinations, in order to work quickly and not
prolong the experience; however, never fail to examine the
heart, throat, ears, lungs, and abdomen.

An attempt to thoroughly describe here the procedure
for examination of the child would result in a review of much
of what has been said during the examination of the newborn,
and what has been said during examination of the adult

throughout the text. A few simple suggestions should suffice in terms of modifications of the basic procedures to the examination of the growing child. Since it would be impossible to include in this text a complete survey of the range of normal findings during each stage of child development, the student is referred to any of the fine pediatric textbooks for further information regarding clinical data.

General Inspection

The examiner should look at the child and evaluate his general appearance. Much of this can be done while playing with the child along with the developmental testing. Does he look ill? Review general state of comfort, cooperation, nutrition, facial expression, consciousness, gait, posture, coordination, activity, and level of intelligence. What is his relationship with parents or guardians? How does he respond to the examination and the examiner?

It is appropriate to take the temperature, pulse rate, respiratory rate, blood pressure, weight, and height during each examination and compare these not only to the previous records, but to standard charts of normal values, remembering the wide variations in patterns. When there is a question regarding progress in height and weight, referral should be made to a pediatrician for evaluation. The mother can be instructed in the office how to take the infant's temperature rectally. This is then a much less frightening experience for both. A rectal temperature up to 37.8°C (100°F) is normal.

Body Systems

Skin

The skin of the infant and young child should, of course, be observed for color, texture, turgor, and lesions. Pallor in the young child may be an indication of anemia, which requires laboratory evaluation. The procedure for office hematocrit is described in Appendix XI. Taking a dietary history (see Chapter 21) will help the clinician in referring for evaluation of anemia when no cardiorespiratory causes are involved, and in outlining a plan for teaching, once therapy is indicated.

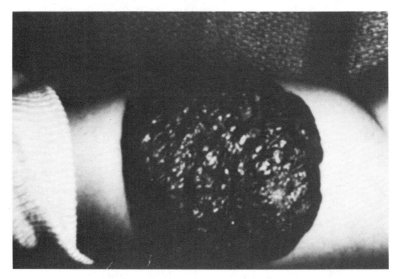

Figure 25.4 Hemangioma.

One or two patches of small, light brown nonelevated
stains (café au lait spots) are within normal range; however,
more than seven may be indicative of fibromas or neurofibro-
matoses (see Chapter 8). The presence of hemangiomas over
the forehead may indicate cerebral angiomatosis, a blood
vessel abnormality of the brain (Figure 25.4). Depigmented
small skin lesions shaped like an aspen leaf are seen as the
earliest sign of tuberous sclerosis, a congenital brain and skin
disorder causing mental retardation and seizures later in
childhood.

In children, turgor may be readily evaluated by feeling
the calf of the leg, which should feel firm. Newborns, premature, and dehydrated infants may have loose, extra skin
at the calf. Pitting edema is always a pathologic sign, usually
associated with long-term heart or kidney disease.

The most common alteration in skin integrity of infancy
is diaper rash. This may range from simple chafing, to mild
erythematous nonraised areas, to bright red, raised papules
which form ulcers when they open, and may even become
infected with organisms such as staphylococci, *Candida albicans,* or streptococci.

There are several skin lesions that occur more often in children than in adults. The practitioner should take a careful history to identify possible causes and then describe the lesions specifically. With experience, characteristic data from history and description provide diagnostic clues that aid the examiner in problem solving. For example, eczema of infancy, occasionally associated with cow's milk sensitivity, reflects itself most often by scaliness on the cheeks, behind the ears, knees, and at the elbows. Flakiness on the head, especially over the fontanelles, is an indication of seborrheic dermatitis, or cradle cap. Infectious conditions such as impetigo frequently are found in areas where children are living in close quarters, such as nursery schools or camps (Figure 25.5). The child usually demonstrates pustules filled with yellowish exudate. Impetigo is a skin infection caused by staphylococci or streptococci that may have their reservoir in the nostrils and pharynx. Scratching breaks the vesicles and infected fluid spreads the infection to other parts of the body and to other persons. It is particularly common during summer, and often occurs in children in summer camps. Prompt treatment and follow-up are of great importance since infection with streptococci can lead to serious complications, such as glomerulonephritis.

Ringworm also occurs frequently in children. It can be identified by its characteristic scaliness. Erythematous lesions may be due to systemic disease. In rheumatoid arthritis, for example, painful, tender, reddened nodules 2-4 cm in diameter along the fibula of the leg or ulnar surface of the arms are known as erythema nodosum. Erythema marginatum is demonstrated by 1-2 cm circular reddened areas with concrete borders and may be seen in children who have rheumatic fever.

The practitioner also must be aware of the significance of bruises. Ecchymoses and hematomas, especially on the extremities, are not unusual in healthy, active children. In fact, the absence of some bruises in a preschooler may be indicative of a hypoactive child. However, when there is a history of weakness, fatigue, general malaise, and spontaneous bruises over the body, blood dyscrasias such as leukemia, platelet disorders, or hemophilia should be suspected. The abused or battered child will also appear with bruises over the body, but there usually is a history of unusual events and peculiar circumstances surrounding their occurrence. The

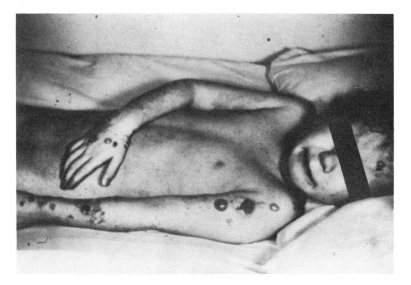

Figure 25.5 Impetigo. Note multiple lesions of various stages from flat, erythematous areas to large vesicles. This is intensely pruritic.

practitioner should be alert to these signs, especially when there are other indications of alterations in parenting.

The heads and hair of children should be examined carefully for signs of lice, mites, or ticks, especially when they live in the country or have animals who roam outdoors. Patches of unusual hair color may indicate pathology. In protein deficiency, the hair tips may have a reddish rust color. The infant with a single patch of white hair may have a condition referred to as Waardenburg's syndrome, which may have an associated condition of congenital deafness.

Head

During the first year the head is regularly measured at its greatest circumference and plotted on a growth chart scale to be compared to normal values (see Appendix VIII). Auscultation of the skull to detect a bruit is useless until the age of six, because many normal children have a bruit over the temporal area until that time. The head should be observed for control, positioning, and movements (Figure 25.6). There should be no head lag past three months. In the event

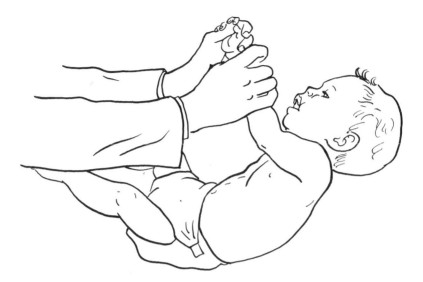

Figure 25.6 Head control.

that the infant cannot control his head after that time, developmental retardation may be suspected. If the infant sleeps on one side, flattening may occur.

Face

The face should be evaluated for symmetry, paralysis, distribution of hair, size of mandible, swellings, and tenderness over sinuses.

Ears

Examination of the ears assumes greater significance in childhood than it does in the adult because of the frequency of infections. Never fail to examine the child's ears. The otoscopic examination is viewed by the young child as particularly intrusive. With otitis it may be painful, therefore the child's reaction may seem out of proportion to any adult examiner who views ear examinations as benign. To examine the ears, gradually insert the largest speculum possible to avoid discomfort. Rest one finger against the head so that any sudden movements will not result in injury. The child can be restrained by laying him on his abdomen. Pull the auricle back and down in infants, back and up in older children. Infants can be tested for hearing and should be when there is any parental concern regarding hearing. Preschool children should have their hearing tested by the practitioner whispering simple commands at a distance of eight feet. Tuning fork of pitches from 512 cps to over 2000 cps also may be used with this age group. A complete screening test with an audiometer should be done on all children before they start first grade. Evaluation of hearing on a regular basis should not be missed, since often even minor problems may result in inability to maintain scholastic activities in school, and false diagnosis of emotional or mental disabilities may be made when, in fact, the problem is one of a sensory-perceptual alteration.

Eyes

The child's eyes should be examined as much as possible, as described in Chapter 10, and the parents questioned about any difficulty they may have noticed, such as stumbling or complaints about double vision. A mild degree of strabismus may be present during the first six months, but is abnormal after that time.

Most infants produce visible tears during the first few days of life. If an infant has tears flowing out onto the cheek when not crying, the tear duct may be blocked, leading to recurrent infections. Referral for evaluation is necessary.

In children over three years of age, a Snellen E chart can be used for testing visual acuity. Once the child knows his alphabet, a regular letter Snellen chart can be used for this testing. Visual acuity at three years is 20/40; at 4-5 years, 20/30; and at six years, 20/20. During the school years, the practitioner can distinguish between simple refractive error and organic ocular disease by asking the child to take his acuity test by looking through a pinhole in a card. When the pinhole card is used, acuity improves if refractive error is the causative factor, but does not when organic disease is present. Fundoscopic examination can be helpful in determining refractive error, since the lens used to focus on the retina corrects for patient lens abnormality. A setting of -4 to -6 D for focusing would be abnormal and warrant referral for evaluation.

Mouth

When you examine the mouth before the throat, you give the child an opportunity to become familiar with the light and tongue blade. Then have him stick out his tongue and say "Ah" louder and louder. Frequently the tongue blade in unnecessary if you have the child tip his head back and open his mouth widely.

The teeth should be examined for their sequence of eruption, number, character, and position during infancy and childhood. Most misalignment of teeth in the young nursery-school-aged child is caused by thumb sucking. If this habit disappears by the time the child is six years old, the problem of misalignment tends to disappear with secondary teeth. Children have their full complement of 20 primary teeth by 2-3 years of age. Eruption of secondary teeth begins about the time the child begins elementary school and ends in late adolescence.

Throat

The child's throat is carefully examined and the size of the tonsils evaluated. Enlarged tonsils may not be significant unless they are a focus of infection or interfere with swallowing and nutrition. The adenoids generally are not visualized unless they are extremely enlarged. Enlarged adenoids may interfere with the child's breathing and speech.

Neck

Neck mobility is an important assessment during childhood because of the possibility of central nervous system disease. Rigidity can be evaluated by placing the weight of the child's head in the examiner's hands while he is supine and flexing it. Small toddlers may be enticed into flexing the neck by holding a toy and lowering it into his lap. Resistance to movement may indicate meningitis.

In the older child, the thyroid gland may be more easily defined with palpation from behind.

Lymphatic System

It is always necessary to evaluate the status of lymph glands in the child. Lymphadenopathy is usually a sign of infection but may be present with no other specific clinical complaints.

The anatomy of the drainage system should be reviewed to locate the infection site. For example, cervical adenitis usually indicates tonsilitis and pharyngitis, while submandibular adenitis usually indicates stomatitis or dental problems.

Thorax and Lungs

The thorax should be examined as in the adult for shape and symmetry, veins, retractions, pulsations, flaring of the ribs, Harrison groove, pigeon breast, funnel shape, size and position of nipple, length of sternum, and intercostal or substernal retractions.

The thoracic wall, in infancy, is very thin, so that ribs and sternum are readily seen. At about one year of age, the ratio of transverse diameter to anteroposterior diameter is 1:1.25. It changes little after age six, when it is approximately 1:1.35, as in the normal adult.

Diaphragmatic breathing predominates in young children with a simultaneous drawing-in of the lower thorax and protrusion of the abdomen on inspiration, and the reverse on expiration. This is known as paradoxical respiration. Any unusual head movement with inspiration indicates severe respiratory disease. The percussion note heard throughout the infant's chest is normally hyperresonant. Any diminution may signify ineffective breathing patterns.

It has been mentioned earlier that breath sounds in infants and children are normally louder and more bronchial in character, with expiration more prolonged than inspiration. than in adults. The clinician should use the bell or a small diaphragm stethoscope to listen to the infant's chest. This will provide for more specific location of sounds. Breath sounds are rarely absent in the infant or child even in the presence of disease because of the small size of the thorax and subsequent ease of transmission of sounds. The small size of the bronchial tube also allows for increased occurrence of rhonchi and rales. To distinguish between these, listen with the bell at the mouth and compare with what is heard at the chest, for while rhonchi can be heard orally, rales cannot.

Cardiovascular System

As the child grows, it will become necessary to examine his blood pressure with a pediatric cuff. These come in a variety of sizes. It should cover two-thirds of the length of the arm from the elbow to the shoulder. The blood pressure is normally 90/60 at about six years of age and about 110/65 at ten, when it begins to reach the normal adult reading. Pulses should be examined, particularly the femorals, since the absence of a femoral pulse may indicate *coarctation of the aorta.* Normally, the newborn pulse of 120/min will drop to 80-90 by 7-9 years of age. In the child, because of the thin chest wall, the PMI is often visible between the fourth and fifth interspaces. It is found left of the MCL before age four, at MCL between four and six years of age, and right of the MCL after seven. The heart sounds are higher in pitch, shorter in duration. S_1 is louder than S_2 at the apex. Splitting of S_2 at the apex may produce an extra heart sound in one-fourth to one-third of all children. S_2 is louder than S_1 at the base and, although splitting here is rarely pathologic, referral may be indicated, especially when accompanied by other clinical findings.

Examine the heart with the child sitting up, lying down, and leaning to the left. Many children have sinus arrhythmias normally and premature ventricular contractions are not rare. Murmurs must be identified, and consultation should always take place when one is suspected. Many children have normal vibratory systolic murmurs. A normal physical examination otherwise suggests a functional murmur, as does the absence of a thrill. Physical signs related to alteration in cardiac output, such as inadequate weight gain, cyanosis, clubbing of fingers and toes, delayed development, tachypnea, tachycardia, heaving precordium, and edema, assist in the evaluation of significance of a murmur.

Any question or suspicion of cardiac disease requires early referral to a pediatrician or pediatric cardiologist. Final determination will require laboratory tests, chest x-rays, electrocardiograms, possibly cardiac catheterization, and other techniques. The clinician needs to assist the parents to understand why referral is indicated and to offer continued support. To encourage compliance with recommended regimens, counseling is of great assistance.

Abdomen

Protuberance of the abdomen may be seen throughout childhood when the child is standing; however, this protuberance should disappear when the child lies down. Infants often demonstrate umbilical hernias, ventral hernias, and diastasis

recti, most often after 2-3 weeks of age. These conditions
are usually noted when the infant is crying. Most disappear
within the first year. Because of the thin nature of the abdominal wall, superficial veins are often noted until puberty.
    In children, light, superficial palpation of all quadrants
should always precede deep palpation to prevent unsuspected
discomfort. The area suspected as the site for pathology or
pain should be examined last. If the child is particularly
ticklish, try placing his hand partially under the examiner's.
This should reduce sensitivity and permit relaxation. Verbal
as well as nonverbal expressions such as facial grimaces will
give clues to tenderness. Examine the spleen and liver, which
are easily palpable in most children.
    In young children, it may be difficult to localize intra-
abdominal inflammation, for tenderness and spasm are rather
diffuse. Pain in the right lower quadrant is frequently a sign
of acute appendicitis, but is not necessarily specific. With
the child supine, ask him to raise his head while you push
down on the forehead. Extend the right leg at the hip as he
lies on the left side, or flex and externally rotate the right
leg at the hip with the knee flexed at 90°. This procedure
should localize the pain in the RLQ. Examination for inguinal
hernia is conducted as for the adult.
    Most nonorganic complaints of abdominal pain are gen-
eralized and/or periumbilical and the more specific the location the more likely to be significant. Constipation is frequently a cause of abdominal pain and fecal masses may or
may not be palpable abdominally. A rectal examination will
be necessary to locate a rectal vault full of stool.

Back and Extremities

    When examining the child for scoliosis, the clinician should
evaluate the range of motion of the spine in all directions and
record impaired physical mobility. Upon forward flexion, the
rotary deformity of the thoracic spine (rib hump) and the thoracic deformity are increased.
    With scoliosis of the thoracic spine, the ribs protrude
backward on the side of the convexity of the curve, the thorax is deviated laterally in relation to the pelvis, and the
shoulder and scapula on the side of the convexity are higher.
The normal contour of the waistline is altered. It is flat on
the side of the concavity, thus the arm on the side of the convexity hangs close to the rib cage and that on the side of the
concavity hangs away from the body.

Scoliosis of the lumbar spine accounts for asymmetry of the hips. The hip on the side of the concavity of the curve is usually more prominent. The extremities should be checked for symmetry, mobility, unusual masses, infections, and joint pain. The wide range of joint motion of infancy diminishes during childhood until it reaches adult status. The foot should be examined for adduction of the forefoot, as in metatarsus adduction. If present, this should be referred to a pediatrician for evaluation.

Until about 18 months of age, there is a distinct bow-legged growth pattern. The appearance then becomes one of knocknees until about 12 years. Twisting or torsion of the tibia inwardly or outwardly is common and usually corrects itself.

When the infant begins to walk, it appears as though he is flatfooted. Actually, this is because his legs are set wide apart and weight is borne on the inside of the feet. There is a degree of pronation of the feet and curving inward of the Achilles tendons. Since the longitudinal arch in infancy is hidden by adipose tissue, the foot appears flat. Watch the toddler and child in several positions, standing upright with the feet together, stooping and standing up to pick up something from the floor, and touching the toes. Have him shift his weight from one leg to the other to observe from behind signs of hip disease. The pelvis will tilt toward a diseased hip when weight-bearing occurs on the affected side, but will stay level with weight-bearing on the good side. Unequal limb signs can indicate blood vessel abnormalities or hip disease. Diminished mobility is generally caused by trauma. Masses, such as ganglions of the tendon sheaths, and growths, such as osteochondromas, should be looked for. Joint pain can indicate trauma or neoplasms. When there is a question of possible growth disturbance, referral should be made to a pediatrician.

Neurologic

We have already discussed much of the screening neurologic examination conducted for the newborn and the infant. Examination during childhood is conducted quite similarly to that for the adult. In essence, throughout the history and physical examination, the clinician is gathering data significant for evaluation of the integrity of the central and peripheral nervous systems.

For review of all neurologic findings, as in the adult, include evaluation of cerebral function, cranial nerves, cerebellar function, motor system, sensory system, and reflexes.

Genitalia and Rectum

During the examination interview, consideration should be given to discussion of elimination habits and control. Many parents need assistance with problems that may exist or clarification of what is normal and what is not. Bedwetting is an anxiety-causing condition both for the child and the parents. It is advisable first to culture the urine to identify possible bladder or kidney infections that may be causing the problem and then explore with the parents other possible sources of stress.

Privacy and modesty should be respected during the examination, even in very young children, when it is often forgotten. The size of the penis before puberty is not significant. In obese boys the fat pad over the symphysis pubis may hide the penis. To evaluate whether the testicles of the young boy have, in fact, descended into the scrotum, have the child sit cross-legged on the table. Palpation in this position will eliminate reflexes that cause apparent undescended testicle.

Examination of the female genitalia in young girls should be accompanied by explanations of organs. The use of a hand mirror is suggested but this should be discussed with the parents and the child before initiating its use, for it may not be congruent with cultural or parental rules of behavior. The practitioner should be alert to signs of sexual abuse even in very young children, which may include extreme anxiety related to this examination, bruises or swelling of the external organs, and vaginal discharge (see Tables 25.2 and 25.3).

Rectal examination may be necessary when there is history of bleeding, pain, and severe constant constipation; however, problems of this type are best dealt with by a specialist.

DEVELOPMENT
(See Appendices VI and VII)

Although we have mentioned the need to evaluate growth and development several times in this chapter, it is recommended again that the clinician become familiar with tests such as the Denver Developmental Screening Test, a method used to evaluate development and detect developmental delays in infancy and preschool years, which is quite simple to administer. There are four categories of testing: gross motor, fine motor — adaptive, language, and personal-social development. This is not an intelligence test, but is a screening instrument for use in clinical practice to determine whether a particular child is within the normal range. If unexplained developmental delays are found, it is important to refer the child for further and more detailed diagnostic study.

We would like to emphasize that careful records of significant findings should be maintained, preferably in the problem-oriented method we have described earlier in the text. This will serve as a method of communicating the developmental changes that will occur, as well as the record of preventive and therapeutic intervention.

POTENTIAL NURSING DIAGNOSES

Weak mother-infant attachment or parent attachment

Potential alteration in parenting

Alteration in parenting

Alteration in growth and development

PATIENT PROBLEM

Liz A. is a 4-month-old, alert, well-developed girl infant brought to the Health Center by her anxious mother because she has been irritable, crying, sleeping, and eating poorly for the past week.

Problem: Fever and Irritability

S: Health record indicates infant low-forceps delivery of
      primiparous mother, age 21; pregnancy normal except
      for urinary tract infection in the fifth month; labor
      16 hr, mother received general anesthesia; Apgar score
      of infant 8; birth weight 3350 g; uneventful neonatal
      period; growth and development patterns normal;
      mother states infant has been sleeping through night,
      taking soybean formula well (eczema since 2 wk), and
      eating prepared fruits and cereals well until 1 wk ago
      when she developed cold symptoms, temp. 38.3°C
      (101°F), Rx with liquid acetaminophen, cool mist vapor-
      izer; condition improved and no respiratory problem
      persists; 2 days ago, began to cry during feeding and
      refused formula; has been difficult to feed and sleeps
      poorly, awakening for formula apparently hungry, yet
      refusing to suck more than an ounce or so; has never
      had penicillin.

O: Well-developed, weight and length appropriate to age
      and birth weight; skin flushed, temp. 38.3°C, crying
      throughout exam. *Mouth:* lower right incisor erupting;
      gums red; no lesions. *Pharynx:* mucosa reddened with
      thin film of white exudate, tonsils enlarged bilaterally.
      Ears: normal placement; right canal with discharge
      (yellowed); right TM — deep red and bulging; light re-
      flex not visible; left TM pink — increased vascular
      markings, light reflex not visible.

ASSESSMENT: Nursing Diagnosis: Potential for sensory
                    perceptual alteration, sleep-pattern
                    disturbance, nutritional deficit.
                    Acute otitis media both ears; possible
                    streptococcal infection pharynx; pain.

PLAN: Goals: Streptococcal infection ruled out,
                    fever reduced, infant eating and sleeping
                    normally.

Nursing Orders:
Diagnostic: Nose and throat culture
stat.
Therapeutic: Per protocol; Infant
Tylenol 0.8 ml qid; Erythrocin 125 mg
p. o. qid x 3 d; encourage feeding
q2h if possible.
Patient Education: Mother advised to
call center in a.m. for throat culture
report; reviewed need to increase
fluid intake and procedure for direct
administration of medications—not
in formula; review proper bottle
feeding methods.

IMPLEMENTATION: Cultures taken.

EVALUATION: Mother called office for culture report.
Fever reduced.
Infant eating and sleeping as before
illness.

chapter 26

Assessment
of the Adolescent

Approach to Evaluation

History

Physical Examination

Potential Nursing Diagnoses

Theoretically, adolescence begins when secondary sex
characteristics appear and ends when the individual completes
somatic growth, is psychologically mature, and becomes an
independent, functioning member of adult society. Essentially, we are dealing with youngsters between the ages of 12
and 18; however, in our increasingly complex society, college
and advanced training programs may extend many adolescent
issues into the mid-20s.

The clinician who relates to the adolescent must know
and understand the special emotional needs of each young
person, the developmental changes undergone, and the physiologic differences true to the age group. When assessing the
health status of the adolescent, the practitioner is not only
concerned with physical problems, but with family constitu-
tion and attitudes, culture of the reference group, and the
educational, recreational, and vocational opportunities available. General psychologic status must be evaluated in terms
of self-acceptance, sense of identity, relationship with family
and peers, and adjustment to society as a whole.

In recent years, we have seen the development of adolescent clinics or medical practices devoted almost exclusively to care of the adolescent as a professional recognition that

adolescents have unique needs that require specially skilled practitioners. The teenage years are ones when there is a great conflict in the self-image between what one would like to be and what one is. It is not unusual for a student with a 93% school average to berate himself because he thought he could get a 95% average. Meanwhile, the pressures for accomplishment, scholarship, peer acceptance, and financial advantages are all around him. At the same time, there are other adolescents who, because of their need simply to survive financially and emotionally, find themselves far away from even considering such issues. For example, the adolescent from an emotionally or economically deprived background may be concerned with "trouble, toughness, smartness, excitement, fate, and autonomy"—six concerns that may offer the adolescent self esteem.[1]

APPROACH TO EVALUATION

The clinician needs to have skill in approaching the adolescent. He must be able to demonstrate interest in him as a total person. Initially, the practitioner must seek to establish a sense of trust and mutual respect. Accomplishing this can be a complex task; but it can be developed by demonstrating honest and genuine interest in what he has experienced in the past, what he is becoming, and what he is hoping for in his life. Some young people may bring unpleasant memories of previous encounters with health care services and personnel to the present evaluation. These feelings may be so strong that the adolescent avoids seeking health care until it becomes a dire emergency. Inexperienced examiners often make the mistake of talking down to the young person as if he were a child, which negates the establishment of a positive relationship and tends to "turn him off." It is unwise to turn to a parent accompanying the adolescent to explain procedures and plans for treatment before providing explanations directly to the youngster, asking his

[1]Miller WE: Lower class culture as a generating milieu of gang delinquency, in Wender AE, Angus DL (eds): *Adolescent Contemporary Studies.* New York, Van Nostrand Reinhold, 1960, pp 189-204.

opinions, and listening to what he is saying or not saying. In fact, for most adolescents, the better situation is to interview parents and adolescents separately, beginning the process of forming a true therapist-patient relationship with the teen. The practitioner dealing with the adolescent needs to be aware of state and local laws regarding confidentiality and also must develop a relationship with the patient's parents that respects the need for this responsibility.

Every adolescent should be knowledgeable about his own health status. He is able to understand explanations about treatments, procedures, illness, and health care preventive measures. The basic problem in many situations is that he is not informed and not educated. His right to knowledge has been ignored and denied. Most adolescents are keenly interested in themselves, their bodies, and the changes occurring therein. The wise clinician will recognize these needs and make an attempt to learn about the individual as a total person, rather than focusing only on his expressed initial complaints. He will take every opportunity to provide the education he needs. Most young people are becoming more interested in their health and they are seeking knowledge about the effects of drugs and alcohol, environmental hazards, and contraceptive devices. Many are anxious to learn about natural foods and about nontraditional healing methods and can respond to much of the scientific literature provided for them. However, the poverty child has learned to block out sensory overload. If the health care worker is not sensitive to and understanding of the deprived youth, or does not attempt to communicate meaningfully, the adolescent who has grown up in poverty may block out well-meaning advice.

The adolescent often needs peers in order to relate to an adult. When someone his own age is present, interactions are more relaxed and spontaneous. Once he begins to know an adult in the presence of peers, establishing individual contact becomes more comfortable.

Adolescents of ethnic groups of color have many conflicts regarding health and illness beliefs and values. They are exposed to one culture at home and then often to another in school among peers from the dominant culture and through the media. It is especially important that the practitioner makes every attempt to learn as much as possible about the adolescent's family and culture, and to acknowledge the values to which the young person has been exposed at home.

HISTORY

Chief Complaint

Many, but not all, adolescents seeking health care have an identifiable physical problem. Some young persons may use a vague minor discomfort such as occasional headaches or gastrointestinal upsets to obtain referrals for social or psychological counseling services. The real problem may be rather serious, or not quite as complicated as the individual believes. Common *complaints* include skin problems (especially acne), muscle pain, fatigue, and menstrual irregularity. Common disturbances often actually relate to drug use or abuse, alcoholism, sexual uncertainties or stress, unanticipated pregnancy, fear of or real signs of venereal disease, depression with or without suicidal tendencies, family adjustment difficulties, need for financial assistance programs, and school-associated behavior problems. The practitioner should keep in mind that the four major causes of death during adolescence are *accidents, suicide, homicide,* and *cancer.* Therefore, the practitioner should be attuned to the issues of violence, depression, and anger which contribute to these fates, as well as preventive measures (seatbelts, motorcycle helmets, gun safety, annual physical exam) which may help to prevent these deaths. Whatever the problem expressed, it should be explored sufficiently to provide a thorough understanding of events leading up to, surrounding, and affecting the present situation. The important responsibility for the practitioner is to establish clearly the nature of the real problem and to plan with the adolescent for education, counseling, treatments, or appropriate referral based upon total needs as an individual. We cannot overemphasize this principle. If the adolescent is disappointed with the relationship established during his health care contact, he may not follow through with referral, or accept the guidance necessary to help cope with physical, social, or psychologic problems.

Evaluate the common complaint of fatigue in the adolescent completely, as for the adult. A careful history and physical examination may or may not reveal a physiologic basis for this problem. Frequently, emotional and social factors are responsible. The pubescent often feels tired and appears to require an extra amount of sleep. Unfortunately, the early adolescent also is anxious to keep up with older peers, wanting to watch late evening television when adult programs, perhaps previously restricted, are available. At the same time, the responsibilities of school work increase with a requirement for more reading and written assignments. All of this is occurring at a time when the need to join groups, social clubs, or, particularly, competitive athletic teams, is at its peak. The daily schedule for the adolescent is often a hectic one. Imagine a 14-year-old suburban boy who responds to the alarm at 5:30 a.m. to deliver the daily newspaper, arrives home in time to shower off the newsprint, grabs a breakfast granola, runs for the 7:10 a.m. school bus, joins the football practice session immediately after school, takes the late bus home in time for 7:00 p.m. dinner, spends a half hour for homework, 15 minutes of push-ups, walks the dog, and then relaxes. No wonder he is tired! The urban child may have just as many individual or group activities, although the focus may be different, to keep him or her rushing.

The complaint of *menstrual irregularity* among girls is a common one, especially during the first years of menstruation. Amenorrhea should be evaluated by an endocrinologist by the time a young woman reaches age 16. Missed periods are not unusual. Dysmenorrhea among American adolescents is a particularly disturbing situation that should never be belittled. Although this may be a time of lessened fertility for a few, the teenager must be aware that pregnancy can occur. Unfortunately, the fear that a missed period is not a normal physiologic process, but rather a result of conception, is a particularly shattering one. The emotional support needed and counsel required on the part of the concerned clinician cannot be overemphasized.

Past Medical History

Prior to the physical examination, review past health history with the adolescent and, if possible, separately with the parents. Whenever possible, time should be provided for

interaction with the young patient alone. There may be significant information he will be unwilling to relate in the
presence of family, such as use of oral contraceptives or
sexual activity. Guidelines to the history in the previous
chapter for infant and child, as well as for the adult, should be
followed during the initial visit. A review of status of physiologic and sexual development is necessary. There may be
concern about delayed or precocious puberty, which requires
evaluation and referral. History of frequent accidents and
injury may indicate emotional problems and crying out for
help. Obtain information about past problems or situations
that may influence the young person's capacities. Devote
special attention to information regarding adjustments with
family, peers of both sexes, school, or work situations.

PHYSICAL EXAMINATION

The examiner should be careful to allow the adolescent
privacy during the physical assessment. Curtains should be
drawn or the examining room door closed when the evaluation
is being done. Young people of both sexes usually want to
disrobe in a private area away from the view of the examiner.
When it is necessary for the young person to disrobe in the
examining room, the practitioner may leave the room and
return when the patient is ready for the physical examination.
Draping is done so that only the part being examined is exposed at a time. Do not be surprised, however, if the adolescent prefers not to be draped. We mentioned earlier that the
young person may be more comfortable during interaction
with adults when a peer is present. This may or may not be
the case during the physical examination. Ask the adolescent
who brings along a friend if she or he prefers to have the
friend stay. Many practitioners make the mistake of insisting
that friends leave the room. Certainly we are not thinking
of a group session in the examining room but having a friend
standing by can be a very important source of support. The
examiner who permits this may be establishing a reputation
as a specially considerate and concerned human being, and
may gain an opportunity for additional health teaching. Of
course, if the adolescent feels comfortable enough with the
friend in the waiting room, the need for privacy may be a
greater need than one for peer support, so it should be
respected.

The following assessment guide is presented to aid the practitioner in the assessment of the adolescent. Its focus is on the special adaptations of the physical examination for the young person. Included in this outline are the common health problems of the adolescent. Procedures or techniques that are the same as those for the adult patient, are for the most part, not included.

It is important to remember that the adolescent is interested in his/her body, and the time of physical examination becomes an excellent opportunity for health teaching. Self-examination may be an area of cultural conflict, however, since some cultures have rules regarding touching or exposing one's body. Be certain to assess the cultural or family background regarding self-examination.

Anticipate that the examination may take longer than that for children or even adults, but it is time well-spent. The practitioner who explains the objectives for each component of the examination may find himself with a cooperative ally who later comes for guidance at the earliest signs of a problem.

Growth and Development

During the year or two preceding puberty and throughout adolescence, rapid changes occur in the rate of growth and the physiology of the body as a result of maturation of the gonads and associated hormonal activities. Every individual grows at his own rate, and there is a wide degree of normal range for body measurements. When body measurements such as height, weight, and head and chest circumference are recorded regularly and plotted on a growth graph, comparisons can be made with the growth identified on standard charts for the general population. The rate of growth and development depends on heredity, constitutional makeup, racial and national characteristics, sex, environment (including prenatal environment), socioeconomic status of the family, nutrition, climate, illness and injury, exercise, position in family, intelligence, hormonal balance, and emotions.

Alterations in established growth patterns that cannot be attributed to physiologic changes expected in this age group require further evaluation. The causes of uneven distribution in growth patterns, e.g., height remaining constant and weight continuing in a upward direction, may indicate endocrine or metabolic disturbance, or may eventually prove insignificant.

Weight and height records vary significantly in all children. As height increases take place due to the elongation of the long bones, so weight gain should also take place. There are frequently many emotional problems associated with the differences in rate of growth. The clinician must be alert to the adolescent's feelings about her/his size and shape. In early adolescence, girls grow more rapidly than boys, but later on boys catch up and pass girls. It is not unusual for boys to reach full adult height after age 21, while rapid growth ceases in girls at the onset of menses. Yet, epiphyseal closure may occur as late as 24 years in both sexes.

Boys are frequently disturbed by either a late start, with short stature, or a rapid start, with the skeletal system growing faster than supporting muscles, which tends to cause clumsiness and poor posture. Since large muscles may grow faster than small ones, the youth often lacks coordination. In addition, the extremities, including the hands and feet, begin to grow before the rest of the body's growth accelerates, which causes more problems in coordination.

Preadolescent and adolescent girls (and boys as well) may experience a rapid increase in weight that is proportionally greater than the gain in height. The result is that obesity may occur and the individual appears stocky. Rarely is hypothyroidism, hypoadrenocorticism, or Cushing's syndrome a factor. Review of dietary habits should be made to evaluate whether the actual cause is overeating, with underlying emotional factors and/or lack of exercise. A severe body-image disturbance may be present or potentially present. Unfortunately, in our society, emphasis upon the desirability of a size 5 figure fostered by the mass media creates even more emotional problems. On the other extreme, extreme efforts to lose weight or stay thin may be manifested by anorexia nervosa and bulimia, eating disorders frequently found in the adolescent, which may actually lead to malnutrition.

Most of the symptoms of physical distress complained of by pubescents and adolescents are the manifestations of normal physiologic changes occurring in their bodies and the inner emotional turmoil surrounding the expectations of them as they approach the responsibilities of adulthood.

Boys should be prepared well in advance for the normal changes in their bodies that generally occur in sequence:

1. Increase in size of genitalia
2. Swelling of the breasts
3. Growth of pubic, axillary, and facial hair
4. Voice changes
5. Production of spermatozoa
6. Rapid growth in shoulder breadth from about age 13 on
7. Occurrence of nocturnal emissions

Girls need preparation for the various changes that will be occurring in their bodies. Changes that occur in girls in the usual order of their appearance are:

1. Increase in transverse diameter of the pelvis
2. Development of the breasts
3. Change in vaginal secretions
4. Growth of pubic and axillary hair
5. Occurrence of menstruation sometime between the appearance of pubic hair and axillary hair

Parents should be advised to prepare their children for the various changes that will occur, as well as the concepts of ovulation, fertilization, pregnancy, and birth. Young people need to know about menstruation as a normal physiologic phenomenon well before it occurs. In our society, girls are experiencing the menarche earlier than in past years. Many have already begun to menstruate by the time they reach junior high school. Some girls experience menarche as early as age 10 years. The clinician should be alert to these needs and should be concerned with facilitating appropriate discussions regarding feelings the adolescent may have about these changes. Adolescents often need an adult outside the family to relate to about problems they are experiencing, both the physiologic changes and the many emotional problems they are faced with during this age.

General Survey

Vital Signs

During the age of adolescent development, the vital signs are affected by the various physiologic changes occurring in the body. The body temperature may be slightly higher normally than in adults, with females higher than males. Temperatures up to 38.3°C taken orally are considered within normal limits. The pulse rate varies significantly depending upon conditioning through physical activity, adaptation to psychologic stress, and normal fluctuations within the age groups. For example, athletes in training have a slower heart rate than their peers. The mean pulse rate is higher in females than in males. Between the ages of 10 and 18 there is a normal drop in pulse rate and respiratory rate, which probably reflects the slowing growth rate as the individual approaches full maturity.

The blood pressure, however, gradually increases to its normal adult level. While the mean blood pressure of the normal 10-year-old is 107/57, and 119/62 at age 15, by the time he reaches 18 years of age it is 122/64. The blood pressure reading is most significant if it varies markedly from these mean scores. A significant elevation correlated with protein in the urine and edema of the face, hands, or feet, may signify glomerulonephritis. In girls, elevation associated with obesity, amenorrhea, and visual disturbances may signify pregnancy with early toxemia. Recently, through hypertension screening sessions, a rise in the detection of teenage hypertension, especially in blacks, has been identified. Early recognition and management can prevent the multiple complications associated with hypertension. A low blood pressure in the adolescent may be insignificant if there are no associated symptoms, or may reflect heredity, poor nutrition, drug or alcohol use, or alteration in cardiac output.

The practitioner should be particularly aware of the effects of drug use upon cardiopulmonary function. Careful monitoring of vital signs, along with observation for other drug-induced manifestations, will help to identify the presence of this problem in individuals.

Skin

Alterations in skin integrity in adolescents are so common that they often are considered normal manifestations of the process of growth, sexual development, and age-related psychologic stresses. Most adolescents have acne to some degree at one time or another during these years. Whiteheads and blackheads (comedones), followed by superficial and deep papules are commonly found on the forehead, chin, and cheeks, and may even extend to the back, shoulders, and chest. When pustules and cysts form, scars will result. It is imperative that referral be made when improvement does not occur as a result of initial diet and hygiene supervision, although there are differences in opinion regarding any effect of elimination diets on acne.

Melasma, a blotchy, symmetrical, nonscaly hyperpigmented macular rash usually on the forehead, cheeks, chin, and upper lip, is very common in postpubescent females, but may rarely be seen in males. It frequently occurs during pregnancy or when the patient has been taking oral contraceptives (Figure 26.1).

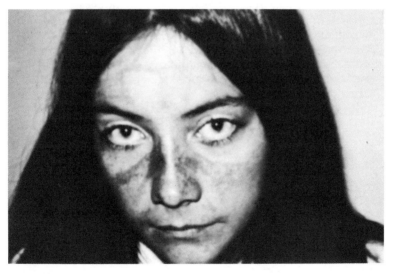

Figure 26.1 Patchy hyperpigmentation in this characteristic distribution in pregnant women or women taking oral contraceptives.

Scars, needle tracks, and bruises are important clues that require detailed historical data to make a full and accurate evaluation. The implications in terms of possible physical abuse at home, drug abuse, or hematologic disorders all are too complex to discuss fully here. Pallor in adolescents, especially girls, is not uncommon. It usually is a reflection of a low hemoglobin level and poor nutritional habits. True anemias may exist so that full assessment through referral for laboratory studies should always be done. Since hepatitis and infectious mononucleosis occur frequently in adolescents, any suspicion of jaundice must be investigated carefully as well. (The procedure for hematocrit is discussed in Appendix II.)

Head, Face, and Neck

Examination of the head, face, and neck is quite similar to that done for children during early adolescence and for adults later on. Any history of head injury should encourage careful palpation for hemorrhagic masses. The scalp and neck often are the sites of sebaceous cysts so these should be looked for. The adolescent who scratches his head often may be communicating the presence of lice or seborrhea. In the presence of fever of unknown origin with or without rash, ticks should be looked for on the scalp.

Alterations in mobility of the neck often occur in adolescent athletes. When accompanied by fever and general malaise, the possibility of meningitis should be considered and investigated.

Mouth

The adolescent in our country who has no caries is probably blessed with good heredity or is the child of a dentist who brushed his teeth for him and a mother who never gave pennies for the gum machine in the A & P. Otherwise, dental caries are a major problem in teenagers. They need frequent dental examinations and constant reminders about oral hygiene. Despite the fact that straight teeth and braces for teenagers are a sort of status symbol in our culture, underneath those braces plaque and decay may be forming. The mouth should therefore be carefully inspected.

Eyes

The adolescent requires frequent eye examinations.
Myopia tends to increase during this age and school demands
for increased reading and studying often result in sensory-
perceptual alterations. Evaluate visual acuity with glasses
and refer for complete examination if deviations from normal
are present. The wearing of glasses fluctuates as an "in" or
"out" vogue. In recent years, more and more teenagers have
been fitted for contact lenses, usually without problems.
Unfortunately, the cases of poor lens hygiene and overuse in
this group are higher than necessary. Corneal abrasion is
common. The practitioner should always refer such cases
immediately to an ophthalmologist to prevent permanent damage.

Lymph Glands

Adolescents develop clinically significant infectious
mononucleosis more often than any other age group. Any
individual with fever and generalized adenopathy should have
full studies to determine the etiology. Refer to Chapter 22,
Laboratory Examination, and Appendix XI, Office Laboratory
Procedures.

Chest and Lungs

The chest and lungs must be examined as in adults.
Respiratory infection and asthma occur frequently in this
age group. Adolescents seem more susceptible to tuberculosis. An abnormally slow respiratory rate may be the first
sign of opiate poisoning or brain tumor. The finding of a
pigeon or barrel shape of the chest may be a reason for referral for evaluation of the pulmonary system.

Nose

The teenager is especially conscious of his appearance.
Often, minor deviations are interpreted as major defects and
the self-image is destroyed. A deviated nasal septum may
not only produce ineffective breathing patterns but, in the
adolescent, when accompanied by malformation and prominence, the shape of the nose becomes a major crisis. The
interest in rhinoplasty today is so common among urban and
suburban adolescents that it is almost considered a therapeutic, not merely a cosmetic, surgical procedure. Many

surgeons and families alike report the occurrence of significant personality changes accompanying the repaired nose.
When a prominent or distorted nose presents a serious problem to the teenager, the practitioner should not hesitate to
refer the family for evaluation by a specialist. However,
teenagers should be discouraged from having rhinoplasty before their facial bones have finished growing, since distortion
may occur.

Breast

The breasts develop and mature during adolescence.
(See Figure 26.2 and Table 26.1.) Asymmetrical early development is not unusual. Some unilateral or bilateral increase
in breast tissue, with or without pain, is expected and normal
in early adolescent males. Patient's with excessive and true
tissue should be referred for evaluation. Now is the time to
begin to teach girls to examine their breasts regularly. When
adolescents are made aware of the importance of this procedure from puberty on, they will usually remember it
throughout their lifetime. In this way, early lesions may be
located and treated promptly. All other previously mentioned
guidelines should be followed when examining the breast;
however, the practitioner should be aware that young girls
may be particularly sensitive about the examination. Breast
size and shape may be related to self-esteem disturbance.

Heart

The apex beat in the adolescent usually is found at the
fifth left intercostal space at the MCL. No murmurs should
be heard. In most cases, functional murmurs will have almost disappeared by the time of young adulthood, although
in some instances they still persist. Any evidence of a previously unknown murmur with or without accompanying cardiovascular signs is a cause for referral.

Abdomen

Examine the abdomen as in the adult. It should be soft
and no pain should be expected with palpation. In the presence
of a history of pain, it is appropriate to carefully elicit rebound tenderness. Appendicitis occurs more frequently in
the adolescent period than during other developmental
stages. Because teenage girls are dieting today, one week

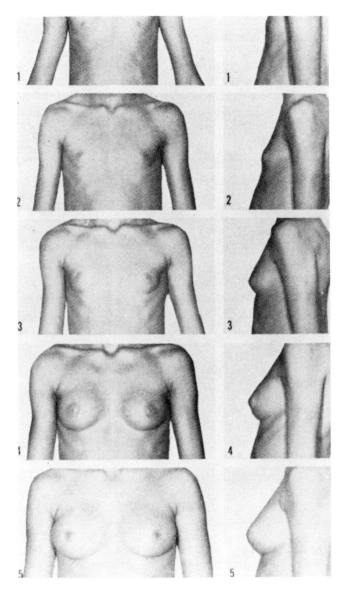

Figure 26.2 Standards for breast development ratings. (Tanner, 1973.)

Table 26.1 Classification of Sex Maturity Stages in Girls

Stage	Pubic Hair	Breasts
1	Preadolescent	Preadolescent
2	Sparse, lightly pigmented, straight, medial border of labia	Breast and papilla elevated as small mound; areolar diameter increased
3	Darker, beginning to curl, increased amount	Breast and areola enlarged, no contour separation
4	Coarse, curly, abundant but amount less than in adult	Areola and papilla form secondary mound
5	Adult feminine triangle, spread to medial surface of thighs	Mature; nipple projects areola part of general breast contour

Source: Adapted from Tanner JM: *Growth at Adolescence,* ed 2. Oxford, England, Blackwell, 1973.

on and one week off, it is not unusual to identify striae over the abdomen due to rapid weight loss or gain.

Genitalia

It is essential to evaluate the presence of the testes in the scrotum in males. Undescended testicles at this age will most often be accompanied by sterility. An estimate of genital and secondary sexual development, as with the system developed by Tanner, is helpful in monitoring developmental changes in both males and females (See Figures 26.3 and 26. 4, and Table 26.2.) (Tanner, 1973.)

While the genital examination usually is limited to examination of the external genitalia, in young girls, if there is complaint of pain, discharge, or delayed menstruation, abdominal-pelvic examination should be performed. In view of the higher incidence of cervical cancer in younger girls today, Pap smears should be done annually on all sexually

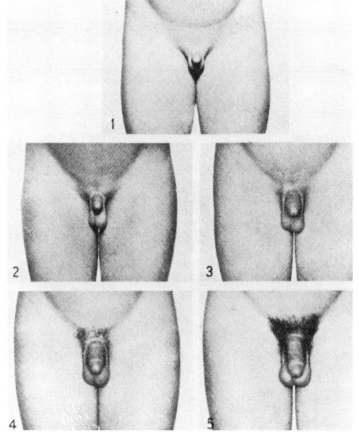

Figure 26.3 Standards for genital maturity in boys. (Tanner, 1973.)

active females. When there is a history of the mother having taken stilbesterol during pregnancy, the adolescent should be examined for vaginal cancer. A few research studies have demonstrated the presence of urinary infections in girls supposedly without subjective or objective signs. It has, therefore, been recommended that urine cultures be taken at intervals during the years 15–18. A nitrate stick culture of a clean catch specimen along with routine urinalysis may be

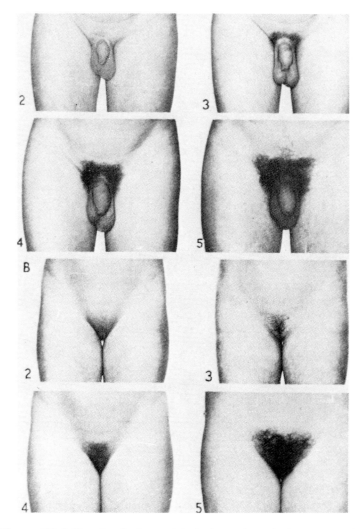

Figure 26.4 Standards for pubic hair ratings in boys and girls (see Tables 1 and 2). (Tanner, 1973.)

Table 26.2 Classification of Genitalia Maturity Stages in Boys

Stage	Pubic Hair	Penis	Testes
1	None		
2	Scanty, long slightly pigmented	Slight enlargement	Enlarged scrotum, pink, texture altered
3	Darker, starts to curl, small amount	Penis longer	Larger
4	Resembles adult type but less in quantity; coarse, curly	Larger, glans and breadth increase in size	Larger, scrotum dark
5	Adults distribution, spread to medial surface of thighs	Adult	Adult

Source: Adapted from Tanner JM: *Growth at Adolesence*, ed 2. Oxford, England, Blackwell, 1973.

sufficient. The incidence of venereal disease, especially chlamydia trachomatis has increased significantly in teenagers due to the lessened use of male prophylactics and increasing sexual activity. Every case of increased vaginal discharge with a history of sexual activity should be evaluated.

Extremities and Back

As we mentioned earlier, the growth of long bones and large muscles during the adolescent period may create uncoordination and posture defects. However, by the end of this time span, the various childhood characteristics should have given way to more mature, adult stature. Knock-knees should have been straightened out and postural slumps corrected. The feet of the adolescent, however, often show corns, calluses, and blisters. Their sizes have also changed rapidly, and they may often be wearing too small or ill-fitting shoes.

Any indication of asymmetry of the neuromuscular system requires early referral. Scoliosis, unfortunately, is common among adolescents, and during careful examination appears as alteration in symmetrical levels of shoulders or hips (refer to Chapter 16, Extremities and Back). If the teenager walks with a limp and there is no history of trauma, consider the possibility of slipped femoral epiphysis. In addition, any persistent severe pain or swelling in the long bones should also be immediately referred for evaluation in view of the possibility of osteosarcoma or Ewing tumor, which occur during this period. Muscle aches, pains, and tenderness are common in adolescents who are active sports participants. It is probably most unfortunate that our society places so much emphasis upon competitive sports in junior and senior high schools when muscle and bone growth is so significant. The Little League pitcher at age 14 may have permanent injury with a lifetime of discomfort. Parents need counseling regarding the pressures placed upon young athletes in schools, and practitioners should not hesitate to assume responsibility for offering suggestions to individual students, teachers, and school board members.

Neurologic and Mental Evaluation

The clinician working with adolescents should evaluate carefully the past developmental history of this system. This evaluation should be as thorough and complete as described in Chapter 19 for adults. Complaints of frequent headaches, loss of consciousness, seizures, episodes of muscular weakness, numbness or loss of feeling in any part of the body, as well as visual disturbances, among others, may indicate serious neurologic problems.

Adolescents may experience a sudden insidious onset of epilepsy, which is most frightening. Brain tumors may result in sudden symptoms with little previous neurologic history. There may have been vague complaints, such as headaches and fatigue, for a period of time that were considered normal for the age group.

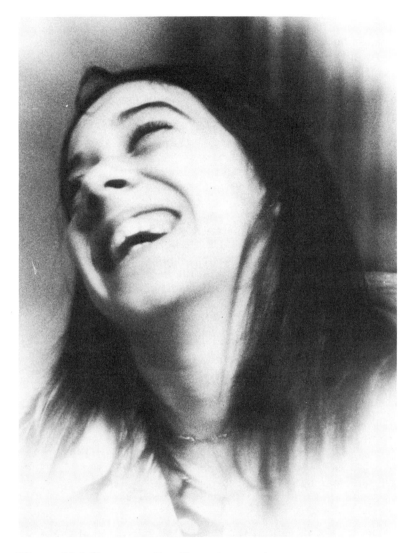

Figure 26.5 Happy, well-adjusted, outgoing young girl.

Evaluate the present mental status. The adolescent should be alert with responses appropriate to the situation, with judgment and insight into problems. Inappropriate behavior, delayed reflexes, lack of ability to think abstractly, and communicate intelligently in the presence of an otherwise unremarkable history may indicate use or abuse of alcohol or drugs. The adolescent must be encouraged to talk about how things are for him: Is he satisfied? What is his general mood or mental outlook (Figure 26.5)? The practitioner must be able to put these signs together with the possible history presented of school work deficiencies, of poor parental relationships, of anxiety about personal abilities, and make an assessment that calls for consultation and counseling. Impaired thought processes and potential for cognitive impairment exist for many adolescents. Particularly be aware of signs of "boredom" and depression, and do not be afraid to question the patient about suicidal ideation, which must always be taken seriously. Suicide has become a major problem of adolescence.

Laboratory Examination

As part of the routine physical examination, specific laboratory tests should be done. An annual urine specimen should be screened for pH, color, and the presence of sugar, protein, and acetone. Menstrual blood, heavy vaginal discharge, and strenuous exercise may result in false positives for protein, and "crash" diets may result in acetone in the urine. A CBC or a hemoglobin and hematocrit should be done routinely since anemias are common. If not screened before, the black adolescent should be screened for sickle cell disease. All sexually active adolescents should have annual serology and AIDS virus screening if at high risk.

Summary

It is obvious that the physical examination of the adolescent is much the same as for the adult. The guidelines presented throughout the text hold true for the young person with essentially the same basic principles we have been emphasizing throughout this text. Essentially, the unique problems are those of growth and development, and of adjustments to psychologic and social stresses placed by family, peers, and society. The skilled practitioner plans professional activities in collaboration with the patient to help him to meet the needs that are his alone.

POTENTIAL NURSING DIAGNOSES

Coping, ineffective individual: due to maturational crisis

Alteration in nutrition, less than body requirements: due to anorexia — emotional stress

Impaired skin integrity: due to developmental and psychogenic factors

Body image disturbance, perceived developmental imperfections

Decisional conflict regarding abortion

Potential for self-directed violence expressed to clinician

Impaired social interaction

Altered sexuality patterns

Altered growth and development

Impaired adjustment

Assessment of the Aged

Lay persons and health professionals alike are aware that the number of people in the "aged" population is increasing significantly. We also are all aware of the development of a much greater interest in the social and health problems of the elderly. It is important for the health professional, however, to recognize that this increased interest in the elderly is relatively recent in history. For example, in this country at the time of its birth, the average life span was about 35 years and the medical focus was largely on acute infectious diseases and trauma in a young agricultural society. Diseases of the elderly were present, of course, but they received only a small portion of the practitioner's attention.

Medicine made great advances in the nineteenth century that provided the basis for more treatment than was possible before. Despite this, the elderly benefited much less than did children and younger adults. Notable among these advances were the development of practical methods for vaccination against smallpox, the prevention of puerperal fever, the use of anesthesia, and the development of antiseptic techniques. Smallpox had always taken its greatest toll among children. For example, in the period before vaccination, about one-third of all children in England died of smallpox before they reached three years of age. Thus, the emphasis in vaccination was on protection of the children. Puerperal fever was a disease of younger women in their childbearing years.

Surgery was an ancient art and was extensively used in treatment of trauma, particularly for military casualties. The discovery of anesthesia and of antiseptic techniques led to an extension of surgical treatment. However, since elderly patients presented greater surgical risks, and since they had a shorter expected life span, the generally healthier and stronger young patients were the principal beneficiaries of the newer surgical procedures.

Thus, the treatment of the aged did not improve significantly. They remained in a less important category in the medical care process, since they were fewer in number and their medical problems were often more complicated and less well understood. This attitude toward the elderly is reflected in a story told by Dr. Paul Dudley White, the famous cardiologist. He pointed out that one of the case records of the Massachusetts General Hospital, about 100 years ago, listed the cause of death of a 45-year-old woman as "old age." (Dr. White died in 1973 at the age of 87.) Out of this situation grew a number of concepts, habits, practices, prejudices, and school curricula that continued to emphasize the care of the young with relative neglect of the aged.

Over the past 40-50 years, however, the situation has taken a distinct change. With better control of infectious diseases, better medications for cure or control of chronic illnesses, advances in clinical nutrition, and accelerated research into the problems of the aged, the life span of our population is now double that of 200 years ago. (On the average, a child born today can expect to live at least 75 years.) The decrease in infant and child mortality, coupled with better care for the aging person, has increased greatly the number of the elderly population. The expectations of our society now include adequate health care for all elements of our population, and this change is reflected in teaching, government support of research, and improved attitudes toward conservation of the health of the elderly.

While there are legal and social definitions of aging, there is no fixed medical criterion for this state. Aging is a highly relative condition. The professional athlete "ages" rapidly in his career and may be forced to change his occupation at 30 or 35. At the other extreme, persons may be active and highly productive for eight or nine decades in literature, the arts, and other intellectual pursuits. For example, Goethe completed *Faust* when he was 82; Titian painted his last masterpiece, *Christ Crowned with Thorns,* at 95; Verdi composed the opera Falstaff at age 87; and Stradivarius was still at work making violins just before he died at 93.

There are numerous examples from many fields similar to the above, indicating that creativity does not cease with the achievement of an arbitrary birthday. As health professionals, we must not assume that any person is senile, incompetent, or of little importance simply because of age.

Gerontologists recognize the great variability in the older population and marked differences in personal resources and needs between persons at the lower and upper ends of the "over 65 year" range. Most important for us, as clinicians, is our *attitude* in the evaluation of the elderly patient. If we feel that anyone over 65 (or any fixed age) is "on his last legs" physically and mentally simply because of his age, the examination and assessment are likely to be skimpy and, therefore, inadequate. The elderly patient requires the same courteous, competent evaluation as does his younger counterpart. In addition, he needs a sensitive examiner who will use all available personal skills and understanding in appraising the patient. A smile, a gentle manner, a slower pace in speaking, patience in eliciting the history, a steadying hand on or off the examining table — all communicate the special caring so supportive to the older patient.

THE AGING PROCESS

General

There are many anatomic and physiologic changes that can be associated with aging. What is not so clear is just which changes are related to factors such as heredity, diet, previous or present illnesses, occupation, "wear-and-tear," and environment. Current research and review of past data will assist in clarifying many features of the process we call aging.

We do know from many studies that aging is not a uniform process, in that there are great variations in aging from individual to individual. It is also known that, in any one person, aging will involve certain organs, systems, or functions and will spare others. Thus, aging does not follow a fixed schedule directly related to the length of life. With this important feature of variability in mind, one can properly consider certain general characteristics of the aging process.

Anatomical Changes

Some examples of the changes in body cells, tissues, and organs that are often seen are the following:

Reduced body weight, but with redistribution of fatty tissue

Shortened stature due to atrophy of intervertebral discs

Reduced bone mineral content (with increased fragility of bones)

Loss of tissue water, e.g., skin, muscle

Reduced number of taste buds

Impaired elasticity of the lens of the eye

Increased AP chest diameter

Loss of and atrophy of muscle fibers

Reduced arterial elasticity

Progressive arteriosclerosis

Fewer kidney glomeruli

Reduced brain weight and number of cortical cells

Reduced number of fibers in nerve trunks

Shifting of center of gravity with postural changes

As a rule, when these changes do occur, they are more distinct and severe after the age of 60.

Physiologic Changes

In the general slowing down process of aging, a number of individual organ functions become less competent. Some of the losses that may occur include:

Lowered visual acuity

Hearing loss, particularly for high frequency tones

Reduced vital capacity of the lungs

Reduced pulmonary ventilation on exertion

Lowered oxygen uptake during exercise

Reduced cardiac output

Reduced secretion of gastric acid and gastric hormones

Decreased renal function

Decreased urinary bladder capacity

Less mobile joints

Reduced strength of muscles

Reduced blood flow to the brain

Slower nerve conduction

Slower reaction time

Reduced basal metabolic rate

Lowered glucose tolerance

Less effective immune protective mechanisms

Decreased pain perception

The presence of a number of these reductions, particularly if some are severe, limits an individual's ability to respond to stresses of various types. He can no longer meet demands for extreme and prolonged physical exertion and cannot tolerate the effects of disease, injury, or emotional upheaval as well as he could several decades earlier.

In general, therefore, as a person ages, he adapts less well to changes from his basal resting state and must live within a narrower range of activities.

Mental Functions

Some general features of change in mental functions are:

Lowered scores on some types of intelligence tests (however, some scores can be raised on subsequent testing)

Fixed habits that are harder to change

Selective slower rate of learning, depending upon interests

Slowed speed of mental activity, e.g., arithmetic

Poorer memory of recent events than for distant events

Retention of memory for distant events, possibly less reliability of content

Selective attention to surroundings

Selective interest in current events

Some of these features may *not* be due to actual lack of intellectual capacity but, rather, to reduced energy level. Elderly persons may also attach less importance to some of these items than do the young.

Several studies have shown that when people remain in stimulating environments through their later years, they seem to retain mental capacity better than those whose environment is dull and uninteresting. This has important implications for prevention and treatment of reduced mental functions in elderly persons. The individual's perception of how he is viewed by others is important for retaining interest and mental functioning.

APPROACH TO THE EXAMINATION

To assess the health care needs of the geriatric patient, the clinician will not need to learn any additional methods for interviewing or physical examination. Basically, the techniques for obtaining a health history and a physical examination are no different from those described for the adult in Chapters 3 through 20. The assessment of the problems of the elderly should be as complete as that for any other person.

The examiner must be acutely aware of the fact that multiple chronic problems are more common in the aged, and that signs and symptoms of one disorder may confuse the manifestations of other problems found in the same patient. Depending on the actual anatomic, physiologic, and psychologic aspects of the individual patient, certain modifications of the examination may be in order. If the patient is fully alert mentally and in good physical condition, there will be little difference in the examination. On the other hand, for a patient who is impatient or inattentive, the history must be abbreviated at the first visit. Similarly, for a patient who seems to tire easily or to be physically weak, the physical examination may need to be curtailed or carried out in several short sessions. In either case, the clinician must be prepared to focus the examination on critical matters first and to aim toward completion at subsequent visits. Knowing how to modify either the history or physical examination is a matter of judgment that will come with knowledge and experience. There are a few guidelines, however, that may be of assistance in changing the pattern of the initial evaluation where indicated by the patient's mental and/or physical status.

First of all, the clinician must make a rapid, general assessment of the patient to judge how alert, attentive, and strong the patient is. This will give the examiner a basis for judging how much of the history and physical he may be able to accomplish at the first visit. The next chapter, on the comatose patient, presents the concept of "shifting gears" as needed. In the examination of the elderly patient, the clinician must frequently resort to such a modification of the routine pattern.

THE HEALTH HISTORY

Several suggestions may guide the interviewer in obtaining the health history:

1. Keep the questions simple, clear, and pertinent.
2. Use language that the patient can understand but do not speak "down" as though to a child.
3. Speak distinctly and directly to the patient and wait for the response. Do not shout.

4. Avoid extensive writing during the interview.
5. Pace the questioning to the ability of the patient to respond.
6. Avoid the appearance of rushing.

Chief Complaint and Present Illness

These remain the most vital portions of the history and, without question, have the first priority. Verification of information through family members or records, where available, is highly desirable. However, do not underestimate the older adult's ability to be a creditable historian.

A most important consideration is that pain perception is often reduced, as noted earlier. This reduction may be minimal or may be nearly total, particularly with visceral pain. Thus, disorders that ordinarily are associated with severe pain (e.g., obstruction of the ureter, perforation of the intestine) may possibly produce only minor symptoms.

Past History

As noted in Chapter 4, this element should consist of diagnosed illnesses that are considered medically important. For the aged patient, medical diseases and surgical procedures, likely to be of long-term significance, are to be asked about. Certainly, diabetes, hypertension, myocardial infarctions, and renal or liver disorders, for example, will be of importance. Surgical removal of organs or tumors and repair of heart valves are key subjects to explore. Of lesser consequence are illnesses or minor surgical procedures of the distant past that are unlikely to influence the patient's current status. Examples are the usual childhood diseases, old extremity fractures, removal of nonmalignant skin lesions, or single bouts of pneumonia.

Information about childhood immunizations is of little consequence. Data about tetanus boosters, and influenza and pneumococcal immunizations, however, is important information.

Drug allergies and a record of current medications are of distinct importance in the history and should not be neglected at this interview. It may be extremely useful to ask the patient to bring in all medications he is taking. Be specific when questioning that you are asking about *both* prescription and over-the-counter medications.

The past history may be reviewed in briefer format, if it is felt necessary, but the examiner should be aware of any pertinent items left out for exploration at a later date.

Review of Systems

Guidelines for a modified review are difficult to provide since the circumstances of the patient's present illness will determine the requirements for questioning. For example, if the chief complaint consists of a generalized, poorly defined problem such as fever, malaise, and weight loss, it is likely that a major diagnostic problem exists and, therefore, a nearly complete review of systems is indicated. Even here, some items relating to problems of the distant past may be eliminated, such as menstrual history (in a woman well past menopause) or pregnancies (unless complicated).

Any current or recent problems, however, must be regarded in detail no matter what the problem may be. If time presents difficulty, the ROS may be broken into two or more sessions. Since the most common medical problems among the elderly relate to pulmonary, cardiac, gastrointestinal disease, and neuropsychiatric disorders, review of these systems should take priority.

Particular attention must be paid to the patient's dietary habits, for disorders of nutrition become far more prominent in older persons. Dental problems such as loss of many teeth or illfitting dentures often interfere with eating an adequate diet. With regard to food, not only "how much" and "what" should be determined, but the patterns of obtaining and preparing foods also should be discussed.

Since complaints about improper bowel function are almost universal, special attention should be given, in the ROS, to this problem. Care must be taken to distinguish abnormalities, such as alternating diarrhea and constipation and tarry or bloody stools, from simple constipation. The patient with the latter should be assured that a bowel movement once a day is *not* necessary, and that proper diet and fluid intake are much to be preferred to constant use of laxatives.

Family History

As indicated in the description of family history in Chapter 5, questioning about first-order relatives generally will be adequate. While most of the familial disorders will have become manifest well before the sixth or seventh decade, information should be obtained for the benefit of other members of the family.

Personal and Social History

Items of particular concern to the clinician relate to the daily living pattern, the social environment, economic status, the physical environment, and self-image of the aged person. Whenever possible, information about significant others and the personal support system should be obtained.

Activities of Daily Living

Particular attention must be paid to nutritional assessment, since dietary disorders become far more prominent in older persons. Factors in the personal and social situation that may have a serious impact on nutrition include reduced income, loss of a spouse, limitation of shopping, and loss of motivation.

The 24-hour food intake recall commonly reveals inadequacies in three major dietary substances: protein, calcium, and iron. If any one of these is suspected, the assistance of a dietitian may be useful in completing the evaluation. Lack of knowledge about foods, misconceptions, dyspepsia, and limited income are factors that also may contribute to the development of malnutrition.

Complaints of inability to sleep at night often are heard from aging patients, especially when they have limited exercise or when they nap during the day. It is important for the clinician to know, however, that the *normal* sleep pattern in the elderly person consists of frequent intervals of awakening and sleeping.

Occupational exposure to dusts or toxins in the past may produce disorders such as pulmonary fibrosis or carcinoma of the lung many years later. Thus, an occupational history is required, even in the retired person, as is a history

certainly of tobacco or alcohol use even in the person who
has quit such habits.

Certainly, the present socioeconomic status of the
patient is of great importance for an adequate evaluation of
the current state. As is well known, poverty and loneliness
are potent influences on any patient's health status, and this
is particularly true of the aged. Although some older people
do not wish to discuss their problems, it is important to know
what financial and social support is available.

The physical conditions of the patient's home, including
space, utilities, stairs, etc., should be determined. In addition,
information about the patient's community and its resources
is of vital importance. Although discharge planning for hospitalized patients should begin at the time of admission,
realistic planning is seldom done unless someone interviewing
the patient upon admission is alert to questioning in this area.
Some homes and communities where the aged live, especially
where they live alone, are not able to provide for their special needs when families are unable to help. With adequate
time to plan, temporary (or permanent) alternate arrange-
ments often can be made that can provide a safer environment and reduce unnecessary hospitalizations or nursing home
stays.

It is in the areas of interpersonal functioning and environment that multiple hidden problems may directly affect
not only the mental status but the physical health and well-
being of the patient.

THE PHYSICAL EXAMINATION

The actual technique of performance of the examination is not essentially different for the aged patient than for
the younger adult. Each element of the examination remains
important for the proper evaluation of the patient; none may
be safely eliminated. Since the examination itself does not
differ from the routine described in previous chapters, the
sections below, on each region, will indicate the pertinent
earlier chapter, so that the student can refer to it readily
as he reviews this material. One may expect to find some
of the features described in the section on the Aging Process
in the examination. It is also valuable to look closely for
signs of malignancy, cardiovascular disease, arthritis, and
malnutrition — all more frequently present in the elderly.

Basic Data (Chapter 7)

As noted earlier, there is a tendency in late age for stature to shorten and for body weight to be somewhat reduced. There are no precise tables to indicate the normally expected changes. However, if the changes simply are due to aging, they should be of small degree and should occur slowly.

Blood pressure probably should *not* increase with age. It is now well known that the adage that "systolic pressure should be 100 plus the patient's age" is grossly incorrect. The standards for normal blood pressures in the aged are no different from those of the fully matured young adult. Elevated pressure usually is the result of disease — not of aging. However, lability of blood pressure seems to increase with aging and, therefore, multiple measurements should be taken before hypertension is determined to be a problem.

Integument (Chapter 8)

Since the water content, the elasticity, and the subcutaneous fat are reduced, it is to be expected that the skin will be drier, more lax, and that it will appear thinner. Therefore, the natural defenses of aging skin are less competent, and more infections may occur. Pruritis may occur, due to dryness and decrease in activity of sebaceous and sweat glands.

Many skin lesions have the same appearance as in younger patients. However, there are several that are common in the elderly, including ecchymoses, senile keratoses, and seborrheic keratoses. The latter are plaques made up of the outer (keratin) layer of skin, raised slightly above the skin surface. They are of varying size and range in color from tan to black. These seborrheic keratoses are often seen on the face and neck and are unimportant lesions unless they undergo distinct changes in size, color, or sensation.

Senile keratoses are nodular in shape, quite firm to the touch, and scaly on the surface. They occur most often on areas of the skin exposed to the sun. Since they occasionally undergo malignant change, they should be described carefully and reported.

Thickening of nails, particularly of toenails, is due to drying of the tissue and to change in circulation. If present, this is likely to be a site of fungal infection.

Head, Face, and Neck (Chapter 9)

While the examination does not differ greatly from that of the younger adult, signs arising from strokes and occlusion of the carotid arteries should be searched for carefully because of their increased incidence. The examination of all cranial nerves should be complete, and palpation plus auscultation of the carotid arteries will aid in detection of possible occlusions that may be surgically corrected.

Eyes (Chapter 10)

Diminution of pupil size may be noted on interview and examination of the older adult. As noted, a frequent change is loss of elasticity in the lens. This leads to inability to focus on near objects, referred to as farsightedness or presbyopia.

Distant vision is tested by use of the Snellen chart, but since presbyopia is almost universally present in the older patient, near vision also should be evaluated. This is simply done by having the patient read from a newspaper, magazine, or book. If the patient wears reading glasses, have him use them for this test. A person with normal near vision, or one with properly refracted reading glasses, should be able to read newsprint at a distance of 15 to 30 cm (6-12 in.). Failure to do this warrants referral for further examination.

A change associated with age is *arcus senilis* (Figure 27.1). While this does appear more often in older persons, it is not pathologic, nor is it associated specifically with arteriosclerosis, as was formerly thought.

Cataracts also are found frequently and can be identified by dark areas in the examination of the red reflex with the ophthalmoscope. In extensive cataract formation, the red reflex may be totally absent. Since cataracts are present in the lens (see Figure 10.1), they will come into sharp focus with the ophthalmoscope lens set from +15 to +10.

Any suggestion of increased firmness of the eyeball is enough to indicate referral for tonometry testing for glaucoma. Many clinicians advocate routine tonometry for all persons over 50 years of age annually.

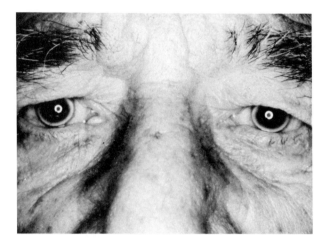

Figure 27.1 Arcus senilis. Here the rings around the limbus are complete.

Peripheral vision may also be diminished in the older adult.

Ear, Nose, Mouth, and Pharynx (Chapter 11)

Hearing loss is commonly a problem for the elderly person, particularly if it involves a loss in the normal conversational range (i.e., 80-2000 cps). Since the tuning fork tests hearing only at a single frequency, it is preferable to test the patient by the whispered voice test. Any indication of hearing difficulty is cause to refer the patient, since such loss can interfere significantly with the patient's ability to keep in good contact with his environment.

Evaluation of teeth or dentures must be careful enough to determine the patient's ability to bite or chew properly—functions that are important for his overall state of nutrition. The swallowing mechanism should be checked carefully.

Cancers of the mouth, tongue, and pharynx increase in frequency with age, so careful inspection and palpation are indicated.

Thorax and Lungs (Chapter 12)

The aging process has direct effects on the chest cage and on the process of ventilation of the lungs. The AP diameter of the thorax is increased, dorsal kyphosis often develops (see Figure 12.8), and there is a reduction in chest expansion. These changes are secondary to degeneration of the intervertebral discs, stiffening of ligaments and joints, and weakened musculature. Arthritis of the spine, a common disorder of the elderly patient, may also interfere with adequate chest expansion. These changes in the chest wall lead to the common findings of hyperresonance on percussion and reduction of the loudness of breath sounds even in healthy lungs.

Chronic bronchitis, emphysema, or chronic obstructive pulmonary disease all are frequently found in the aged, particularly in smokers and those who have been exposed to dust or fumes in their occupation.

These disorders produce somewhat different physical findings, but all have the effect of increasing the air content of the lungs and making expiration more difficult. Thus the hyperresonance and diminished breath sounds, noted earlier as a result of aging, are exaggerated. In addition, auscultation often reveals prolonged expiratory breath sounds and rhonchi in one or both phases of respiration.

Carcinoma of the lung increases in frequency up to the seventh decade of life and should be searched for diligently. Often, there are no physical findings unless a bronchus becomes partially or completely obstructed. Although signs are variable, partial obstruction often will cause a localized, unilateral wheeze (sibilant rhonchi), while complete obstruction of a bronchus leads to collapse of the lung peripheral to the obstruction. In this situation, depending upon the size and location of the collapsed (atelectatic) lung, there may be diminished expansion of the chest on the side of the lesion, an area of dullness, diminished breath sounds, and reduced voice transmission.

Breast (Chapter 13)

There is a change in the texture of the female breast arising from involution of the milk glands and ducts and increase in fatty tissue. There will be a reduction in breast size, and the ducts will become stringy and fibrous to palpation.

The examination of the breast, however, will not differ from that described, and the search for masses must be as detailed in the elderly as in the younger woman. The detection of a lump may be of greater significance in the older woman because cystic mastitis is not common after menopause. Male breasts should also be examined for any masses or nipple discharge.

Heart (Chapter 14)

The heart may be expected to be of normal size, or smaller, due to some degree of muscle atrophy secondary to the aging process. With changes in the AP diameter of the thorax and some emphysema that often occurs, percussion of the left border of cardiac dullness becomes less accurate, and the PMI frequently cannot be palpated. Displacement of the PMI may be due to kyphosis, or scoliosis or both, so that this finding should not be used as an index of cardiac enlargement under such conditions.

Heart valves become thicker and more rigid, due to fibrosis, and often do not shut completely, leading to the production of murmurs. The heart sounds themselves are not as loud, and they are sometimes difficult or nearly impossible to hear if emphysema is present.

Atrial fibrillation is much more common in the elderly, so careful attention should be paid to cardiac rate and rhythm, presence of pulse deficit, and varying intensity of S_1.

Abdomen (Chapter 15)

Physical examination of the abdomen must take into account the fact that the diaphragm is frequently low in the thorax, being flattened by aging changes or by emphysema, as noted earlier in this chapter. Because it is low, the diaphragm can move only a short distance between inspiration and expiration.

This depression of the diaphragm will push the liver downward so that it is frequently palpable in the abdomen. The student has been cautioned previously not to assume that a palpable liver is an enlarged liver, and special caution must be observed in the elderly in whom the liver is frequently palpable. Percussion of the upper border of the liver under the ribs and palpation of the lower border in the abdomen will give the clinician a measure of the span of the organ, and that span is the most reliable index of liver size on physical examination.

There are no other important differences in the physical findings on abdominal examination of the elderly. However, special attention should be given to the search for masses, since neoplasms increase in frequency with advancing age. Duodenal and gastric ulcers, diseases of the gallbladder and biliary system, hiatus hernia, and diverticulosis of the colon all are commonly present also, but more often their presence is suspected by symptoms, rather than physical signs.

Aneurysms are more frequent in the aged and should be searched for here as well as in other palpable arteries. In the abdomen, aneurysm of the aorta may be detected on physical examination if careful deep palpation is done along the midline from the epigastrium down to the inferior portion of the umbilical region.

The femoral arteries are most conveniently palpated while the patient is supine for the abdominal examination. It is recommended that auscultation of these arteries be routinely performed in the elderly patient since aneurysms or occlusion of the vessels may be present.

Extremities and the Back
(Chapter 16)

With the degeneration of intervertebral discs, the frequent presence of arthritis of the spine, and the dominance of flexor muscles over extensors, there is a change in the posture of aging patients. The head is thrust forward, kyphosis of the dorsal spine is exaggerated, the arms are carried in slight flexion, and there is some flexion of the leg on the thigh as the body's center of gravity shifts. The ideal posture of the younger person (see Figure 16.1) is infrequently maintained.

Gait may be influenced by any of the disorders noted in Table 16.1 but, in addition, poor vision, arthritis, and the characteristic flexed posture may also cause a loss of the easy, "loose-jointed" gait of the younger adult.

Loss of balance, however, is not a direct consequence of the aging process, but follows disorders of the semicircular canals, loss of proprioceptive sense, cerebellar disease, muscular weakness, or medication effect.

Lack of regular exercise, as well as the aging process, leads to reduction in muscle bulk often seen in the elderly patient. Muscle strength often is found to be fairly well preserved despite the reduction in bulk.

Decreased range of motion (ROM) of the neck, back, and extremities is to be anticipated. This limitation is due to stiffening of ligaments and joints arising from the aging process, as well as to the development of arthritis.

It is important to determine whether any limitation in ROM is primarily due to painful joints or to mechanical difficulties in motion, since the pain of arthritis is often more readily treated. A useful technique is to palpate joints for pain before testing the ROM by movement.

Osteoarthritis is found commonly in the spine and in peripheral weight-bearing joints such as hips, knees, and ankles, and also in hands and feet.

Examination of veins and arteries is carried out in the same detail as for other adults. Since peripheral arterial disease is more commonly present, it may be expected that weaker pulses will be found. Of particular importance is the determination of differences in pulse strength from one side to the other, for this may identify localized areas of partial arterial occlusion. Such findings warrant referral, for appropriate therapy may prevent the development of gangrene.

Male Genital and Rectal Examination
(Chapter 17)

While tumors of the testes are more frequently seen in young men, they are not to be overlooked in the elderly, so bimanual palpation of the scrotal contents is to be done routinely. Often the testes will be soft, small, and somewhat atrophic in older males.

The knee-chest position may be quite uncomfortable for patients with arthritis of the spine, shoulders, hips, and knees, so the less stressful lateral or lithotomy positions are preferred for the rectal examination.

Benign prostatic hypertrophy, carcinoma of the prostate, and carcinoma of the rectum, are all lesions more commonly found in the aged and should be searched for diligently.

Female Genital Examination (Chapter 18)

With loss of estrogen production, several changes in the genitalia are to be expected. The external genitalia will show a loss of vulval hair, subcutaneous fat is reduced, producing flattened labial folds, and the introitus is smaller.

In the vagina, the epithelium thins, the wall becomes less elastic, and secretions are much reduced, producing a smooth, shiny, and dry vaginal canal. The cervix becomes small, as does the entire uterus.

The position for speculum examination, most often performed with the patient in the dorsolithotomy position in stirrups, may need to be modified if arthritis is present. The simple lithotomy position or lateral Sims position will allow for a thorough examination without stressing the patient unduly. Due to the narrowing of the introitus and vagina referred to above, it is desirable to use a pediatric speculum to avoid pain or the induction of bleeding, which may follow use of the standard adult instrument.

While uterine myomas are less frequent in postmenopausal women, the incidence of uterine cancer remains high, so careful inspection and regular Pap smears are always in order.

Because the uterus is significantly smaller and more mobile in elderly women, bimanual examination is often more difficult to interpret, but the critical characteristics of size, mobility, position, consistency, and contour should all be identified and reported. Unless an ovary is enlarged due to disease, it is rarely palpable, since it should become smaller after menopause.

Neurologic and Mental Status Examination (Chapter 19)

Keeping in mind the expected changes due to the aging process, the clinician will proceed in the manner used for the adult examination. Deep tendon reflexes are likely to be hypoactive, but should not be absent. Comparison of reflexes from right and left sides is most important for proper interpretation of this examination. The plantar reflex may be absent without signifying an abnormality but, as with younger patients, dorsiflexion of the great toe and spreading of the toes is distinctly abnormal.

Since the incidence of stroke and peripheral neuropathy increases with aging, and since both may produce weakness of specific muscle groups and loss of reflexes and/or sensory perception, the examiner must accurately describe and record these abnormal neurologic findings to allow the cause to be identified.

Great care must be taken in this evaluation of the aged patient so that the events associated with the experiences of living and aging are not misinterpreted as evidence of psychologic or organic disorders.

POTENTIAL NURSING DIAGNOSES

Any one of the approved nursing diagnoses may be descriptive of the problems older adults may experience. However, the following list may represent those found more commonly:

Health maintenance alteration

Noncompliance

Potential for infection

Potential for injury

Alteration in nutrition, less than body requirements

Potential skin breakdown

Alteration in bowel elimination, constipation

Impairment of urinary elimination, incontinence

Impaired physical mobility

Hopelessness

Self-toileting deficit

Sleep-pattern disturbance

Uncompensated sensory deficit, hearing loss

Potential cognitive impairment

Impaired thought process

Powerlessness

Dysfunctional grieving

Social isolation

Spiritual distress

Part Six

SPECIAL
SITUATIONS

chapter **28**

Psychiatric Mental Health Assessment

Dynamics of the Interview

Psychiatric/Mental Health Assessment Guide

Anxiety

Depression

Summary

In the general care setting, psychosocial needs and problems of patients may not always be readily identified because some patients and their family members may be reluctant to report "nonmedical" problems or fears. They do not believe these should be shared with strangers or that they are within the nurse's concern. However, when behavior indicates that problems or needs may exist, a purposeful and planned, goal-oriented psychiatric/mental health assessment may be helpful regardless of the setting. The practitioner must recognize that assessment of the patient's current level of psychiatric functioning expands upon the Mental Status Evaluation described earlier (in Chapter 19) and usually requires advanced skills of focused observation, listening, and questioning by a specialist.

Psychiatric/mental health hypotheses are explored through history, interview, various psychiatric assessment

This chapter was prepared by Sandra Jaffee-Johnson, R.N., Ed.D., School of Nursing, State University of New York at Stony Brook, Stony Brook, New York.

tools, such as psychiatric tests, and the Mental Status examination. Under certain circumstances, or in emergencies, the nurse generalist may be called upon to evaluate the situation before consultation is available or referral made. Therefore, in this chapter we present examples of some tools developed to assess more specifically the level of emotional distress, anxiety, and depression. The following assessment guide and rating scales can be used selectively or adapted to elicit information beyond that obtained during the screening interview. They can further expand questions related to the patient's personality style and pattern of response to others, dynamics of unresolved conflicts (e.g., early relationships), maturational or situational crises, self-image, body-image, and physical dependence on alcohol or other drugs.

The depth of history is determined by the problem area and the purpose of the assessment. It can help clarify nursing diagnoses and assist in the development of the nursing care plan by identifying priorities and probable responses to potential therapeutic interventions.

DYNAMICS OF THE INTERVIEW

Creating an atmosphere in which the patient feels liked, respected, understood, and senses the possibility of being helped is particularly vital to the establishment of a trusting relationship when there are emotional problems. The examiner should make a special effort to demonstrate interest in the patient and his history by asking questions, explaining meanings, encouraging precise detailed descriptions in the here and now, and by making no assumptions without confirming with the patient what is being said. The establishment of this dynamic and cooperative environment is not only supportive to the interview process, but therapeutic to the patient because it helps him take more responsibility during the process of obtaining help.

PSYCHIATRIC/MENTAL HEALTH
ASSESSMENT GUIDE

The following guide is suggested as a tool for collection of data specifically related to mental health problems. Much

of the information would be the same as that collected during a general screening examination; however, now it is
focused upon the mental or emotional signs and symptoms.
The elements of the mental status examination are for the
most part, generally the same, however, since disturbance
in mental content may be more evident, greater attention
needs to be paid to this part of the physical examination.
A list of nursing diagnoses most commonly used for psychia-
tric/mental health problems is included within the assessment
guide.

Date: _____

PSYCHIATRIC/MENTAL HEALTH ASSESSMENT GUIDE

Name: _____   Source of Referral:

Address (home): _____   (B)
                                     (B)
_____

Telephone (home): _____   Marital Status: _____

Sex: _____   Age: _____
Date of Birth: _____

The following items may be explored through open-ended
questions (e.g., "Tell me about . . .") later in the interview
when rapport is established.

Significant Others: _____   Living Arrangement: _____
_____   _____

Position in Family: _____   Occupation: _____
_____   _____

Roles in Family: _____   Religion: _____
_____   _____
_____   _____

Parenthood Experience: _____   Education: _____
_____   _____
_____   _____

Socio-cultural: _____
_____

I. History: Present Condition
   A. What has brought you here (or to a psychiatric facility or to seek psychotherapy, if seen in clinic or private setting) at this time? (Patient's primary concern and perception of current situation.)
   B. How long have you been feeling this way — does any recent stress contribute to the problem? (The nature of problem and disruption caused by the problem.)
   C. How did you previously handle your feelings and/or current situation? (The time and context, or circumstances when first noticed problem.)
   D. What are the situations in which your problem bothers you (a) the most, (b) the least?
   E. What are your specific fears related to your problem and the kinds of changes that are becoming evident?
   F. When was the last time you sought any kind of counseling? Have you had prior hospitalizations (psychiatric and medical?)

Date(s)	Name	Place

   G. Were medications ever prescribed to relieve your anxiety or depression?
   H. Do you take any over-the-counter drugs or nonprescription medications to help you to relax?
   I. 1. When was the last time you visited a physician? Why?
      2. Are there any biologic or neurologic illnesses, etc., that may be contributing to your current problem?
      3. What previous major illnesses have you had?
   J. Usual sleep pattern (present and past):
      1. How long do you sleep at night? Is it interrupted — do you wake up? What happens then?
      2. What kind of dreams do you have?
      3. Have you experienced changes in your pattern recently?
   K. Nutrition and eating habits:
      1. How is your appetite?
      2. Have you experienced a change in your pattern (gain, loss, etc.)?
      3. What foods do you prefer? What is your typical diet during the day? (Habits.)
      4. Do you have any food allergies or any restrictions on the food you can eat?

II. Interpersonal Relationships:
   A. 1. Do you have close friends? Who are they?
      2. How often do you see them?
      3. Can you exchange thoughts and feelings with them?
      4. What activities, people and things give you a boost?
   B. Describe your relationships with your co-workers and co-leaders. (One's expectations.)
   C. How do you feel when you are in social situations? (View of others.)
   D. What do you like most about yourself? (Assess negative statements about self that increase anxiety, fear, hopelessness.)

III. Motivation and Lifestyle:
   A. How do you spend your mornings/evenings? (Assess recent loss or change in social system.)
   B. What do you do for fun? (Leisure time activities.)
   C. Are you ever lonely? What do you do? (Who lives with client?)

IV. Use of Alcohol and Other Drugs:
   A. Alcohol History
      1. At what age did you start drinking alcoholic beverages?
      2. What do you like to drink?
      3. When did you have your last drink?
      4. What is your pattern of drinking?
        (a) daily
        (b) weekends
        (c) periodic
        (d) holidays and special occasions
        (e) binges (1-2 weeks and then stop for a while)
        (f) abstinent
      5. Have you ever used efforts to control the amount you are drinking by
        (a) cutting down?
        (b) stopping briefly?
        (c) switching type of alcohol, e.g., Scotch or beer or vodka?
      6. Has anyone ever said anything to you about your drinking?
        (a) Has a doctor told you to quit?
        (b) Has a close friend, spouse, children, boss, co-worker complained about your drinking?

      7. Do you ever take a few shots of alcohol in the morning to feel more relaxed?

      8. Do you drink more than you usually intend to and feel quilty afterward?

      9. Have any of your family been "drinkers" and caused problems for self and other family members?

B. Drug Taking Other Than Alcohol

    1. What drugs do you take?

      (a) prescribed drugs

      (b) over the counter drugs

      (c) drugs obtained on the street, e.g., cocaine, pot, amphetamines, etc.

    2. How do you administer the "street" drugs? (e.g., mainlining [intravenous], snorting, smoking, skin popping [subcutaneous], orally.)

    3. What is your usual manner of taking drugs?

      (a) as directed

      (b) more than directed

      (c) less than directed

      (d) according to what you feel you need

    4. Have you experienced any of the following problems as a result of your use of "street" drugs?

      (a) weight loss

      (b) drug overdose (nausea and vomiting)

      (c) jaundice or hepatitis

      (d) septic arthritis (joint pain)

      (e) endocarditis (chest pain)

      (f) anemia (thin blood)

      (g) pneumonia (respiratory infection)

      (h) abscesses (skin infections)

      (i) thrombophlebitis (blood clot)

      (j) depressions

      (k) auditory and/or visual hallucinations

      (l) suicide attempt or ideas

    5. Are you allergic to any drugs?

V. Sex Life

A. Who do you prefer to have sexual relations with?

B. How often do you have sex with your partner(s)?

C. Are you satisfied with your sexual activity?

D. How often do you masturbate?

VI. Vocational History
    A. Are you working now?
    B. What is your current position on the job?
    C. Have you experienced any recent loss of status, disappointment at work?
    D. Are you satisfied with your current work status? Any future plans?
    E. What kinds of work have you done in the past?
    F. Experience in high school/college:
       1. How much education have you had?
       2. Did you experience a lot of stress?
       3. How did you cope with it?

PHYSICAL EXAMINATION

I. General Observation and Behavior:
  Appearance
    Posture
    Gait
    Dress
    Jewelry, make-up
    Facial expression
  Behavior
    Motor activity
    Eye contact
    Purposeful or goal-directed actions
  Communication
    Verbal (amount, rate, flow of speech)
    Nonverbal (gestures, body language)
  Clarity of communication
    Communication of feelings
    Communication with family or significant others present

II. Mental Status:
    A. Mood: Depressed   Elated   Angry
                    Anxious   Agitated
       Comments:
    B. Emotional Reactions (affect):

Appropriate:	Inappropriate:	
Labile	Pressured	Flat
Constricted	Blunted	Animated
Broad		
Comments:		

C. Memory: Intellectual Performance
    Recent: Math:
      Repeat a series of 3 digits
      Repeat a series of 7 digits – frontward and backward
      Count backward from 100 by 7
      Multiply 5 x 17 = 85
    Past: Name past three presidents of the United
           States
D. Abstract Reasoning – (How appropriate is the
    response?)
      What does the saying "A rolling stone gathers no
      moss" mean?
      "People who live in glass houses shouldn't throw
      stones"?
      "A stitch in time saves nine"?
E. Oriented:
    Time:
      What day of week is this?
      What is the date?
    Place:
      What place is this?
    Person:
      Who am I?
F. Speech and Stream of Mental Activity?
    Logical (normal)   Concrete   Loosening
    Flight of ideas   Circumstantial   Scattering
G. Mental Content — Major Themes:
    1. Suspicious   5. Delusional   9. Phobias
    2. Ambivalent   6. Paranoid   10. Obsessions
    3. Flight of ideas   7. Grandiose   11. Homicidal
    4. Hallucinating   8. Depersonalizing 12. Suicidal
III. Client Functioning and Problem Areas (Summary)
    Expresses Anxiety or Concerns during Interview
      Being seen as crazy
      Being rejected
      Loss of control
      Falling apart
      Lack of support
      Being powerless (victim)
      Being seen as helpless
    Character Defenses
      Constant explanation
      Justification

Rationalization
Projection
Intellectualization
Avoidance
Withdrawal
Denial
Diagnostic Impression (List of nursing diagnoses most commonly used for psychiatric/mental health nursing.) (Check which apply.)
Nursing diagnoses approved by the North American Nursing Diagnoses Association (5th Conference) (NANDA):

Activity intolerance
Anxiety
Communication, impaired:
  verbal
Coping, ineffective, family:
  potential for growth
Coping, ineffective, family:
  compromised
Coping, ineffective, family:
  disabling
Coping, ineffective, individual
Family process, alteration in
Fear
Grieving, anticipatory
Grieving, dysfunctional
Injury, potential for

Knowledge deficit (specify)
Noncompliance
Parenting, alteration in:
  actual or potential
Powerlessness
Self concept, disturbance
  in body image, self-esteem,
  role performance,
  personal identity
Social isolation
Spiritual distress
Thought processes,
  alteration in
Violence, potential for:
  self-directed or directed
  at others

Identified Needs and Resources

Disposition — Intervention

Plan
  Short-term goals
  Long-term goals

ANXIETY

When symptoms appear to indicate that the patient is anxious, the nursing diagnosis needs to be established based upon a thorough description of what the patient is experiencing. The following Anxiety Rating Scale was adapted from Hamilton's work in the British Journal of Medical Psychology. The score derived from a careful exploration of the patient's signs and symptoms provides a key to the degree of anxiety present.

ANXIETY LEVEL (circle one)

| 0 Not Present | 1 Mild + Senses alerted | 2 Moderate ++ Perception narrowed; Attention narrowed | 3 Severe +++ Focus on detail | 4 Very Severe ++++ Detail distorted |

HAMILTON RATING SCALE FOR ANXIETY STATES

Assess Degree of Anxiety
using scale above: 0 (not present) to very severe 4

Suggested Scoring
43–56 Very Severe
29–42 Severe
15–28 Moderate
1–14 Mild

Item	Score	Symptoms
Anxious mood		Worries, anticipation of the worst, fearful anticipation, irritability
Tension		Feelings of tension, fatigability, startle response, moved to tears easily, trembling, feelings of restlessness, inability to relax
Fears		Of dark, of strangers, of being left alone, of animals, of traffic, of crowds
Insomnia		Difficulty of falling asleep, broken sleep, unsatisfying sleep and fatigue on waking, dreams, nightmares, night terrors
Intellectual (cognitive)		Difficulty in concentration, poor memory

Depressed mood	Loss of interest, lack of pleasure in hobbies, depression, early waking, diurnal swing
Somatic (muscular)	Pains and aches, twitchings, stiffness, myoclonic jerks, grinding of teeth, unsteady voice, increased muscular tone
Somatic (sensory)	Tinnitus, blurring of vision, hot and cold flushes, feelings of weakness, pricking sensation
Cardiovascular system	Tachycardia, palpitations, pain in chest, throbbing of vessels, fainting feelings, missing beat
Respiratory system	Pressure or constriction in chest, choking feelings, sighing, dyspnea
Gastrointestinal system	Difficulty in swallowing, wind, abdominal pain, burning sensations, abdominal fullness, nausea, vomiting, borborygmi, looseness of bowels, loss of weight, constipation
Genitourinary system	Frequency of micturition, urgency of micturition, amenorrhea, menorrhagia, development of frigidity, premature ejaculation, looseness of bowels, loss of weight, constipation
Autonomic system	Dry mouth, flushing, pallor, tendency to sweat, giddiness, tension headache, raising of hair
Behavior at interview	Fidgeting, restlessness or pacing, tremor of hands, furrowed brow, strained face, sighing or rapid respiration, facial pallor, swallowing belching, brisk tendon jerks, dilated pupils, exophthalmos

Adapted with permission from Hamilton M: The assessment of anxiety states by rating. *British Journal of Medical Psychology*, 1959, 32:54–55.

DEPRESSION

The nurse may recognize signs and/or symptoms of potential or actual depression that need to be evaluated further. A variety of clinical tools may be helpful in determining the degree of depression, such as the Beck Depression Inventory, included here with permission.

Level of Depression (Beck Depression Inventory)

The Beck Depression Inventory is an easily administered questionnaire that can be completed by the patient in about 10 minutes. Scoring consists of adding up the encircled numeral values. The total score provides an estimate of the degree of severity of depressed mood. The total scores can be interpreted as follows:

Total Score	Levels of Depression
0-9	These ups and downs are considered normal
10-15	Mild depression
16-19[a]	Mild-moderate depression
20-29	Moderate-severe depression
30-63	Severe depression

[a]A persistent score of 17 or above indicates the need for professional consultation.
Subjective experience of depression is highly variable.

Beck Inventory

On this questionnaire are groups of statements. Please read each group of statements carefully. Then pick out the one statement in each group which best describes the way you have been feeling the PAST WEEK, INCLUDING TODAY! Circle the number beside the statement you picked. If several statements in the group seem to apply equally well, circle each one. *Be sure to read all the statements in each group before making your choice.*

1. 0 I do not feel sad.
   1 I feel sad.
   2 I am sad all the time and I can't snap out of it.
   3 I am so sad or unhappy that I can't stand it.

2. 0 I am not particularly discouraged about the future.
   1 I feel discouraged about the future.
   2 I feel I have nothing to look forward to.
   3 I feel that the future is hopeless and that things cannot improve.

3. 0 I do not feel like a failure.
   1 I feel I have failed more than the average person.
   2 As I look back on my life, all I can see is a lot of failures.
   3 I feel I am a complete failure as a person.

4. 0 I get as much satisfaction out of things as I used to.
   1 I don't enjoy things the way I used to.
   2 I don't get real satisfaction out of anything anymore.
   3 I am dissatisfied or bored with everything.

5. 0 I don't feel particularly quilty.
   1 I feel guilty a good part of the time.
   2 I feel quite quilty most of the time.
   3 I feel guilty all of the time.

6. 0 I don't feel I am being punished.
   1 I feel I may be punished.
   2 I expect to be punished.
   3 I feel I am being punished.

7. 0 I don't feel disappointed in myself.
   1 I am disappointed in myself.
   2 I am disgusted with myself.
   3 I hate myself.

8. 0 I don't feel I am any worse than anybody else.
   1 I am critical of myself for my weaknesses or mistakes.
   2 I blame myself all the time for my faults.
   3 I blame myself for everything bad that happens.

9. 0 I don't have any thoughts of killing myself.
   1 I have thoughts of killing myself, but I would not carry them out.
   2 I would like to kill myself.
   3 I would kill myself if I had the chance.

10. 0 I don't cry any more than usual.
    1 I cry more now than I used to.
    2 I cry all the time now.
    3 I used to be able to cry, but now I can't cry even though I want to.

11. 0 I am no more irritated now than I ever am.
    1 I get annoyed or irritated more easily than I used to.
    2 I feel irritated all the time now.
    3 I don't get irritated at all by the things that used to irritate me.

12. 0 I have not lost interest in other people.
    1 I am less interested in other people than I used to be.
    2 I have lost most of my interest in other people.
    3 I have lost all of my interest in other people.

13. 0 I make decisions about as well as I ever could.
    1 I put off making decisions more than I used to.
    2 I have greater difficulty in making decisions than before.
    3 I can't make decisions at all anymore.

14. 0 I don't feel I look any worse than I used to.
    1 I am worried that I am looking old or unattractive
    2 I feel that there are permanent changes in my appearance that make me look unattractive.
    3 I believe that I look ugly.

15. 0 I can work about as well as before.
    1 It takes an extra effort to get started at doing something.
    2 I have to push myself very hard to do anything.
    3 I can't do any work at all.

16. 0 I can sleep as well as usual.
    1 I don't sleep as well as I used to.
    2 I wake up 1-2 hours earlier than usual and find it hard to get back to sleep.
    3 I wake up several hours earlier than I used to and cannot get back to sleep.

17. 0 I don't get more tired than usual.
    1 I get tired more easily than I used to.
    2 I get tired from doing almost anything.
    3 I am too tired to do anything.

18. 0 My appetite is no worse than usual.
    1 My appetite is not as good as it used to be.
    2 My appetite is much worse now.
    3 I have no appetite at all anymore.

19. 0 I haven't lost much
       weight, if any,
       lately.
     1 I have lost more than
       5 pounds.
     2 I have lost more than
       10 pounds.
     3 I have lost more than
       15 pounds
     I am purposely trying to lose
     weight by eating less
          Yes ___ No ___

20. 0 I am no more worried
       about my health than
       usual.
     1 I am worried about
       physical problems
       such as aches and
       pains, or upset sto-
       mach or constipation.
     2 I am very worried
       about physical
       problems and it's
       hard to think of
       much else.
     3 I am so worried about
       my physical problems
       that I cannot think
       about anything
       else.

21. 0 I have not noticed any
       recent change in my
       interest in sex.
     1 I am less interested in
       sex than I used to be.
     2 I am much less interested
       in sex now.
     3 I have lost interest in
       sex completely.

SUMMARY

The guidelines for collecting data relative to an individual's personal, social, and cultural background, such as lifestyle, habits, interpersonal relations, self-image, and coping abilities, were provided in Chapter 5. During the neurological screening examination, mental functioning is explored through the mental status examination. Within most other chapters, signs and symptoms are identified that may represent mental or emotional rather than physical illness. When such problems become evident or are suspected, further assessment of mental functioning, anxiety, and depression are necessary. Therefore, in this chapter we have provided a series of tools the clinician may find helpful for the development of a nursing diagnosis, establishment of patient goals, and creation of a course of nursing activities.

chapter 29

Examination of the Comatose Patient

Patient Status

Approach

History

Physical Examination

The major emphasis of this textbook has been on the examination under optimum conditions, i.e., adequate time for the examiner and a fully cooperative patient. There will be many situations in which these ideal circumstances will not pertain, where it will be necessary for the practitioner to "shift gears" — to increase his speed and/or to eliminate certain portions of the examination. Situations such as the evaluation of an uncooperative patient, a weak elderly patient, an acutely ill, or severely injured patient, obviously demand modification of the history taking process and the physical examination. An extreme example of such a situation is the evaluation of an unconscious person.

PATIENT STATUS

The first, and by far the most important, step in the evaluation of the comatose patient is the requirement to judge rapidly the adequacy of the patient's respiratory and circulatory systems to sustain life and integrity of the brain. The essential ingredients are a patent airway and adequate ventilation to provide *oxygen,* enough blood glucose to avoid permanent *metabolic brain damage,* and a pulse rate and systolic blood pressure sufficient to provide *circulation* of the oxygen and glucose to the brain.

Priority, therefore, must be given to examination of the pharynx, to the vital signs, and to the level of blood glucose. A significant abnormality of any of these calls for deferment of further examination until emergency treatment is initiated. A team is urgently required under these circumstances, for the workup must be continued while treatment is in progress.

APPROACH

While there are many conditions that may produce coma, there are far fewer than the total list of conditions which cause illness in general. Familiarity with common causes of coma narrows the list of possibilities and thereby makes certain parts of the "routine" examination more important and others unnecessary. One classification of the causes of coma is the following:

Supratentorial structural lesions: cerebral trauma, cerebral or subarachnoid hemorrhage, encephalitis, acute stroke (uncommon)

Posterior Fossa structural lesions: basilar artery thrombosis, acute cerebellar or pontine hemorrhage, occasionally tumors

Metabolic-toxic disorders: exogenous poisons, cardiac arrest arrhythmias, diabetic keto-acidosis, hepatic or uremic syndromes, epilepsy, postictal state

Psychogenic: conversion, malingering, catatonic state

Review of this classification, and of some of the specific causes, will help the examiner to concentrate his attention on certain elements of the history and the physical examination. Despite the urgency of the situation, jumping to conclusions is more dangerous than a deliberate appraisal. The history and physical examination must be abbreviated but not carelessly performed.

HISTORY

Since the comatose patient cannot give a history, this element of evaluation is often totally neglected to the detriment of the patient. Questioning people who brought the patient in, or relatives and friends who can be reached quickly, may be lifesaving. Examination of the patient's clothing and purse or wallet may reveal important clues, such as a diabetic identification card, a bottle (full or empty) of medication, or a suicide note. Information from previous medical records should be obtained if available promptly.

PHYSICAL EXAMINATION

In the immediate assessment of the patient's status, the respiratory and cardiovascular systems took first priority, but that examination was performed quickly to evaluate the viability of the patient. These systems should now be re-evaluated in more detail when searching for clues as to the etiology of the coma. Since coma is a manifestation of a serious neurologic disorder, the neurologic system must be carefully examined. A suggested order for this type of physical examination is:

Vital Signs: Nearly continuous monitoring of pulse, respiration, blood pressure, rectal temperature, and urine output is obviously mandatory.

Head: Inspect and palpate for skull trauma. If blood is detected in the hair, the scalp should be shaved rapidly to allow for careful examination.

Face: Inspect for symmetry of facial muscles.

Eyes: Inspect for pupillary size, equality, and reaction to light, nystagmus, or "wandering" of the eyeballs. Pupillary reaction and eye movements are important indices to vital brain-stem functions. A funduscopic examination should be done for evidence of papilledema.

Ears: Inspect for blood or spinal fluid in the canals or behind the eardrum. Inspect for bulging or rupture of the drum.

Nose: Inspect for leakage of spinal fluid or blood.

Mouth: Smell the breath for odor of alcohol, acetone, or hepatic fetor. Inspect the tongue for bite marks and the palate for bleeding.

Neck: Flex the head to detect resistance or rigidity.

Chest: Inspect for rate, rhythm, and depth of respiration. Percuss and auscultate for signs of consolidation or lung collapse.

Heart: Recheck rate and rhythm. Auscultate for murmurs.

Abdomen: Inspect for bruising. Auscultate for bowel sounds.

Extremities: Inspect for evidence of trauma, for needle tracks on the forearm, and for puncture marks on the thighs. Assess for muscle tone. (This may be done by raising and dropping both arms or legs at the same time.) Attempt to obtain reactive movement by jabbing a pin into each hand and foot. Examine tendon and plantar reflexes. These evaluations are done to detect inequality of responses from one side to the other.

Level of Consciousness: This is evaluated by the patient's responsiveness to stimuli. The more vigorous the stimulus needed to obtain a response, the deeper is the coma. Thus, spoken words, shouted words, mild pain stimuli (slapping or pinprick), deep pain stimuli (pressure over the medial portion of the upper orbital ridge and pressing a pencil over a fingernail bed) are progressively severe stimuli. The patient's level of consciousness should be reevaluated regularly during the comatose state based on responses to such stimuli.

Glasgow Scale

This is a practical recording of eye opening, verbal response, and motor response according to a specific code that serves to assure consistent evaluation when observations are made by different observers (Table 29.1). This sequence of examination is given as a guide to the areas of the examination most likely to produce information related to the etiology of coma. The full evaluation of the comatose patient requires the selection of appropriate laboratory studies, a review of which is beyond the scope of this text.

Table 29.1 Neurological Assessment (Glasgow Coma Scale)

A

Eyes open spontaneously	(4)
to verbal command	(3)
to pain	(2)
no response	(1)

B

Best verbal response

oriented and converses	(5)
disoriented and converses	(4)
inappropriate words	(3)
incomprehensible sound	(2)
no response	(1)

C

Best motor response to verbal command

obeys	(6)
localizes pain	(5)
flexion withdrawal	(4)
flexion —abnormal (decorticate rigid)	(3)
extension (decerebrate rigidity)	(2)
no response	(1)

continued

Table 29.1 (continued)

Date		:/7/8?												
Time		$\frac{15}{P}$					7P							
A	4						✓							
	3													
	2													
	1	✓												
B	5						Intubated ✓							
	4													
	3													
	2													
	1	✓												
C	6						✓							
	5													
	4													
	3													
	2													
	1	✓												
Total		3					/45							

PUPIL GAUGE (mm) 1· 2• 3● 4● 5● 6● 7● 8●

Pupils: N — normal;   S — sluggish;   F — fixed

continued

Table 29.1 *(continued)*

Extremity Movement

4. Normal

Grasps hands firmly to command. Able to raise both arms and legs completely off the bed against pressure and retain raised position for indefinite period of time

3. Sl. Weakness

Grasps hands with guarded strength to command. Raises arms and legs completely off the bed against pressure but retains raised position for shorter period of time

2. Mod. Weakness

Grasps hands with decreased power. Has difficulty raising arms and legs off the bed against pressure. Unable to retain raised position for one minute

1. Minimal

Grasps hands slightly on command. Unable to raise arms and legs off the bed against pressure or retain a raised position for any length of time

0. None

No movement

continued

Table 29.1 *(continued)*

Date	5/7/86									
Time	1'⁵⁄ₚ					7P				
SIZE Rt.	2					3				
SIZE Lt.	2					3				
REACT Rt.	S					3				
REACT Lt.	S					3				
Rt. ARM	0					N				
Lt. ARM	0					N				
Rt. LEG	0					N				
Lt.. LEG	0					N				

     As stated at the beginning of this chapter, the evalua-
tion of a comatose patient is reviewed not so much as a
pattern for this examination, but as an illustration of the
variation from the routine when circumstances are not
optimal.
     Thus for the comatose patient discussed above, the
history is condensed, therapy is begun, and the initial physical examination is limited to areas of immediate concern
for the patient's survival. On the other hand, with a patient
who demonstrates an urgent need to talk, the entire time of
a visit may need to be spent discussing a chief complaint and
a psychosocial history.
     The principle should be clear — that the clinician's
judgment must be used to set priorities in the patient assessment process based on the *immediate* needs of the patient.
Subsequent visits are often necessary to piece together a
complete history and physical examination.

Epilogue

In this text we have been trying to express a philosophy that we believe must serve as a guide throughout the practitioner's professional life. The best modality for comprehensive assessment and development of a dynamic and effective nursing care plan for each patient is a competent, caring clinician who looks upon each patient as a unique person and who aims to diagnose and treat that person's response to illness — not a disease.

Since the phenomenon of illness is the process of interaction of one or more problems in a specific host, assessment of any person's health status requires the synthesis of knowledge about the individual, his problems, and the illness. Absence of adequate information about any of these elements leads, inevitably, to less than optimum patient care.

Information about the patient is primarily dependent upon obtaining an adequate health history with accurate data about past health history, family history, personal and social history, and functional health patterns. The careful review of current or potential dysfunctional patterns, a thorough physical examination, and selected laboratory information form the data base for evaluation of response to the disease — i.e., the patient's illness.

An important step in comprehensive assessment is the establishment of a nursing diagnosis, or, in terms of the problem-oriented record, the refinement of the problem.

The establishment of a nursing diagnosis depends upon two major processes: the collection of data from the patient and the analysis of the data. This textbook is principally a guide to the collection of data from the health history and the physical examination. Analysis of data can only be made if the data base is complete and without error. Failure to elicit the fact that there have been several deaths from coronary heart disease in the patient's immediate family will interfere with the clinician's interpretation of the anxiety state in the middle-aged man with mild chest pain. Failure to observe a lesion on the tongue that interferes with chewing and speaking will mislead the practitioner to believing the 75-year-old widow is apathetic due to depression or dementia. Failure to ascertain that in the past the patient had a rash after receiving an injection for a vaginal infection could lead to shock after administration of penicillin in the emergency room. It is obvious that a careful, thorough, and accurate data base must be constructed before the process of data analysis. The practitioner will be able to perform this accurate type of examination through practice over time.

The second phase of the diagnostic process — the analysis of data — is a logical evaluation of the facts accumulated in the initial data base. The practitioner selects those abnormalities in the data base which seem most important and then tries to associate these abnormalities with the various dysfunctional health patterns, diagnostic entities, and risk factors. If clinical data are insufficient for diagnosis, signs and symptoms are documented and further assessment is planned. The nursing diagnosis is used as a basis for projecting outcomes (goals), planning intervention, and evaluating outcome attainment. The ability to do this well is based upon knowledge of human behavior, basic sciences, pathophysiology, a typology of functional health patterns, and experience. Knowing one's limitations and knowing when referral is in order are normal expected parts of the process of evaluation and management of the patient's response to illness.

As indicated in Chapter 3, the establishment of rapport with the patient is a major goal in the assessment process. It should be clear by now that adequate assessment of the patient and of his symptoms and signs depends upon good interchange between the clinician and patient. This rapport is also a significant factor in the nurse's ability to carry out the nursing care plan or manage the patient's illness effectively. It must never be forgotten that the taking of a history and performance of a careful physical examination are parts of the therapeutic process as well as of diagnosis. Every health professional who comes in contact with the patient has a role to play in reducing the patient's anxiety and uncertainty, but the clinician who initiates the evaluation can provide the best therapeutic support for the patient in his anxious state by a careful, thoughtful assessment of the whole person.

 . . . . *for the secret of the care of the patient is in caring for the patient.* [Peabody, 1927]

The Process of Nursing Assessment Questionnaire Guide for Nursing History

ADELPHI UNIVERSITY
MARION A. BUCKLEY SCHOOL OF NURSING[1]
N420/425
Spring 1986
QUESTIONNAIRE GUIDE FOR NURSING HISTORY
AND PHYSICAL ASSESSMENT BASED ON GORDON'S
FUNCTIONAL HEALTH AREAS[2]

1. *Health Perception:* Description

   Includes the individual's perception of health status and its relevance to current activities and future planning. Also included is the individual's general level of health care behavior, such as adherence to preventive health practices, medical or nursing prescriptions, and follow-up care.

[1]These assessment tools were adapted for use in the educational setting by Catherine Windmer, PhD, RN, Erma Barenburg, EdD, RN, and Barbara Krainovich, MS, RN, from Levin RF, Crosby JM: Focused data collection for the generation of nursing diagnoses, *J Staff Development,* 1986;2(2). The forms are in the process of evaluation and revision.

[2]Adapted from Gordon M: *Nursing Diagnosis: Process and Applications,* ed 2, New York, McGraw-Hill, 1987, by permission.

Focus Questions

a. What is your major problem? When did the problem start?
b. What do you think caused this problem? How does this affect you? Why did you seek help?
c. Does anything alleviate the complaint?
d. Medications now taking?
e. Do you experience pain? How do you usually deal with pain?
f. Have you been able to follow the advice/suggestions of doctors and nurses?
g. How has general health been? Any colds or illness in past year?
h. Any known allergies? Management?
i. Most important things done to keep health? Think these things make a difference to health? (Include family folk remedies, if appropriate.) Use of cigarettes, alcohol, other drugs, caffeine, coffee, tea? Breast self-exam?
j. Concerns about present illness? Present hospitalization? Previous hospitalizations?
k. Family health history — health problems of living and deceased (grandparents, parents, siblings).

2. *Nutritional-Metabolic Pattern:* Description

Includes the individual's patterns of food and fluid consumption, daily eating times, the types and quantity of food and fluids consumed, particular food preferences, and the use of nutrient or vitamin supplements. Reports of any skin lesions and general ability to heal are included. The condition of skin, hair, nails, mucous membranes, and teeth, and measures of body temperature, height, and weight are included.

Focus Questions

a. Typical daily food intake? (Describe.) Supplements? Frequency of meals?
b. Special diets.
c. Typical daily fluid intake? Coffee, tea, soda, alcohol. (Describe.)

d. Weight loss/gain? (Amount.)
e. Appetite
f. Food or eating? Discomfort? Diet restrictions?
g. Heal well or poorly?
h. Skin problems? Lesions, dryness, temperature?
i. Dentures, dental problems, condition of mouth?

3. *Elimination Pattern:* Description

Includes the individual's perceived regularity of excretory function, use of routines or laxatives for bowel elimination, and any changes or disturbances in time-pattern, tenemus, mode of excretion, quality, or quantity. Also included are any devices employed to control elimination.

Focus Questions

a. Bowel elimination pattern. (Describe.) Frequency? Character? Discomfort? Aids? When was your last rectal exam?
b. Urinary elimination pattern. (Describe.) Frequency? Discomfort? Problem in control? Aids?
c. Excess perspiration? Odor problems?

4. *Activity/Exercise:* Description

Includes the usual pattern of daily living activities, such as personal hygiene, exercise tolerance, and leisure activities. This area also includes perception of problems related to activities of daily living and ways in which the patient deals with these perceived problems.

Focus Questions

a. What is your usual day like?
b. Usual grooming habits? Oral care? Bathing? Hair washing?
c. Do you engage in regular exercise (e.g., jogging, swimming, walking)? (Note type and frequency.)
d. Use of assistance devices, paralysis, weakness, coordination?
e. Do you have sufficient energy to carry out required and/or desired activities?

    f. What do you do in your spare time?
    g. Has your present health problem interfered with your usual activities? If so, how?

5. *Sleep/Rest:* Description

Includes patterns of sleep, rest and relaxation periods during the 24-hour day. Includes the individual's perception of the quality and quantity of sleep and rest, and perception of energy level. Included also are aids used to sleep, such as medications or sleeptime routines.

Focus Questions

    a. What hours do you usually sleep?
    b. Do you, in general, take naps? How many hours?
    c. Do you feel rested after sleeping?
    d. Is your sleep interrupted?
    e. Do you have trouble falling asleep?
    f. What do you do if you cannot get to sleep? (Aids?)
    g. Do you have dreams? Nightmares?
    h. What helps you relax?

6. *Sexuality/Reproductive:* Description

Includes collection of information describing individual's perception of their sexuality, sexual concerns and reproductive capability or incapability.

Focus Questions

    a. Females: When was menarche, last menstrual period? Any menstrual problems?
       Males: Onset of erection, emission?
    b. Pregnancy history? Parity? Gravida? Problems? Birth control method, problems?
    c. Depending on the client's age: Questions pertinent to male/female menopause.
    d. Any gynecological or urological problems? Discharges? Pruritus? Surgery?
    e. When was last physical exam? (Pap smear, breast exam, prostate exam?)
    f. Do you perform breast self-exam regularly?

g. Do you experience any pain or discomfort during sexual relations? If yes, how?
h. Has your health problem affected your sexuality? If yes, how so?

7. *Cognitive/Perceptual:* Description

Includes level of consciousness and the adequacy of sensory modes, such as vision, hearing, taste, touch or smell and the compensation or prosthetics utilized for disturbances. Reports of pain perception are also included when appropriate. Also included are the cognitive functional abilities, such as language memory, and decision-making.

Focus Questions

a. Level of consciousness?
b. Orientation to person, place, time?
c. Convulsions?
d. Hearing difficulty? Aids?
e. Vision? Aids?
f. Alteration in any other senses? (Specify.)
g. Changes in memory lately?
h. When you want to learn, how do you usually go about it?

8. *Role Relationships:* Description

Includes the individual's perception of the major roles and responsibilities in current life situation. Satisfaction or disturbances in family, work, or social relationships and responsibilities related to these roles are included.

Focus Questions

a. Occupation, educational background, age.
b. Ethnic/cultural/spiritual background.
c. Family membership.
d. Recreation.
e. Do you belong to social groups?
f. How will your hospitalization affect you and your family, work, school?

9. *Self-Perception/Self-Concept:* Description

Includes individual's attitudes about himself or herself, perception of abilities (cognitive, affective, or physical) body image, identity, general sense of worth, and general emotional patterns. Body posture and movement, eye contact, voice, and speech patterns are included.

Focus Questions

a. How would you describe yourself?
b. Strengths/weaknesses.
c. Have you experienced any physical or emotional changes? How have they affected you? How have you dealt with them?
d. Description of facial expression, body posture, tone of voice?

10. *Coping-Stress Tolerance:* Description

Includes the patient's perception of his level of stress and its management in general and at this particular time.

Focus Questions

a. Usual response to stress? (Calm, slightly anxious, moderately anxious, very anxious.)
b. Who is most helpful in talking things over? Available to you now?
c. Any big changes in your life in the last year or two?
d. Do you frequently get angry? Annoyed? Fearful? Anxious, depressed?
e. When you perceive problems in your life, how do you handle them?
f. Response to stress now (same as a.)

11. *Value/Belief:* Description

Includes what is perceived as important in life and any perceived conflicts in values, beliefs, or expectations that are health related.

Focus Questions

a. What kinds of things are important in your life?
b. Is religion important in your life? If appropriate: Does this help when difficulties arise?
c. Will being here interfere with any religious or cultural practices?

Nursing Diagnoses

The purpose of this text is to guide in the development of history taking and physical examination skills. Subjective and objective data to support nursing diagnoses are identified through the procedures described herein. Analysis and interpretation of data about individual patients by nurses for determination of nursing diagnoses, care planning, and evaluation will need to be made by the individual nurse within the context of her basic and advanced education, clinical experiences, and the system of health care delivery (i.e., institutional policies and procedures).

APPROVED THROUGH THE FIRST TO SIXTH NATIONAL CONFERENCES OF THE NORTH AMERICAN NURSING DIAGNOSIS ASSOCIATION

Activity/Rest

Activity intolerance

Activity intolerance, potential

Diversional activity, deficit

Sleep pattern disturbance

Circulation

Cardiac output, alteration in: decreased

Tissue perfusion, alteration in

Elimination

Bowel elimination, alteration in: constipation

Bowel elimination, alteration in: diarrhea

Bowel elimination, alteration in: incontinence

Urinary elimination, alteration in

Emotional Reactions

Anxiety

Coping, ineffective individual

Fear

Grieving, anticipatory

Grieving, dysfunctional

Powerlessness

Rape trauma syndrome

Self-concept, disturbance in: body image; self-esteem; role performance; personal identity

Social isolation

Spiritual distress (distress of the human spirit)

Violence, potential for

Family Pattern Alterations

Coping, family: potential for growth

Coping, ineffective family: compromised

Coping, ineffective family: disabled

Family process, alteration in

Parenting, alteration in: actual or potential

Food/Fluid

Fluid volume, alteration in: excess

Fluid volume, deficit, actual

Fluid volume, deficit, potential

Nutrition, alteration in: less than body requirements

Nutrition, alteration in: more than body requirements

Nutrition, alteration in: potential for more than body requirements

Oral mucous membranes, alteration in

Hygiene

Self-care deficit (specify level: feeding, bathing/hygiene, dressing/grooming, toileting)

Neurologic

Communication, impaired verbal

Sensory-perceptual alteration

Thought processes, alteration in

Pain

Comfort, alteration in: pain (acute and chronic)

Safety

Injury, potential for

Mobility, impaired physical

Skin integrity, impairment of: actual

Skin integrity, impairment of: potential

Sex

Sexual dysfunction

Teaching/Learning

Health maintenance, alteration in

Home maintenance management, impaired

Knowledge deficit (specify) [Learning need (specify)]

Noncompliance (specify) [Compliance (specify)]

Ventilation

Airway clearance, ineffective

Breathing pattern, ineffective

Gas exchange, impaired

APPROVED AT THE 1986 SEVENTH NATIONAL CONFERENCE

Elimination

Stress incontinence

Reflex incontinence

Functional incontinence

Total incontinence

Urge incontinence

Urinary retention

Emotional Reaction

Impaired social interaction

Unilateral neglect

Posttrauma response

Hopelessness

Impaired adjustment

Food/Fluid

Impaired swallowing

Safety

Potential for infection
Altered comfort: chronic pain
Hypothermia
Hyperthermia
Ineffective thermoregulation
Potential alteration in body temperature
Impaired tissue integrity
Altered growth and development

Sex

Altered sexuality patterns

During this conference several existing approved diagnoses were made more specific (e.g., listing five forms of
incontinence instead of merely listing "Alteration in elimination, urinary). Defining characteristics cited in previous
approved lists as "subjective" and "objective" data were now
identified as "Major" or "Minor" or "Related Factors," while
"Risk Factors" were identified when a problem was listed as
"Potential." It is apparent that changes in these approved
lists will continue to occur annually until greater specificity
can be accomplished and criticism regarding this issue is
diminished.

Nursing Health Assessment Form and Nursing Care Plan

NURSING ASSESSMENT FORM

UNIVERSITY HOSPITAL

17-year-old white male Catholic in acute distress.

DATE: _8/8/90_ TIME: _2 p.m._ FROM: _ER_

Home: _x_ Other: _____

Unit of Admission: _Neurology_

Admitting Nurse: _Judith Metcalf,_ RN, MN

ALLERGY BAND IN PLACE Y (x) N ( )

NAME BAND IN PLACE Y (x) N ( )

VIA: Ambulatory _____ Wheelchair _____ Stretcher _____

Information From: _____

Accompanied by: _Parents_

Disposition of Valuables: _None_

DENTURES WITH PATIENT Y ( ) N (x)

GLASSES Y ( ) N (x) *CONTACTS* Y ( ) N (x)

PROSTHETICS Y ( ) N (x) *HEARING AIDS* Y ( ) N (x)

VS: BP _116_/_70_P _72_RR _20_ T _98_ HT _5'9"_ WT _160_

From SUNY Stony Brook, New York, 1986, by permission.

ALLERGIES: _penicillin & sulfa drugs_

REASON FOR VISIT: _Head injury 4 hours DTA "My head is killing me." "I feel sick to my stomach."_

TRANSFUSION HX: Prior Transfusion: Y ( ) N (x)
Reaction: Y ( ) N (x)

HISTORY OF PRESENT ILLNESS: _Pt was well and_
Description of chronology, duration
of sx., treatments & pt. response, _active until_
pt. understanding of illness.

about 10 a.m.

when he fell from his "dirt bike." Sustained head injury, but denies awareness of loss of consciousness. Sustained several bruises over body, but able to get up from ground and walk home. Complained of mild pain over forehead progressively increasing. Now "terrible throbbing." Complains of feeling "sick to my stomach," tired, weak, and wanting to lie down to sleep. Examined in ER. Skull X-rays revealed fracture with possible epidural hematoma. Two episodes of vomiting.

EXPECTATIONS FOR _Diagnose and treat head_
TREATMENT:
injury pain & discomfort.

Able to return home & to school.

PAST ILLNESS/   _T & A age 4, no sequelae._
HOSPITALIZATIONS:
     Appendectomy age 16, no

       sequelae.

IMMUNIZATIONS: _All childhood diseases with_

     boosters.

FAMILY Hx/RISK   _Mother 45 L & W no problem._
FACTORS:
     Father 46 L & W mild

       hypertension

Two male siblings 1.0 & 1.4 L & W.

HEALTH PERCEPTION,
HEALTH MAINTENANCE:
Allergies, ADLs,   _Allergic to penicillin,_
hygiene practices,
smoking, alcohol use,   _sulfa. Does not smoke,_
drug use, appearance,
perceptions of previous _occasional beer and wine,_
hospitalizations/illness.
       denies drug use. Appears

drowsy-unable to _interview._ _Mother denies_

problems relating to previous hospitalization.

MEDICATIONS:
Names, types, dosages,
frequency, last dose
taken, compliance,
overcounter, home
remedies, disposition
of medications.

No over-the-counter or

prescribed medication.

INTESTINAL
INTEGRITY:
Pain, constipation,
diarrhea, tarry
stools, change in
bowel habits,
blood per rectum,
hemorrhoids, col-
ostomy appliances.

NORMAL PATTERN: *One BM*

each day.

LAST B.M.: *This AM.*

AIDS FOR BOWEL FUNCTIONING:

None.

HX: *Appetite good normally.*

Complains of "Sick to my stomach."

EXAM OF ABDOMEN: *Abdomen*

flat, no skin lesions, no hernia, no

pulsations. No tenderness or masses.

Spleen, kidney not palpated.

Uncooperative for liver location.

ACTIVITY/EXERCISE:
Respiratory Integrity:
shortness of breath,
dyspnea on exertion,
paroxymal nocturnal
dyspnea, orthopnea,
cyanosis, barrel
chest, cough, sputum
production, breath
sounds, fatigue,
tracheostomy, aids
to breathing, TB
exposure, TB test-
ing, exposure to
environmental
agents.

HX: _No cough, SOB, wheeze;_

has colds 1-2x year, chest
X-ray for school physical
negative

THORAX: Inspection:_Symmetrical_
full expansion equal
bilaterally;

AP _diameter not increased._

Palp: _No tenderness;_

no axillary adenopathy.

EXAM OF LUNGS: Palp: _Fremitus_

equal bilaterally.

Perc: _Lung fields resonant_
throughout.

Ausc _No adventitious breath_

sounds,vocal sounds normal.

CIRCULATORY
INTEGRITY: rhythm,
pulse deficit, chest
pain, palpitations,
intermittent claudica-
tion, color of
extremities, edema,
neck veins, varico-
sities, shunts,
fistulas, peripheral
veins, broviacs,
HTN.

HX: _No chest pain,_
palpitations,
hypertension, or vascular
problems.

EXAM OF HEART AND BLOOD VES-

SELS: _Inspection: No heave._

Palp: _No heave, thrill, or_
rib retraction.
PMI 5th LICS medial to MCL.

Perc.: _LBCD at MCL in 5th ICS._

Ausc: _Rate 72/min reg; sounds_
normal; S₂ (aort)>S2 (pulm); S₂ split on
inspiration; no murmurs, gallop, rubs.

MOBILITY: gait, muscle weakness, paralysis, deformities, physical tolerance, muscle atrophy, tremors, range of motion, range of ambulation, set-up at home to assist mobility, prosthetics.

LEVEL OF INDEPENDENCE: _____

USE OF AIDS: None (x) Walker ( )

Cane ( ) Wheelchair ( )

With Patient? Yes ( ) No ( )

HX: *No problems in past.*

PE: MOTOR: Arms: R.U.E. *-Can lift and hold against resistance; handgrasp normal.*
L.U.E. *- Can lift but not maintain position. Significant downward drift noted. Weakened hand grasp*

Legs: R.L.E. *- Can lift and hold against resistance; dorsi and plantar flexion normal.*
L.L.E *-Can lift and hold only momentarily; dorsi and plantar flexion both weakened.*

No atrophy or involuntary body movements

noted.

Tendon Reflexes: *Positive Babinski sign noted.*

DT reflexes somewhat depressed.

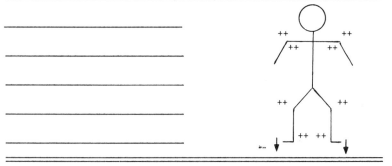

NUTRITIONAL/METABOLIC:
Food and Fluid Intake
dysphagia, anorexia, nausea,
vomiting, abdominal pain,
distention, weight gain or
loss, bowel sounds, changes
in taste, food preferences,
dietary patterns, special
diet.

DENTURES None (x)
     Upper ( )
     Lower ( )
     Both ( )
With Patient? Yes ( ) No ( )

HX: _Well nourished,_
good appetite. Feels
"sick to my stomach";
Two episodes of
vomiting.

PE: _No jaundice._

METABOLISM:
Weight gain or loss,
polydipsia, polyuria,
hair loss, lethargy,
increased activity,
heat or cold
intolerance.

HX: _No major weight_

changes, no glycosuria,

polydipsia, or sweating.

PE: _Normal hair_

distribution.

SKIN INTEGRITY:
Color, swelling, turgor,
abrasions, scars, decubiti,
temperature, pruritis.

HX: _Has had acne for_
four years, treated by
dermatologist with
varying agents.

PE: _Acne on cheeks_
(macular, papules,
pustules, comedones). No deformity of
hair or nails.
Small abrasion noted over mid-forehead.
Swelling of scalp & tenderness over
right temporoparietal region.

HEMATOLOGICAL
INTEGRITY:
Bleeding tendencies.

HX: _No bleeding history._

PE: _No adenopathy._

ELIMINATION:
Genital-Urinary
Integrity: frequency,
burning, hematuria,
nocturia, retention,
polyuria, inconti-
nence, flank pain,
aids to urination,
dialysis, appliances,
catheter.

HX: _No dysuria, hematuria,_

Nocturia, UD.

PE: _Deferred._

COGNITIVE-PERCEPTUAL
Sensory Integrity:
Level of consciousness,
pupillary response,
orientation, memory
loss, retention, syncope,
vertigo, convulsions,
headache, seizures, numb-
ness, tingling,
alterations in heat and
cold sensation.

HX: _C/O pounding_
headache over top of
head, says he wants to
sleep, closing eyes.

Cerebral Function: _Very drowsy._
Spontaneous eye opening
to loud verbal stimuli,
occasionally vigorous shaking
of shoulder required. Affect
flat. Occasional moaning.
Speech clear but slow.
Oriented to person and place.
Confused to time and date.
Glasgow Coma Score = 13.

COGNITIVE-PERCEPTUAL (cont'd)

Cranial Nerves: CN 1 - _Recognizes alcohol._
                  CN 11 - _Refuses to cooperate._
CN 111) _Right pupil 4 mm. Reactive sluggishly_
)   _to light._
    1V)_Left pupil 3 mm. Reactive briskly_
)   _to light._
    VI)_Direct and consensual light reflex_
       intact. Both eyes move conjugately.
       Extraocular movement normal. No
       nystagmus, no ptosis.
CN V - _Sensory intact, jaw closure OK._
CN V11 - _Facial muscles symmetrical, no weakness._
CN V111 - _Hearing intact, Weber no_
          lateralization.
CN 1X - _Swallowing and gag reflex intact;_
CN X - _Uvula in midline._
CN X1 - _Unwilling to cooperate_
CN X11 - _Tongue protrudes in midline, slight_
         tremor.

Sensory: Bilateral sensory exam within

          normal limits.

Cerebellar Function: Balance Tests: _Too drowsy to_

                      test.

                      Coordination Tests: _Finger to_

                      nose slightly off.

                      Alternating Motion: _Unable to_

                      evaluate.

VISION:
Visual disturbances,
diplopia, blurring,
excessive tearing,
cataracts, glaucoma.

GLASSES/CONTACTS: Yes ( ) No (x)

With Patient? Y ( ) N ( )

GLASS EYE? Yes ( ) No (x)

With Patient? Yes ( ) No ( )

DEGREE OF VISUAL ACUITY:

Grossly normal.

HX: _No visual problems. No_
family history of glaucoma
or cataracts.

PE: _See above._

SEXUALITY/
REPRODUCTIVE:
Menses, contracep-
tion, breast changes,
pregnancies, dis-
charge, gynecomastia,
sexual impotence,
venereal disease.

LMP: _N/A_

LAST PAP SMEAR: _N/A_

HX: _Not available at this_
time.

PE: _Not available at this_
time.

ROLE/
RELATIONSHIPS:
Support systems,
social skills.

Marital Status: (S) M D W Sep

Years:

Children: —

ROLE/ RELATIONSHIPS: (cont'd)	Occupation: _High School Student._ Education: _Grade 11._ _Average student per parents'_ _report._
SELF PERCEPTIONS: Anxiety, self-esteem, body image.	_Appears frightened and_ _anxious, "Do I have to stay_ _in the hospital?"_
COPING/STRESS TOLERANCE: Effective/ ineffective coping skills, life stressors, referrals to other agencies.	_Parents describe well-adjusted_ _adolescent._ _No major problems._ RN MD
VALUE/BELIEF: Cultural/religious practices, spiritual needs.	_Catholic, American-born of_ _Italian descent. Attends_ _Mass occasionally with family._ Referral to Clergy:

EARS AND HEARING:
Tinnitus, pain, discharge.

HX: _No history of hearing problems._

PE: _No masses, lesions of auricles or canal. No blood or fluid in ear canal. Both TM pearly gray. No perforations._

SPEECH:
Mouth, throat, face.

HX: _No speech problem._

PE: _Speech slow._

MENTAL STATUS:
Illogical thinking,
delusions, hallucinations,
perception of reality,
suicidal thoughts,
homicidal thoughts,
elated, agitated,
depressed.

HX: _No history of problems._

PE: _Sleepy and poorly oriented to time & date due to head injury._

COMFORT:
Pain (include location,
duration, periodicity,
severity, relief measures),
positioning, diversional
activity, environment.

HX: _See CC and HPI._

PE:

SLEEP/REST: HX: *No history of problems.*
Hours of sleep,
difficulty falling   PE: *Drowsy now.*
asleep, sleep aids.

LEARNING NEEDS: *Safety rules, need to wear*
Health maintenance,
illness teaching,   *helmet when biking.*
coping skills training.

CONTINUITY OF   Type of Residence: *Private home.*
CARE NEEDS:
Social service   Phone #
referral, equipment
for home care.   With whom does patient live? *Parents.*

                     Known to agency? *No.*

                     Contact person: *Mother.*

                     Phone #   *555-1234*

NURSING CARE PLAN

Nursing Diagnosis:

1. *Alteration in thought process secondary
    to a decrease in level of consciousness
    related to skull fracture - epidural
    hematoma.*
    Short Term Goal:

    *Patient's level of consciousness will
    improve during hospitalization.*

    Implementation:
    *Assess and monitor neurological vital signs
    and neurological assessment.*

*Promote nursing measures to reduce
intracranial pressure.
*Assess & monitor homeostatic balance:
   Body fluids
   Electrolyte
   Acid base levels
*Provide environment to promote patient
safety.

Evaluation:

Patient experienced progressive decrease
in level of consciousness.
Epidural hematoma evacuated.
Patient level of consciousness improving -
recovery normal.

Nursing Diagnosis:

2. Alteration in family process secondary to
   diagnosis of epidural hematoma and rapid
   nature of life-threatening treatment.
   Short Term Goal: Family will verbalize
   awareness and knowledge of all plans for
   nursing care and treatment modalities.

Implementation:
* Assess family level of understanding of
  son's neurological diagnosis.
* Assess and identify family coping
  mechanisms and strengths.
* Include family in plan of care and discuss
  daily all pertinent information with
  opportunity for questions.
* Encourage participation in family support
  group.

Evaluation: Family verbalizing adequate
understanding and actively participating
in family support group.

Sample Case Report: Medical Model

This report is presented as a sample of a complete writeup of a patient's history and physical examination. It incorporates all of the elements of the data base expected from our students in a suggested order and format. As recommended throughout, the recording makes minimal use of the terms *negative* or *normal* but emphasizes, by use of specific entries, what information was sought on history, and what was observed or tested in the examination.

The patient's history in this example incorporates several problems. The physical findings, however, have been extracted from the sections entitled "Recording" in the chapters on physical examination and are, therefore, all within normal limits. The order of the reporting varies slightly from that of the text and is presented here in a more convenient order.

BASIC DATA

Mrs. J.H.A.   Date of Examination
1234 Middleville Road
Stony Brook, N.Y.
Date of Birth: 9/24/1941, Washington, D.C.
Source: Patient; history seems reliable

HISTORY

CC: "headache for 20 yr"

PI: Mrs. A. had only infrequent headaches through childhood and adolescence, but beginning at about age 25 (2 yr after her marriage) she noted the beginning of a right-sided temporal headache which at first seemed to be present once or twice a year, particularly in hot weather. For the past 4 yr she has had these headaches at 2-3 mo intervals, but for the past week has had nearly daily bouts which have become much more severe, accounting for her visit to the office today.

Characteristically, the headache begins as a spot of pain on her right temple, becomes penetrating and seems to bore right into her skull. Within a 2-3 min period the pain spreads to the whole right side of her face and neck. The headaches vary in severity from moderate to so severe that Mrs. A. must stop what she is doing to lie down. She has vertigo with severe headache only. Usually they last from 2-3 hr. She knows of nothing that will bring on or relieve an attack although she is aware of the fact that they usually occur after 2 or 3 p.m. and do not awaken her at night. She has had anorexia and nausea with severe attacks but has never vomited. She has seen no "flashes" or "sparks" prior to or during these attacks.

A brother, aged 40, has had a similar problem which is under treatment as migraine. Her case was considered by her brother's doctor (J.P.M_____, M.D.) *not* to be migraine and she was given some tablets (type unknown) last year which did no good since her attacks were generally over within 3 hours whether she took the tablets or not. Now takes three aspirin tablets at onset of headache. She had an EEG as part of her workup which was said to be normal.

Past History

Medical: Pneumonia, right 1960; duodenal ulcer 1980; no difficulty in past 5 yr

Surgical: Appendectomy 1961; no sequelae

Injuries: None

Allergies: Penicillin, manifested by drug fever and urticaria — 1960; none known to foods, other drugs, pollens, or contact materials

Immunizations: Smallpox, typhoid, and one other (type unknown) before going abroad in 1969

Current medication: None other than in PI

REVIEW OF SYSTEMS

General: Overall state of health is good; no major weight changes; can carry out normal ADL except when headache is severe

Integument: No eruptions, rashes except for urticaria (see PH); no disorders of hair or nails

Head: See PI; no history of trauma

Eyes: No vision problems; wears glasses past 5 yr only for reading; no diplopia; no eye exam for past 5 yr

Ears: Normal hearing, no tinnitus, no infections

Nose: No epistaxis, discharge, or sinusitis

Mouth, teeth, gums: Visits dentist 2x/yr; no major problems

Throat and neck: Infrequent sore throat, no neck stiffness or pain, no hoarseness

Breasts: No masses, discharge, bleeing

Resp.: No wheeze, cough, SOB; has colds about 3x/yr; no Rx other than aspirin; last x-ray 1 yr ago — neg.

CV: No chest pain, palpitation, hypertension, or vascular problems

GI: Appetite good; one BM every day; no jaundice; ulcer (see PH) requires no Rx; no nausea — except as in PI

GU: No dysuria, hematuria, nocturia, VD

GYN: Grav 0 para 0; no contraception; no reason known for lack of conception; onset menses age 12, q. 25-28 days; LMP 5 days ago; no dysmenorrhea; Pap smear done 6 mo ago at routine checkup — negative

Musc.: No weakness, joint pains, cramps

NP: No syncope, vertigo (except with severe headache — see PI), dizziness; intelligent and well-oriented in 3 spheres; sensorium intact; no paresthesias; affect seems good but there is a sense of rigidity and "perfection seeking" about her responses which seems inconsistent with her attempt to be friendly and helpful; no apparent depression

Lymph-hemat: No adenopathy, bleeding disorders

Endocrine: Prefers cold weather, but is tolerant of heat; no glycosuria, polydipsia, excessive sweating

FAMILY HISTORY

M. died at age 67 — heart attack

F. died at age 70 — pulmonary embolism

1 sister d. age 3 mo of congenital heart dis

1 brother in good health except for headaches (see PI)

No history of diabetes, cancer, hypertension, or other familial disease

ACTIVITIES OF DAILY LIVING

Occupation: Real estate salesperson — 15 yr; hours vary so has little time for recreation; combined family income adequate

Recreation: Little to none; occasional swimming

Diet (24-hour recall):

Time	Food/Fluid	Approx. Amount
8 a.m.	Juice	4 oz
	Toast	1 slice
	Coffee (milk & sugar)	1 C
11 a.m.	Coffee (milk & sugar)	1 C
1 p.m.	Roast beef sandwich;	
	vegetable soup;	1 C
	tea	1 C
4 p.m.	Fruit salad	1 C
7 p.m.	Pork chops	2
	Mixed vegetables	1 C
	Baked potato	1
	Tossed green salad	Small bowl
	Chocolate cake	1 slice
	Coffee (milk & sugar)	1 C

Habits: Does not touch alcohol, cigarettes; no over-the-counter drugs except aspirin (see PI)

Geographic: Has lived on Long Island all her life; travelled to Europe once with husband in 1969; did not like it

Marit/sexual: preferred not to discuss since she sees gynecologist regularly

Interpersonal relationships: Lives with husband (postal worker); married 22 years — unwilling to discuss relationship; would like to open her own business but husband does not support the idea; has friends at work; socializes only occasionally

Intrapersonal functioning: Says she is satisfied with limited social and recreational activity as she works hard and needs rest; yet has indicated wish for own business in real estate "where I can prove myself"; recognizes that she is rigid and highly self-controlled.

PATIENT PROFILE

This is a pleasant but highly rigid, self-controlled woman who seems unhappy but denies problems, who has no apparent financial or social difficulties. Lives with her husband.

PHYSICAL EXAMINATION

Vital signs and measurements:

Ht: 163 cm (5'4")
Wt: 63.6 kg (140 lb)
Temp: 37° C (98.6°F) oral
Pulse: 80 reg.
Resp: 16 reg.
BP RA: 135/80
  LA: 130/80 supine
  LA: 130/80 upright

General: Mrs. A. is an alert, well-developed, moderately obese, 45-year-old white woman appearing about stated age in no acute distress; no speech defects

Skin: Pink; good turgor; warm; no excoriations or lesions

Hair: Normal distribution and consistency

Nails: No deformities, nail beds pink, no clubbing

Head: Symmetrical, normocephalic; normal hair distribution

Face: No muscle weakness; appropriate facial expression; light touch intact

Eyes: Lashes and brows present; no stare or ptosis; normal ocular tension; conjunctivae clear; sclerae white; no defects of cornea or iris; pupils equal, round, react to light and accommodation (PERRLA); Snellen 20/20 OD, 20/20 OS; color intact for red green; fields normal by confrontation; extraocular movements (EOM) normal, no nystagmus or strabismus

Fundi: Red reflex: Clear

   Discs: Flat with sharp margins; cup normal

   Vessels: Arterioles and venules normal; no AV nicking

   Retina: No hemorrhage or exudates; macula normal, foveal reflex present

Ears: No masses, lesions of auricles or canals; no discharge; both TM pearly gray, no perforations, light reflex present; watch ticking heard bilaterally; Weber test, normal

Nose: Patent bilaterally; no septal deviation or perforation; mucosa pink; can identify alcohol

Mouth: Can clench teeth; mucosa and gingivae pink, no lesions or masses; teeth in good repair; tongue protrudes in midline; no tremor

Pharynx: Mucosa pink, no lesions; tonsils absent; uvula rises in midline on phonation; gag reflex present, bilaterally

Neck: Full ROM; veins not distended; carotid pulsations equal and of good quality; thyroid not palpable; trachea in midline; no lymphadenopathy

Thorax:

   Insp: Symmetrical, full expansion equal bilaterally; AP diameter not increased

   Palp: No tenderness; no axillary adenopathy

Lungs:

Palp: Fremitus equal bilaterally

Perc: Lung fields resonant throughout

Ausc: Breath sounds normal; vocal sounds normal; no rales, rhonchi, rubs

Breasts: Symmetrical; contour and consistency appropriate for age and parity; no retraction or nipple discharge; no masses or tenderness

Heart:

Insp: No heave; apical impulse in 5th LICS medial to MCL

Palp: No heave, thrill or rib retraction

Perc: LBCD at MCL in 5th ICS

Ausc: Rate 80/min regular; sounds normal; S_2 (aort) > S_2 (pulm); S_2 split on inspiration; no murmurs, gallop, rubs

Abdomen:

Insp: Abdomen flat, no skin lesions, no hernia, no pulsations

Ausc: Normal bowel sounds q. 10 sec; no bruits

Palp: No tenderness or masses; spleen, kidneys not palpated, liver edge at costal margin, nontender

Perc: Normal abdominal tympany; liver 12 cm long

Back: Normal curvature, no spinal tenderness, no CVA tenderness

Extremities: No skin, hair, or nail abnormalities; full range of motion (ROM); normal gait; Romberg negative; muscle strength intact; no venous dilation; radial, femoral, dorsalis pedis, and post tibial pulses all palpable and equal; no lymphadenopathy

Genitalia:

External: Normal pubic hair, no labial swellings or lesions; normal clitoris; introitus admits two fingers; no urethral redness, swelling, or discharge; Skene's and Bartholin's not inflamed; perineum intact, no scars

Internal: Vagina: No bulging or masses, mucosa intact and pink

Uterus: Anterior, average size, regular shape, mobile, normal consistency

Cervix: Compatible with nullipara, posterior position, 0.5 cm erosion 3 o'clock

Adnexa: Tubes not palpated, ovaries not enlarged, slight tenderness

Cul-de-sac: No bulging, tenderness, or masses

Discharge: Clear, mucoid, 1+, no odor

Pap: To lab

Rectal: No external or internal hemorrhoids, no fissures or fistulae; sphincter tone good; no masses or tenderness; no stool or visible blood on glove

Neurologic:

Cerebral function: Alert and responsive, memory and orientation intact; appropriate behavior and speech

Cranial nerves:

I: Identifies alcohol

II: Vision 20/20 both eyes; color intact; visual fields by gross confrontation normal

III, IV, VI: EOM intact; no ptosis; no nystagmus; PERRLA

V: Sensory intact, jaw closure normal

VII: Facial muscles symmetrical; no weakness

VIII: Hearing intact; Weber no lateralization

IX-X: Swallowing and gag reflex intact; uvula in midline

XI: Head movement and shrug of shoulders normal

XII: Tongue protrudes in midline, no tremor

Cerebellar function: Finger to nose, heel to shin coordination intact; gait normal; Romberg neg.

Motor system: no atrophy, weakness, or tremor

Sensory system: Intact to light touch, vibration; pin-prick, hot-cold, deep pain not tested.

Reflexes

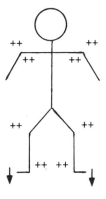

PROBLEMS

1. Headache — probably migraine
2. Sterility — patient or husband
3. Penicillin allergy
4. Inactive duodenal ulcer
5. Moderate obesity

_____

Signature

INITIAL NOTE

Problem: Headache

S: Headache for 20 yr. Began at about age 25 (2 yr after marriage). Characteristically begins as pain in right temple, spreads within minutes to right side of head and neck, lasting 2-3 hr. Pain is boring and seems to penetrate skull; occasionally requires her to stop work and lie down; had 4-5/yr but now almost daily; no known cause or relief; always afternoon; no scotomata, has nausea with severe attacks; one brother (age 40) has migraine.

O: Head, face, neck, ears, mouth, eyes, neurologic within normal limits.

A: The pain and attack features are characteristic of migraine. Pt. is tense, rigid, overly neat, which fits the typical personality pattern. Migraine in brother is also typical.

P: Dx: Per protocol, therapeutic trial of ergotamine, then referral to physician.

Rx: 2.0 mg ergotamine tartrate at start of attack, then repeat 2 mg at 30 min and again at 1 hr if necessary; Pt. will phone results.

Pt. Ed.: Schedule revisits to explain in more detail this syndrome and its relationships to behavior and interpersonal relationships. Pt. told that medication for longer term use (methysergide) may be useful, but that alteration of life patterns and behavior is required. Further counseling may be scheduled with psychologist or psychiatrist in future.

_____
Signature

Maternal-Child Health Care Index

Name: _____ Date: _____

EDC: _____ Hospital: _____ & Number: ____

The scoring system below attempts to categorize the degree of maternal and fetal risk based on the information available at the initial history and physical examination upon registration in our obstetric clinics. Please circle the numbers under each of the eight categories you feel apply and, at the bottom of this sheet, add up these numbers and subtract from a perfect score of 100.

I. Maternal age

Under 15	20
15-19	10
20-29	0
30-34	5
35-39	10
Over 40	20

II. Race and marital status

White	0
Nonwhite	5
Single	5
Married	0

III. Parity

0	10
1-3	0
4-7	5
Over 8	10

IV. Past obstetric history:

Abortions		Prematures		Fetal death	
1	5	1	10	1	10
3+	30	2+	20	2+	30

Neonatal death		Congenital anomaly		Damaged infants	
1	10	1	10	Physical	10
2+	30	2+	20	Neurologic	20

V. Medical-obstetric disorders and nutrition:

Systemic illnesses

Acute, mild	5
Acute, mild	15
Chronic, nondebilitating	5
Chronic, debilitating	20

Specific infections

Urinary:
Acute	5
Chronic	25

Syphilis:
Treated	0
Untreated	20
At term	30

Diabetes
Pre	30
Overt	30

Chronic
hypertension

Mild	15
Severe	30
Nephritis	30

Heart disease

Class I or II	10
Class III or IV	30
History prior failure	30

Endocrine disorders

Definite adrenal, pituitary, or thyroid problem	30
Recurrent menstrual dysfunction	10
Involuntary sterility:	
Less than 2 years	10
More than 2 years	20

Anemia

Hb, 10-11 g	5
Hb, 9-10 g	10
Hb, less than 9 g	20

Rh problem

Sensitized	30
Prior infant affected	30
Prior ABO incompatibility	20

Nutrition

Malnourished	20
Very obese	30
Inadequate diet but not malnourished	10

VI. Generative tract disorders

Prior fetal malpresentations		10
Prior cesarean section		30
Known anomaly or incompetent cervix		20
Myomas: Over 5 cm	20	
Submucous	30	

Contracted pelvis:
Borderline   10
Any contracted
plane   30
Ovarian masses: Over
6 cm   20
Endomet-
riosis   5

VII. Emotional survey (grade 0-20 based on):

Fears, attitudes, biases, hostilities, motivations, and behavioral patterns; prior pregnancies without supervision;
time of registration; standard of child care and responsibilities; family unit, marital relationship; history of
psychiatric illness in family

VIII. Social and economic survey (grade 0-10 based on):

Employment — husband, patient; annual income adequacy, public assistance; education — husband, patient;
housing — location, quality, facilities, and neighborhood
environment

Total score of all eight categories   _____

100 less above score equals MCH Care Index   _____

Nesbitt-Aubry scoring index to emphasize leading causes of
pregnancy risk and to identify those who should be assigned
to high-risk group. (Nesbitt REL, Aubry RH: *Am J Obstet
Gynecol* 1969;103:972, with permission.)

Clinical Estimation of Gestational Age

Examination First Hours

WEEKS GESTATION

PHYSICAL FINDINGS		20–27	28	29	30	31	32	33	34	35	36	37	38	39	40	41	42	43	44–48
Vernix		Appears	Covers body, thick layer										On back, scalp, in creases	Scant, in creases		No vernix			
Breast tissue and areola			Areola and nipple barely visible no palpable breast tissue						Areola raised		1–2 mm nodule		3–5 mm	5–6 mm	7–10 mm		≥12 mm		
Ear	Form	Flat, shapeless							Beginning incurving superior		Incurving upper 2/3 pinnae		Well-defined incurving to lobe						
	Cartilage	Pinna soft, stays folded						Cartilage scant, returns slowly from folding			Thin cartilage, springs back from folding			Pinna firm, remains erect from head					
Sole creases		Smooth soles without creases						1–2 anterior creases		2–3 anterior creases	Creases anterior 2/3 sole		Creases involving heel		Deeper creases over entire sole				
Skin	Thickness & appearance	Thin, translucent skin plethoric, venules over abdomen, edema						Smooth, thicker, no edema		Pink		Few vessels	Some desquamation pale pink		Thick, pale, desquamation over entire body				
	Nail plates	Appear		Appears on head		Nails to finger tips							Nails extend well beyond finger tips						
Hair		Appears		Eye brows and lashes		Fine, woolly, bunches out from head					Silky, single strands, lays flat				?Receding hairline or loss of baby hair, short, fine underneath				
Lanugo		Appears	Covers entire body					Vanishes from face			Present on shoulders		No lanugo						
Genitalia	Testes					Testes palpable in inguinal canal					In upper scrotum		In lower scrotum						
	Scrotum			Few rugae							Rugae, anterior portion		Rugae cover	Pendulous					
	Labia & clitoris			Prominent clitoris, labia majora small, widely separated							Labia majora larger, nearly cover clitoris		Labia minora and clitoris covered						
Skull firmness		Bones are soft			Soft to 1" from anterior fontanelle					Spongy at edges of fontanelle, center firm		Bones hard, sutures easily displaced		Bones hard, cannot be displaced					
Posture	Resting	Hypotonic, lateral decubitus		Hypotonic		Beginning flexion, thigh	Stronger hip flexion		Frog-like		Flexion, all limbs		Hypertonic		Very hypertonic				
	Recoil leg	No recoil					Partial recoil				Prompt recoil								
	Arm	No recoil						Begin flexion, no recoil			Prompt recoil, may be inhibited		Prompt recoil, may be Prompt recoil after 30" inhibition						

Modified from Lubchenco LO: *Pediatr. Clin. North. Am.* 1970;17:125.

582   Guide to Patient Evaluation

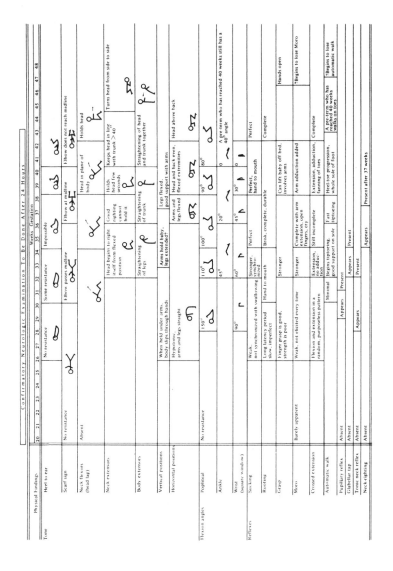

Reproduced with permission from Kempe CH, Silver HK,
O'Brien D (eds): *Current Pediatric Diagnosis and Treatment,*
ed 6, Los Altos, California, Lange Medical Publications,
1980.

Denver Developmental Screening Test

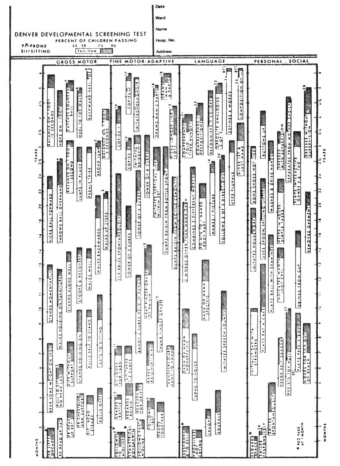

Courtesy of William K. Frankenburg, M.D., and Josiah B. Dodds, Ph. D., University of Colorado Medical Center, copyright 1969. Reproduced with permission.

1. Try to get child to smile by smiling, talking or waving to him. Do not touch him.
2. When child is playing with toy, pull it away from him. Pass if he resists.
3. Child does not have to be able to tie shoes or button in the back.
4. Move yarn slowly in an arc from one side to the other, about 6" above child's face. Pass if eyes follow 90° to midline. (Past midline; 180°)
5. Pass if child grasps rattle when it is touched to the backs or tips of fingers.
6. Pass if child continues to look where yarn disappeared or tries to see where it went. Yarn should be dropped quickly from sight from tester's hand without arm movement.
7. Pass if child picks up raisin with any part of thumb and a finger.
8. Pass if child picks up raisin with the ends of thumb and index finger using an overhand approach.

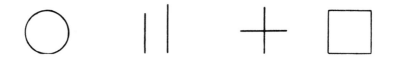

9. Pass any enclosed form. Fail continuous round motions
10. Which line is longer? (Not bigger.) Turn paper upside down and repeat. (3/3 or 5/6)
11. Pass any crossing lines.
12. Have child copy first. If failed, demonstrate.

When giving items 9, 11 and 12, do not name the forms. Do not demonstrate 9 and 11.
13. When scoring, each pair (2 arms, 2 legs, etc.) counts as one part.

14. Point to picture and have child name it. (No credit is given for sounds only.)

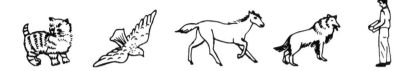

15. Tell child to: Give block to Mommie; put block on table; put block on floor. Pass 2 of 3. (Do not help child by pointing, moving head or eyes.)
16. Ask child: What do you do when you are cold? . . . hungry? . . . tired? Pass 2 of 3.
17. Tell child to: Put block *on* table; *under* table; *in front* of chair; *behind* chair. Pass 3 of 4. (Do not help child by pointing, moving head or eyes.)
18. Ask child: If fire is hot, ice is ?; Mother is a woman, Dad is a ?; a horse is big, a mouse is ? Pass 2 of 3.
19. Ask child: What is a ball? . . lake? . . desk? . . house? . . banana? . . curtain? . . ceiling? . . hedge? . . pavement? Pass if defined in terms of use, shape, what it is made of or general category (such as banana is fruit, not just yellow). Pass 6 of 9.
20. Ask child: What is a spoon made of? . . a shoe made of? . . a door made of? (No other objects may be substituted.) Pass 3 of 3.
21. When placed on stomach, child lifts chest off table with support of forearms and/or hands.
22. When child is on back, grasp his hands and pull him to sitting. Pass if head does not hang back.
23. Child may use wall or rail only, not person. May not crawl.
24. Child must throw ball overhead 3 feet to within arm's reach of tester.
25. Child must perform standing broad jump over width of test sheet. (8-1/2 in.)
26. Tell child to walk forward, heel within 1 inch of toe. Tester may demonstrate. Child must walk 4 consecutive steps, 2 out of 3 trials.

27. Bounce ball to child who should stand 3 feet away from tester. Child must catch ball with hands, not arms, 2 out of 3 trials.
28. Tell child to walk backward, to within 1 inch of heel. Tester may demonstrate. Child must walk 4 consecutive steps, 2 out of 3 trials.

DATE AND BEHAVIORAL OBSERVATIONS (how child feels at time of test, relation to tester, attention span, verbal behavior, self-confidence, etc.):

Growth and Development Charts

PERCENTILE CHART FOR MEASUREMENTS OF INFANT BOYS

THIS CHART provides for infant boys standards of reference for body weight and recumbent length by month from birth to 28 months and for head circumference by week from birth to 28 weeks. It is based upon repeated measurements at selected ages of a group of more than 100 white infants of North European ancestry living under normal conditions of health and home life in Boston, Mass. The distribution of the measurements obtained from the infants at each age is expressed in percentiles, each percentile giving a value which represents a particular position in the normal range of occurrences. The number of the percentile refers to the position which a measurement of the given value would hold in any typical series of 100 infants. Thus, the 10th percentile gives the value for the tenth in any hundred; that is, 9 infants of the same sex and age would be expected to be smaller in the measurement under consideration while 90 would be expected to be larger than the figure given. Similarly the 90th percentile would indicate that 89 infants might be expected to be smaller than the figure given while 10 would be larger. The 50th percentile represents the median or midposition in the customary range. Here, the 10th and 90th percentiles are presented in heavy lines to show the limits within which most infants remain. The lighter lines in the graphs divide the distributions into segments for ready recognition and description of individual differences as well as of the "regularity" of progress. The 3rd and 97th percentiles represent unusual though not necessarily abnormal findings.

In line with common usage in the United States, the charts are ruled on a scale in pounds to represent weight. They are ruled, however, in centimeters to represent length and head circumference, because this scale facilitates accuracy in measuring and recording and centimeter rules and tapes are readily available. For the convenience of those preferring them, scales for kilograms and inches are placed outside of the principal scales and paralleling them. Therefore, if weights are taken in kilograms and lengths and head circumferences in inches, they may be plotted directly without conversion by placing a ruler at the appropriate points on the outer scales of the charts.

To determine the percentile position of any measurement at a given age, the vertical age line is located and a dot is placed where this intersects the horizontal line representing the value obtained from the measurement. Vertical lines give age by one-month intervals for weight and length and one-week intervals for head circumference; horizontal lines give ½-pound, 1-cm. and 0.5-cm. intervals respectively. This permits by interpolation accurate placement for age to weeks, for weights to 2 ounces and for centimeters to 0.5 cm. Recognition of the position within or outside of the range held by an infant in respect to each measurement recorded calls attention to the relative size and build of the individual at the time. More importantly, comparisons of percentile positions held by these measurements at repeated periodic examinations indicate adherence to or possibly significant deviation from previous percentile positions. Under normal circumstances, one expects an infant to maintain a similar position from age to age — that is, on or near one percentile line or between the same two lines. Occasional sharp deviations or gradual but continuing shifts from one percentile position to another call for further investigation as to their causes. In all cases, readings of measurements should be checked and care should be taken to secure the same position of the infant at all examinations. The following procedures were used in obtaining these norms and therefore are recommended:

Body Weight — The infant is weighed without clothing, preferably on special infant scales.

Recumbent Length — The infant lies relaxed on a firm surface parallel to a centimeter rule or on a special infant measuring board which permits the following procedure. The soles of the feet are held firmly against a fixed upright at the zero mark on the rule, and a movable square is brought firmly against the vertex. Care must be taken to secure extension at the knees, and the head should be held so that the eyes face the ceiling.

Head Circumference — This measurement is more satisfactory if taken with the infant lying on his back. The tape is passed around the head from above and placed anteriorly over the lower forehead just above the supraorbital ridges. With the position of the tape thus fixed anteriorly, the largest circumference is obtained by passing it posteriorly over the most prominent part of the occiput.

To obtain original copies of the following Anthropometric charts, please write to MEDIFORM SYSTEMS, 32 Jameson Road, Newton, Massachusetts 02158

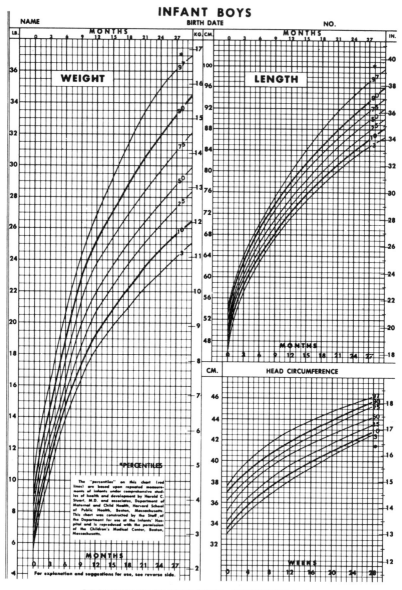

THE CHILDREN'S MEDICAL CENTER, BOSTON - ANTHROPOMETRIC CHART

PERCENTILE CHART FOR MEASUREMENTS OF BOYS

THIS CHART provides for boys standards of reference for body weight and recumbent length at ages between 2 and 6 years and for weight and standing height from 6 to 13 years. It is based upon repeated measurements at selected ages of a group of more than 100 white boys of North European ancestry living under normal conditions of health and home life in Boston, Mass. The distribution of the measurements obtained from these children at each age is expressed in percentiles, each percentile giving a value which represents a particular position in the normal range of occurrences. The number of the percentile refers to the position which a measurement of the given value would hold in any typical series of 100 children. Thus, the 10th percentile gives the value for the tenth in any hundred; that is, 9 children of the same sex and age would be expected to be smaller in the measurement under consideration while 90 would be expected to be larger than the figure given. Similarly the 90th percentile would indicate that 89 children might be expected to be smaller than the figure given while 10 would be larger. The 50th percentile represents the median or midposition in the customary range. Here, the 10th and 90th percentiles are represented in heavy lines to show the limits within which most children remain. The lighter lines in the graphs divide the distribution into segments for ready recognition and description of individual differences as well as of the "regularity" of progress. The 3rd and 97th percentiles represent unusual though not necessarily abnormal findings.

In line with common usage in the United States, the charts are ruled on a scale in pounds to represent weight. They are ruled, however, in centimeters to represent length under 6 years and height thereafter, because this scale facilitates accuracy in measuring and recording and centimeter rules and tapes are readily available. For the convenience of those preferring them, scales for kilograms and inches are placed outside of the principal scales and paralleling them. Therefore, if weights are taken in kilograms and lengths and heights in inches, they may be plotted directly without conversion by placing a ruler at the appropriate points on the outer scales of the chart.

To determine the percentile position of any measurement at a given age, the vertical age line is located and a dot is placed where this intersects the horizontal line representing the value obtained from the measurement. Vertical lines give age by 2-month intervals and horizontal lines by 2-pound and 2-cm. intervals. This permits by interpolation accurate placement for age to ½ month and for measurements to ½ pound or 0.5 cm. Recognition of the position held by a child within or outside of the range in respect to each measurement recorded calls attention to the relative size and build of the individual at the time. More importantly, comparisons of percentile positions held by these measurements at repeated periodic examinations indicate adherence to or possibly significant deviation from previous percentile positions. Under normal circumstances, one expects a child to maintain a similar position from age to age — that is, on or near one percentile line or between the same two lines. Occasionally encountered sharp deviations or more gradual but continuing shifts from one percentile position to another call for further investigation as to their causes. In all cases, readings of measurements should be checked and care should be taken to secure the same position of the child accurately at all examinations. The following procedures were used in obtaining these norms and therefore are recommended:

Body Weight — The child is weighed without clothing except light undergarments.

Recumbent Length — The child lies relaxed on a firm surface parallel to a centimeter rule. The soles of the feet are held firmly against a fixed upright at the zero mark on the rule, and a movable square is brought firmly against the vertex. The head is held so that the eyes face the ceiling.

Height — The child's heels should be near together, and heels, buttocks and occiput should be against a firm vertical upright mounting the measuring stick. The eyes should be horizontal and approximately in the same plane as the external auditory canals. A right angle triangle or other movable device should be placed firmly on the head at right angles to the measuring stick and the measurement read after a satisfactory position has been adopted.

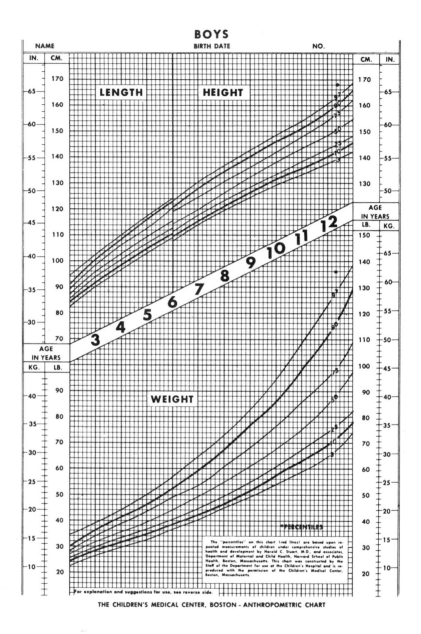

BOYS

NAME   BIRTH DATE   NO.

LENGTH   HEIGHT

WEIGHT

PERCENTILES

The "percentiles" on this chart (red lines) are based upon repeated measurements of children under comprehensive studies of health and development by Harold C. Stuart, M.D. and associates, Department of Maternal and Child Health, Harvard School of Public Health, Boston, Massachusetts. This chart was constructed by the Staff of the Department for use at the Children's Hospital and is reproduced with the permission of the Children's Medical Center, Boston, Massachusetts.

For explanation and suggestions for use, see reverse side.

THE CHILDREN'S MEDICAL CENTER, BOSTON - ANTHROPOMETRIC CHART

PERCENTILE CHART FOR MEASUREMENTS OF INFANT GIRLS

THIS CHART provides for infant girls standards of reference for body weight and recumbent length by month from birth to 28 months and for head circumference by week from birth to 28 weeks. It is based upon repeated measurements at selected ages of a group of more than 100 white infants of North European ancestry living under normal conditions of health and home life in Boston, Mass. The distribution of the measurements obtained from the infants at each age is expressed in percentiles; each percentile giving a value which represents a particular position in the normal range of occurrences. The number of the percentile refers to the position which a measurement of the given value would hold in any typical series of 100 infants. Thus, the 10th percentile gives the value for the tenth in any hundred; that is, 9 infants of the same sex and age would be expected to be smaller in the measurement under consideration while 90 would be expected to be larger than the figure given. Similarly the 90th percentile would indicate that 89 infants might be expected to be smaller than the figure given while 10 would be larger. The 50th percentile represents the median or midposition in the customary range. Here, the 10th and 90th percentiles are presented in heavy lines to show the limits within which most infants remain. The lighter lines in the graphs divide the distributions into segments for ready recognition and description of individual differences as well as of the "regularity" of progress. The 3rd and 97th percentiles represent unusual though not necessarily abnormal findings.

In line with common usage in the United States, the charts are ruled on a scale in pounds to represent weight. They are ruled, however, in centimeters to represent length and head circumference, because this scale facilitates accuracy in measuring and recording and centimeter rules and tapes are readily available. For the convenience of those preferring them, scales for kilograms and inches are placed outside of the principal scales and paralleling them. Therefore, if weights are taken in kilograms and lengths and head circumferences in inches, they may be plotted directly without conversion by placing a ruler at the appropriate points on the outer scales of the charts.

To determine the percentile position of any measurement at a given age, the vertical age line is located and a dot is placed where this intersects the horizontal line representing the value obtained from the measurement. Vertical lines give age by one-month intervals for weight and length and one-week intervals for head circumference; horizontal lines give ½-pound, 1-cm. and 0.5-cm. intervals respectively. This permits by interpolation accurate placement for age to weeks, for weights to 2 ounces and for centimeters to 0.5 cm. Recognition of the position within or outside of the range held by an infant in respect to each measurement recorded calls attention to the relative size and build of the individual at the time. More importantly, comparisons of percentile positions held by these measurements at repeated periodic examinations indicate adherence to or possibly significant deviation from previous percentile positions. Under normal circumstances, one expects an infant to maintain a similar position from age to age — that is, on or near one percentile line or between the same two lines. Occasional sharp deviations or gradual but continuing shifts from one percentile position to another call for further investigation as to their causes. In all cases, readings of measurements should be checked and care should be taken to secure the same position of the infant at all examinations. The following procedures are used in obtaining these norms and therefore are recommended:

Body Weight — The infant is weighed without clothing, preferably on special infant scales.

Recumbent Length — The infant lies relaxed on a firm surface parallel to a centimeter rule or on a special infant measuring board which permits the following procedure. The soles of the feet are held firmly against a fixed upright at the zero mark on the rule, and a movable square is brought firmly against the vertex. Care must be taken to secure extension at the knees, and the head should be held so that the eyes face the ceiling.

Head Circumference — This measurement is more satisfactory if taken with the infant lying on his back. The tape is passed around the head from above and placed anteriorly over the lower forehead just above the supraorbital ridges. With the position of the tape thus fixed anteriorly, the largest circumference is obtained by passing it posteriorly over the most prominent part of the occiput.

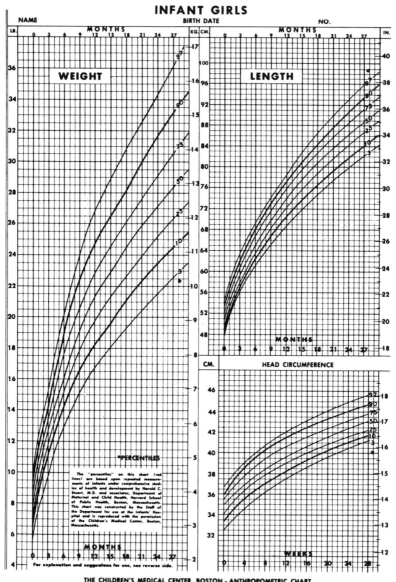

INFANT GIRLS

THE CHILDREN'S MEDICAL CENTER, BOSTON - ANTHROPOMETRIC CHART

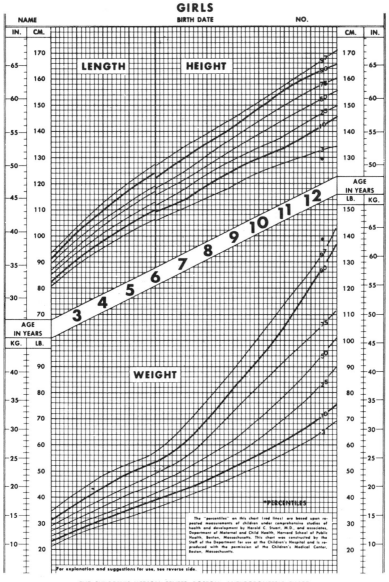

GIRLS

THE CHILDREN'S MEDICAL CENTER, BOSTON - ANTHROPOMETRIC CHART

PERCENTILE CHART FOR MEASUREMENTS OF GIRLS

THIS CHART provides for girls standards of reference for body weight and recumbent length at ages between 2 and 6 years and for weight and standing height from 6 to 13 years. It is based upon repeated measurements at selected ages of a group of more than 100 white girls of North European ancestry living under normal conditions of health and home life in Boston, Mass. The distribution of the measurements obtained from these children at each age is expressed in percentiles, each percentile giving a value which represents a particular position in the normal range of occurrences. The number of the percentile refers to the position which a measurement of the given value would hold in any typical series of 100 children. Thus, the 10th percentile gives the value for the tenth in any hundred; that is, 9 children of the same sex and age would be expected to be smaller in the measurement under consideration while 90 would be expected to be larger than the figure given. Similarly the 90th percentile would indicate that 89 children might be expected to be smaller than the figure given while 10 would be larger. The 50th percentile represents the median or midposition in the customary range. Here, the 10th and 90th percentiles are represented in heavy lines to show the limits within which most children remain. The lighter lines in the graphs divide the distribution into segments for ready recognition and description of individual differences as well as of the "regularity" of progress. The 3rd and 97th percentiles represent unusual though not necessarily abnormal findings.

In line with common usage in the United States, the charts are ruled on a scale in pounds to represent weight. They are ruled, however, in centimeters to represent length under 6 years and height thereafter, because this scale facilitates accuracy in measuring and recording and centimeter rules and tapes are readily available. For the convenience of those preferring them, scales for kilograms and inches are placed outside of the principal scales and paralleling them. Therefore, if weights are taken in kilograms and lengths and heights in inches, they may be plotted directly without conversion by placing a ruler at the appropriate points on the outer scales of the chart.

To determine the percentile position of any measurement at a given age, the vertical age line is located and a dot is placed where this intersects the horizontal line representing the value obtained from the measurement. Vertical lines give age by 2-month intervals and horizontal lines by 2-pound and 2-cm. intervals. This permits by interpolation accurate placement for age to ½ month and for measurements to ½ pound or 0.5 cm. Recognition of the position held by a child within or outside of the range in respect to each measurement recorded calls attention to the relative size and build of the individual at the time. More importantly, comparisons of percentile positions held by these measurements at repeated periodic examinations indicate adherence to or possibly significant deviation from previous percentile positions. Under normal circumstances, one expects a child to maintain a similar position from age to age — that is, on or near one percentile line or between the same two lines. Occasionally encountered sharp deviations or more gradual but continuing shifts from one percentile position to another call for further investigation as to their causes. In all cases, readings of measurements should be checked and care should be taken to secure the same position of the child accurately at all examinations. The following procedures were used in obtaining these norms and therefore are recommended:

Body Weight — The child is weighed without clothing except light undergarments.

Recumbent Length — The child lies relaxed on a firm surface parallel to a centimeter rule. The soles of the feet are held firmly against a fixed upright at the zero mark on the rule, and a movable square is brought firmly against the vertex. The head is held so that the eyes face the ceiling.

Height — The child's heels should be near together, and heels, buttocks and occiput should be against a firm vertical upright mounting the measuring stick. The eyes should be horizontal and approximately in the same plane as the external auditory canals. A right angle triangle or other movable device should be placed firmly on the head at right angles to the measuring stick and the measurement read after a satisfactory position has been adopted.

Child Health Data Base

I. Chief Complaint

   Brief statement of patient's reason for admission; use patient's or parents' own words.

II. Diagnosis/es

III. History of Present Illness

   To include:

   A. Preceding events to onset of illness
   B. Date of onset and initial signs and symptoms
   C. Duration and description of changes in course of illness from onset to present
   D. Factors which increase or decrease signs and symptoms
   E. Current status of illness
   F. Current medication and treatment regimen
   G. Sequential description of *other* current complaints or *illness not* related to present illness described in A through F

IV. Past Health History

   (When appropriate, include date of onset, duration, therapeutic regime, and outcome or residual)

   A. Childhood illnesses: Rubella, rubeola, mumps, chickenpox, frequent colds, sore throats, flu, pneumonia, ear infections, vomiting, diarrhea, seizures, constipation, bronchitis, exposed to any of the above during the last month

This child health data base is from Emory University, Nell Hodgson Woodruff School of Nursing, 1982, by permission.

B. Other illnesses: Rheumatic fever, diabetes, juvenile arthritis, scarlet fever, TB, heart disease and abnormalities, chorea, kidney disease, jaundice, hepatitis, meningitis, hypertension
C. Injuries: Accidents requiring stitches, fractures, dislocations, sprains, location of child at time of accident; burns, poisons, sequelae
D. Hospitalizations: Date, cause, duration, adjustment to hospitalization, treatment, outcome, operations, transfusions, reactions
E. Immunization status
F. Allergies: Food, hay fever, eczema, asthma, rashes, other, age of onset, describe reaction
G. Physical exam previous to admission: Date, handicaps, congenital abnormalities, special concerns
H. Maternal history
   1. Prenatal history
      a. Medical supervision
      b. Diet, nutrition
      c. Illnesses, infections, complications
      d. Medications taken during pregnancy
   Natal history of this child
   1. Length of gestation
   2. Course of labor and delivery
   3. Sedation/anesthesia required (cry immediately)?
   4. Birth weight, length, FOC
I. Development: How does child compare with sibs? latest development task; milestones (age attained): head control, roll from back to stomach, sitting without support, pulled up, crawling, walking without support, self-feeding, climbing, dress and undress self; does child need assistance with dressing, bathing, combing hair, brushing teeth? bladder control during day and night; bowel control, babbling, words, sentences of two to three words, speak well? teeth, age of eruption, number at 1 year
J. Medications at home: What taken, how much, how administered, what and how much is given for fever?
K. Prognosis: For present illness and parents/patient's awareness of

V. Family History

Draw pedigree, include close blood relatives (horizontal = marriage; vertical = descendant; male = ; female =). Record age, state of health, presence of any familial conditions for other family members, i.e., diabetes mellitus, cardiovascular disease (murmurs, rheumatic fever), TB, asthma, hay fever, hypertension, blood dyscrasia, pneumonia, sinus problems, glaucoma, cataracts, myopia, strabismus, ulcers, colitis, kidney or bladder infections, arthritis, muscular dystrophy, clubfoot, congenital dislocated hips, convulsions, mental retardation, epilepsy, mental problems, deafness, blindness, cancer, thyroid, congenital anomalies, any other medical problem in the family that the mother thinks is important

VI. Sociocultural

A. Birthplace
B. Residence duration for this city
C. Language spoken in home (primary, secondary, regional, dialect, slang)
D. Cultural pattern (subculture(s); traditions, superstitions)
E. Family: Role in; type — nuclear, extended, responsibilities; description of members — names, ages (include sibs), sex, roles; changes that have occurred recently in home — illness, births, deaths, etc. What sort of people do parents characterize themselves as being; pets
F. Recreational activities: Does family seem to be happy, chaotic, sad, depressed, violent, general relationships of family; activity they enjoy doing together; religious activities; type of play most enjoyed; favorite games and TV shows, books, radio programs, favorite toy — was it brought with child? hobbies, special interests; parent definition of play and how much importance is placed on it — as a family, with peers, with sibs; play area allotted for play
G. Occupation: Who in family employed; how employed; past, present, and description of
H. Family's economic status (rent/own home, apartment; income meets needs; receiving public assistance
I. Home environment (type dwelling, number of rooms, number of people residing there, specific housing problems, sleeping conditions, play areas)
J. Transportation
K. Education
   1. Parents: Level of education; attitude toward education

2. Child: Nursery school, day care, grade in school, district, grade appropriate? favorite teacher; best friend; grade average; performance; adjustment; problem areas; what like to do in school; social adjustment; special aptitudes; how get along with teachers; any problems with reading, speech, hearing, seeing in school

L. Current daily activities
   1. Usual activities prior to admission: 6 a.m.–6 p.m.
   2. Sleeping: Hours/night — bedtime — times — naps — times, hours snoring, restlessness, type of bed, night terrors or nightmares, awaken during night? enuresis, diapers, whom sleeps with, crib, bed with sides, adult bed; does child climb out of bed? special bedtime routine, security object

M. Significant persons or objects to child (in agency; in home)

N. Availability of family, what time of day and how often will parents be able to visit?

O. Safety: What medications and other poisons in the home and where kept

P. Public Health Nurse or clinic? Names

VII. Psychological Data

A. General appearance: Clothing, posture, hygiene
B. General facial and bodily expressions: Nonverbal; eye contact; activity, talkative, inquisitive, energetic, friendly, aggressive, hostile, dependent, independent, lethargic, apathetic, shy, clinging to mother, irritable, disturbed, anxious, alert, confused, hyperactive, animated, monotone, answers questions promptly or after delay
C. 1. Child's response to interviewer: Verbal response, emotional tone; Does child answer questions directed toward him or does mother answer for him?
   2. Parents' response to interview
D. Response to others in immediate environment
E. Communication patterns:
   1. Articulation: Any substitution, omission, distortion of sounds
   2. Language: Problems in understanding or using language, faulty sentence structure, grammatical errors, limited vocabulary

3. Rhythm: Repetition of sounds, words or phrases, hesitating, blocking
4. Voice: Hoarseness, breathiness, weak or loud voice, high- or low-pitched, voice with nasal quality
F. Orientation level: Time, place, person
G. Concept of time family: Past — present — future oriented
H. Response to current health status:
   1. Parents' response to current health status; understanding of illness/hospitalization
   2. Child's response to current health status; understanding of illness/hospitalization
   3. Expectation of parents in present health situation; of health team members; child
   4. Expectation of child in present health situation; of health team members; of self; of family
   5. Does child know he is being admitted?
   6. Does child have special fears about the hospital; needles; people in white, other?
   7. Child's reaction to life stresses, frightened, angry, worried; regarding success, failure; accepts variations in others? rigid, flexible, narrow-minded
I. Readiness and willingness to learn: Parent; child
J. Unusual behavior/habits: Thumbsucking (which thumb?), nail biting, breath holding, temper tantrums, tics, nervousness, masturbation, pacifier, head banging, pica, accident proneness, rocking, clumsiness
K. Discipline: When does child need to be disciplined, how often does it occur? What kind does he respond to? What does child do that is irritating? Gives good information on parenting skills?
L. How would parent describe child? talkative, energetic, inquisitive, aggressive, friendly, hostile, dependent, withdrawn, cautious, shy
M. How does child see himself: Good, bad, hateful, guilty, mean, shy, insecure, loving, secure, dependent
N. Body image

VIII. Review of Systems — History of:

   A. Physical competency
     1. Neonatal status — Apgar (obtain from chart), congenital abnormalities
     2. Postnatal course
     3. Developmental assessment
       a. Denver Developmental Screening Test or Washington Guide, or other (i.e., Piaget, Erikson)
       b. Recent weight gained or lost
   B. Integument: Hair, scalp, skin changes; pruritus, infection, lesions; scars; calluses
   C. HEENT
     1. Head: Pain[1]: All descriptions of pain regardless of which system involved should include:
       a. Location
       b. Onset
       c. Duration
       d. Characteristics
       e. Alleviating and worsening factors
     2. Eyes: Last vision exam; changes in vision; pain; infection; corrective lenses
     3. Ears: Last hearing exam; changes in hearing pain; infection; aides; tinnitus; itching; myringotomy; tubes
     4. Nose: Epistaxis; discharge; changes in ability to smell; sinus problem
     5. Mouth and throat: Gingivitis; last dental exam; infection; pain; dysphagia; frequency of colds; sore throat; mouth breathing; adenitis
   D. Cardiovascular
     1. Heart: Chest pain; SOB; palpations, murmurs, cyanosis; sweating; fatigue or exertion
     2. Vessels: Changes; pain; extremity numbness
     3. Hematopoietic: Anemia, abnormal bleeding, excessive bruising

[1] Neurosurgery abnormalities are frequently evidenced in other systems. If a neurologic abnormality has been noted in another system, i.e., lowered muscle strengths, lowered hearing, refer reader to appropriate system and avoid repetitious recording.

E. 1. Muscles: Abnormalities; changes in strength; pain; use; postural deformities
   2. Joints: Changes in mobility; pain; gait; co-ordination; exercise tolerance; braces
F. Neurosensory: Sensation changes, numbness; sensitivity to heat; cold; dizziness; fainting; convulsions
G. 1. Chest: Cough productive; sputum character-istics, orthopnea; dyspnea, infection; last chest x-ray; last TB test, hemoptysis, fre-quency of colds; sweat test
   2. Breast: Discharges from nipples, changes in size; contour symmetry
H. Abdomen: Changes in size; contour; pain
   1. Bowel pattern: Preadmission and current; bowel training; constipation; encopresis
   2. Digestion: Changes; nausea; vomiting; diarrhea
   3. Diet: Type; restrictions; food intolerance; food allergies; cultural influence
      Nutrition: Usual appetite (good, poor, varied)

      One day diet: breakfast
      (type and amount)   lunch
                           dinner
                           snacks

      Number of times/week eats meats _____ white

      or dark _____ vegetables _____ fruit _____

      milk _____ eggs: yolk _____ white _____

      sweets _____ types of snacks and when

      eaten _____ fluid

      preferences (juice preference) _____

      utensils used: spoon _____ fork _____

      knife _____ cup _____ bottle _____

Child feed self alone or need assistance; reaction of child to eating; idiosyncrasies, major formula changes; time of weaning, difficulties, vitamin supplements: type, amount, duration; food allergies, nighttime bottle; feeding routines of aids?

I. Genitourinary
1. Reproductive system:
    a. Female: Last menstrual period (LMP); menarche; contraception; last Pap smear; pain; vaginal bleeding; discharge; infections
    b. Male: Genital pain, discharge
2. Urinary system: Polyuria; dysuria; oliguria; hematuria; frequency of nocturia, bedwetting; terms for urination and bowel movement; bladder training

IX. Physical Assessment

A. Ht _____ _____%; wt _____ _____%; FOC _____ _____%;

arm circumference _____; chest circumference

_____ T _____ P _____ R _____

B. Integument (circle any and all appropriate)
Inspect: Color; lesions; scars; dermatitis, reddened areas; calluses, hygiene; mottling; temperature; vernix caseosa — present and if discolored; congenital skin anomalies and tumors; cysts or clefts, lanugo, milia, jaundice, pallor, erythema, lesions, texture, eruptions, hydration, edema, hermorrhagic manifestations, and nevi, Mongolian (blue black) spots, pigmentation, turgor, elasticity, and subcutaneous nodules; striae, wrinkling, sensitivity; hair distribution, and desquamation, texture, parasites
C. HEENT
Inspect:
Face: Color, cosmetics, complexion.

Head: Molding and shape, fontanels and suture
lines, bosses, craniotabes, caput succedaneum,
cephalhematoma, dermal sinuses, FOC/chest ratio,
dilated veins, control
Eyes: Pupils — equal, round, react to light; iris —
color, shape; use of eyebrows; lids; excessive
tearing; exudate; opacity, sclera; conjunctivae;
photophobia; Brushfield spots, nystagmus, Mongolian slant, epicanthic folds
Ears: External ear — brachial cleft, cysts, sinuses,
evidence of hearing problem, exudate, swelling,
position of head for hearing, pulling at ears, pain,
canals, tympanic membranes
Nose: Nares — flaring; discharge; shape; mucosa,
patency, pressure over sinuses
Lips: Color, condition, lesions, cleft
Mouth: Breath, odor, lesions, dental caries, problems with mastication, number of teeth, gingiva —
presence of tooth buds; malocclusion, notching,
tongue, hard and soft palates, uvula, sucking, pads,
Epstein pearls
Throat: Ability to swallow; pharynx; tonsils;
voice hoarseness, stridar, grunting, character of
cry
Neck: Length, mobility, webbing distended veins,
position (torticollis, opisthotonos)
D. Cardiovascular
Inspect: Nail bed — color; bruises, puncture
wounds, edema; varicosities; neck vein distention
Palpate: Pulse — rate, rhythm, volume, peripheral
pulses, BP; extremities — temperature; capillary
refill nail bed
Auscultate: Heart sounds — S_1 S_2 — apical pulse;
murmurs, rate, rhythm, force, quality of sounds
E. Musculoskeletal
Inspect: Bilateral strength — extremities: muscular development and tone, paralysis, dexterity;
movement characteristics, gait, posture, asymmetry, right or left handed; obvious deformities,
palmar creases, edema, spinal bifida, tufts of hair,
dimple or cyst
Palpate: Joints (range of motion); limitations;
temperature; tenderness, hip abduction
Palpate: Spine straightness, tenderness

F. Neurosensory
    Inspect: Orientation — time, place, person; asso-
    ciative functions — speech, writes, reads; level of
    consciousness; judgment; temperature _____F;
    seizures; reflexes — Moro, palmar, plantar grasp,
    suck, rooting, startle, tonic neck, Babinski, para-
    chute stepping

G. Chest
    Inspect: Respirations — rate, rhythm, depth; spu-
    tum characteristics, audible wheezing, retractions
    xyphoid, subcostal, intercostal
    Inspect: Breast size, contour, symmetry
    Palpate: Rib tenderness; PMI; location, intensity
    Auscultate: Breath sounds — clear vs. noisy,
    wheezing

H. Abdomen
    Inspect: Size; contour; symmetry; visible peri-
    stalsis; scars; wounds describe size, location,
    drainage — color, amount, odor; umbilicus abnor-
    mal staining, oozing of blood, redness around cord,
    pulsations; inspect for inguinal hernia
    Auscultate: Bowel sounds — presence or absence
    of

I. Genitourinary
    Inspect: Intake and output (I and O) for character-
    istics, volume/observation duration; urine — color,
    odor, blood, incontinence, catheter-type; normalcy
    of external genitalia; discharge bleeding
    1. Male: Circumcision, meatal opening, hypo-
       spadias, phimosis, adherent foreskin, size of
       testes, cryptorchidism, scrotum, hydrocele,
       hernia, pubertal changes
    2. Female: Vagina, discharges, adhesions, hyper-
       trophy of clitoris, pubertal changes
    Palpate: Bladder distention, scrotum and testes,
    edema

J. Rectum and anus
    Inspect: Anus for structure, sphincter tone, irrita-
    tion, fissures, prolapse, imperforate anus

2Describe any body excretions for: amount, color, consistency,
odor.

X.   Laboratory Findings
     Record relevant laboratory data (i.e., CBC, ECG, EEG,
     lead, sickle cell, chest x-ray, electrolysis, blood sugar)

XI. Results of Screening Test
     1. DDST
     2. Visual acuity (Snellen)
     3. Age and performance guideline
     4. Etc.

Normal Laboratory Values of Common Tests

These tables represent normal values for some commonly used laboratory tests. They are collected from several sources (references 1, 2, 3, and 6), and are therefore "average normals." It must be remembered that the normal range for one laboratory will be approximate, but not necessarily identical, to that of another laboratory. The tables include some commonly used tests with average values for adults being listed. The dynamic changes taking place in infants and children make it necessary to learn a separate set of normal values for these age groups. References 4 and 5 should be consulted if the student is interested in values for the pediatric patient population.

A. Abbreviations (for singular and plural use)
  1. General
U	=	unit
IU	=	international unit
Vol	=	volume
%	=	percent; per hundred
<	=	less than
>	=	more than; greater than
Hg	=	mercury
m	=	milli- (prefix for one thousandth; 1×10^{-3})
μ	=	micro- (prefix for one millionth; 1×10^{-6})
p	=	pico- (prefix for one trillionth; 1×10^{-12})
k	=	kilo- (prefix for 1000)

  2. Weight units
g	=	gram
kg	=	kilogram
mg	=	milligram
pg	=	picogram
μg	=	microgram
Eq	=	equivalent
mEq	=	milliequivalent

607

3. Volume units
    L   =   liter
    ml   =   milliliter
    cc   =   cubic centimeter (equivalent to ml)
    cumm=   cubic millimeter
4. Units of length
    m   =   meter
    mm   =   millimeter
    μ   =   micron
5. Pressure units
    mmHg=   millimeter of mercury
    Osm =   osmol
    mOsm=   milliosmol

B. Normal Values, Adults
    1. Blood
        Red blood cell count (RBC)
            Men   4.2-5.9 million/cu mm
            Women   4.2-5.4 million/cu mm
        Reticulocyte count 0.5-2.5% of total RBC
        White blood cell count (WBC) 4500-11,000/cu mm
            Differential count
                Segmented neutrophils   54-62%
                Bands   0-5%
                Lymphocytes   25-40%
                Monocytes   2-7%
                Eosinophils   1-3%
                Basophils   0-1%
        Platelets   150,000-350,000/cu mm
        Hemoglobin (Hb)
            Men   14-18 g/100 ml
            Women   12-16 g/100 ml
        Hematocrit (Hct) (also called packed cell volume,
        PCV)
            Men   45-52% of whole blood
            Women   37-47% of whole blood
        Iron (serum)   50-150 μg/100 ml
        Iron binding capacity (TIBC)   250-400 μg/100 ml
        Red blood cell indices
            Mean corpuscular volume (MCV) 86-98 cu μ
            Mean corpuscular hemoglobin (MCH) 27-31 pg
            Mean corpuscular hemoglobin
                concentration (MCHC)   32-36%

Erythrocyte sedimentation rate (ESR)
  Wintrobe technique
    Men   0-5 mm/hr
    Women   0-15 mm/hr
  Westergren technique
    Men   0-15 mm/hr
    Women   0-20 mm/hr
  Coombs' test, direct   Negative
  Coombs' test, indirect Negative
2. Blood coagulation
  Bleeding time (Duke)   1-5 min
  Bleeding time (Ivy) <   5 min
  Clot retraction time — begins 30 min-1 hr
                  completed < 24 hr
  Coagulation time (Lee-White)   5-15 min
  Partial thromboplastin time (PTT)   35-60 sec
  Prothrombin time (PT)   12-14 sec
3. Liver function
  Ammonia   12-55 μ mol/L
  Bilirubin
    Direct   0.1-0.4 mg/100 ml
    Indirect   0.2-0.6 mg/100 ml
    Total   0.3-1.0 mg/100 ml
  Bromsulphalein (BSP)   < 5% retained in 45 min
  Enzymes
    Alkaline phosphatase
                5-13   King-Armstrong U
                0.8-2.3 Bessey-Lowry U
    Gamma glutamyl transpeptidase
      (GGTP)   2-30 mU/ml
    Glutamic oxaloacetic
      transaminase (GOT) 7-27 Karmen U/ml
    Glutamic pyruvic
      transaminase (GPT) 1-21 U/ml
    Lactic dehydrogenase (LDH)
      150-450 Wroblewski U
    5' Nucleotidase 1-11 U/L (Arkesteijn)
  Serum proteins
    Albumin   3.5-5.0 g/100 ml
    Globulins   2.3-3.5 g/100 ml
    Total   6.0-8.4 g/100 ml

4. Cardiac enzymes
Creatinine phosphokinase (CPK)   0-50 mU/ml
Lactic dehydrogenase (LDH)   45-90 U/L
Glutamic oxaloacetic
transaminase (GOT)   7.0-27.0 Karmen U/ml

5. Pancreatic enzymes
Amylase (serum)   4-25 U/ml
Amylase (urine)   35-250 Somogyi U/hr
(urine)   800-5000 Somogyi U/24 hr
Lipase (serum)   0-2.0 Cherry-Crandall U

6. Cerebrospinal fluid (CSF)
Cells   < 5/cu mm
Chloride   120-130 mEq/L
Glucose   50-75 mg/100 ml
Protein   15-50 mg/100 ml

7. Urine

Specific gravity (SG)	1.003-1.030
pH	4.6-8.0
Glucose	< 250 mg/24 hr
Protein	10-150 mg/24 hr
Creatinine	15-25 mg/kg body weight/24 hr
Osmolality	38-1400 mOsm/kg water

8. Respiratory/blood gases

Bicarbonate (plasma)	21-28 mEq/L
CO_2 content (serum)	25-30 mEq/L
CO_2 pressure (pCO_2)	35-45 mm Hg
Oxygen pressure (pO_2)	75-100 mm Hg
Oxygen saturation (arterial)	96-100%
pH (arterial)	7.35-7.45

9. Miscellaneous blood chemistry
Cholesterol   120-220 mg/100 ml
Creatinine   0.6-1.5 mg/100 ml
Electrolytes, serum

Cations

Sodium	140 mEq/L
Potassium	4 mEq/L
Calcium	5 mEq/L
Magnesium	2 mEq/L
	151 mEq/L

Anions

Bicarbonate	25 mEq/L
Chloride	103 mEq/L
Proteins	14 mEq/L
Organic Acid	9 mEq/L
	151 mEq/L

Glucose (fasting)	70-110 mg/100ml
Insulin (immunoassay)	6-26 μIU/ml (fasting)
Phosphatase, acid	1.5-4.5 Bodansky U
	0.8-2.3 Bessey-Lowry U
Triglycerides	40-150 mg/100 ml
Urea nitrogen	8-25 mg/100 ml
Uric acid	3-7 mg/100 ml
Vitamin A	0.15-0.6 μg/ml
Vitamin B_{12}	160-600 pg/ml
Vitamin C	0.6-1.6 mg/100 ml

REFERENCES

1. Halstead JA: The Laboratory in Clinical Medicine. Philadelphia, WB Saunders, 1876.

2. Conn RB: Laboratory reference values of clinical importance, in: Conn HF, Conn RB: Current Diagnosis, WB Saunders, ed 6, Philadelphia, 1980.

3. Davidson I, Henry JB: Todd-Sanford Clinical Diagnosis by Laboratory Methods, ed 16, Philadelphia, WB Saunders, 1979.

4. Vaughan VC, McKay PJ, Behrman RE (eds): Nelson's Textbook of Pediatrics, ed 11. Philadelphia, WB Saunders, 1979, Tables 30-2, 30-3, 30-4, 30-5, 30-6, 30-7, 30-8, 30-9, pp 2076-2094.

5. Chapter 8, Normal values in infants and children, in: Garb S: *Laboratory Tests in Common Use,* ed 6. New York, Springer Publishing Co, 1976.

6. Scully RE et al: Normal reference laboratory values (Massachusetts General Hospital). *NEJM* Jan 2, 1986; 314:39.

Office Laboratory Procedures

CULTURES

Cultures are performed to determine the nature of microbial infection. Secretions of material from the mucous membranes of certain body parts may be transferred to a medium that encourages growth of microorganisms.

Throat Culture for *Streptococcus Pyogenes*

Equipment Needed:

Tongue blade, sterile cotton swab, blood agar plate or transport medium, adequate light source

Procedure

A. Have client open his mouth wide. Direct maximum lighting toward back of throat
B. Grasp tongue blade so that the thumb pushes the end upward while the fingers push the middle section downward. Depress the client's tongue in this manner with the tongue blade so that the posterior pharynx and tonsillar areas are clearly visualized
C. Vigorously rub the cotton swab over each tonsillar area and posterior pharynx
D. Immediately streak the swab on a blood agar plate, or follow directions of the laboratory for transport medium

Endocervical Culture for Gonococcus

Equipment Needed:

Vaginal speculum, sterile cotton swab, cotton balls, ring forcep, selective culture medium (e.g., modified Thayer-Martin)

613

Procedure:

A. Moisten speculum with warm water. *Do not* use any other lubricant
B. Remove excessive cervical mucus, preferably with a cotton ball held in ring forceps
C. Insert sterile cotton swab into endocervical canal. Move swab from side to side. Allow 10-30 seconds for absorption of organisms onto swab
D. Roll swab in a large 2-pattern on selective medium. Cross-streak immediately with a sterile wire loop or the tip of a swab in the clinical facility
E. Place the culture plate in CO_2-enriched atmosphere (e.g., candle jar) within 15 minutes of inoculation. Be sure to light the candle each time the jar is opened. Do not place the candle on top of the inoculated plates. Place candle at the bottom of the jar, otherwise the lid may extinguish the candle before an adequate CO_2 atmosphere has been created. Deliver the jar to the laboratory as soon as possible
F. Incubate plates within 1-2 hours at 35-36°C
G. If CO_2 generating tablets are used, follow the directions of the laboratory for proper use

Anal Canal Culture

Equipment Needed:

Sterile cotton swab, culture medium

Procedure

A. Insert sterile cotton swab approximately 1 in. into the anal canal
B. Move swab from side to side in the anal canal to sample crypts; allow 10-30 seconds for absorption of organisms onto the swab. Then move the swab along the wall of the rectum while rotating the swab
C. Place on culture medium same as above (see Endocervical Culture)

Vaginal Culture

Equipment Needed:

Same as for endocervical culture

Procedure:

Same as for endocervical culture except specimen obtained from the posterior vault

Urethra (Female)

Equipment Needed:

Sterile loop or cotton swab, culture medium

Procedure:

A. Strip the urethra toward the orifice to express exudate
B. Use a sterile loop or cotton swab to obtain the specimen
C. Apply to culture medium (see procedure for endocervical culture)

Urethra (Male)

Equipment Needed:

Sterile calcium alginate urethral swab or a sterile bacteriologic loop, culture medium
A standard cotton swab is not recommended for this procedure since it is too large to insert as far as required for a good specimen and results in excessive pain

Procedure

A. Insert the swab or loop no more than 2 cm into the urethra
B. Gently scrape the anterior urethral mucosa
C. Apply to culture medium (see procedure for endocervical culture)

Wound Culture

Equipment Needed:

Sterile gloves, sterile syringe and needle, culture tube or medium, sterile cotton swab

Procedure

A. Don sterile gloves
B. If fluid present in wound, aspirate a generous amount of liquid material into syringe; inject into anaerobic tube
C. If thick, purulent material present, swab with sterile cotton swab; apply on selective culture medium (follow laboratory recommendations)

Culture of Nipple

Equipment Needed:

Same as for wound culture procedure

Procedure:

A. Gently squeeze nipple to express fluid; swab with sterile cotton swab
B. Apply to selective culture medium (follow laboratory recommendations)

Reference:

Criteria and Techniques for the Diagnosis of Gonorrhea. Atlanta, U.S. Dept. of Health, Education and Welfare, Public Health Service, Center for Disease Control, Venereal Disease Control Center.

HEMATOCRIT BY CENTRIFUGATION

Hematocrit is the volume of packed red blood expressed as percent volume of blood. The measurement is used as a screening test for anemia due to blood loss, increased destruction of, or reduced capacity to produce red blood cells.

Equipment Needed:

Alcohol swabs, clean gauze pads, microlancets, capillary tubes (heparinized), crito-seal clay trays, microhematocrit centrifuge

Procedure:

The fingertip is most often used. The ear lobe may be used. The heel is used on an infant

1. Wipe off tip of middle finger with alcohol; wipe clean with gauze; put gauze under the finger
2. Holding the finger firmly, use the microlancet with a quick in-out motion and stick the tip of the finger; wipe away first drop of blood
3. Milking the finger gently along the sides, fill the heparinized capillary tube with blood. Do not squeeze the finger too hard. Hold the tube horizontal, or slightly higher. Seal the dry end with clay
4. Have the client apply pressure at the tip of the finger with gauze
5. Place the tube in the centrifuge, sealed end out. Balance the centrifuge with an empty tube, if necessary
6. Spin down for 5 minutes; read and record results
7. The duration and speed of centrifugation must be controlled to assure consistent results

Normal Lab Values:

Age	Male	Female
1 year	35 ±3	35 ±3
4 years	37 ±3	37 ±3
8-12 years	41 ±3	41 ±3
Adult	40-54%	38-47%

While the centrifuge method is more readily applicable for office practice, the more common laboratory method is based on electronic counting and sizing. On the Coulter S,

red cells are counted and the mean cell volume determined
electronically; the hematocrit is derived based on red cell
size and number. White cells are counted and blood hemoglobin concentration is measured simultaneously.

WET MOUNT

The wet mount is a simple method to aid in the diagnosis of vaginitis caused by *Trichomonas, Candida albicans,* and
corynebacteria.

Equipment Needed:

Normal saline (NS) or 10% potassium hydroxide (KOH)

Glass slide and cover slip

Small test tube and cotton swab (only when making a
suspension)

Pap smear paddle, handle of standard applicator, or wire
loop

Microscope

Procedure:

Wet mount can be prepared directly on a slide or by
first making a suspension of the specimen

A. For trichomonas:
   1. Prepared directly on slide
      a. Obtain specimen from the pool of discharge in the
         posterior vaginal fornix during speculum examina-
         tion with Pap smear paddle, handle of standard ap-
         plicator, or wire loop. Do *not* use cotton swab
         since the cotton may absorb the saline from the
         slide
      b. Place a drop of warm NS on glass slide
      c. Add a drop of specimen onto slide and mix NS
         and specimen together well with wooden stick
      d. Place cover slip over specimen on slide
      e. Observe slide under microscope; first under 10x
         power then under 40x power

2. Suspension of specimen
   a. Place 0.5-1.0 ml of warm NS into a small test tube
   b. Obtain specimen as stated above. Cotton swab *may* be used in this case
   c. Introduce specimen into NS with a swirling motion to suspend specimen. When using cotton swab, carefully express excess fluid by firmly rotating swab against the wall of the test tube above the NS level
   d. Place a drop of suspension on a slide and apply coverslip
   e. Observe slide for trichomonads
3. Results indicative of infection
   a. Trichomonads have a pear-shaped body with four anterior and one posterior flagella, a undulating membrane, a nucleus, and independent movement
   b. A preparation is positive if any trichomonad is seen
4. Cautions
   a. Motility of trichomonads is increased in warm temperatures. Keep specimen warm by storing in an incubator or briefly holding over a lightbulb
   b. When trichomonads dry up they are difficult to distinguish from polymorphonuclear leukocytes. Therefore, *examine the wet mount as soon as possible after preparation*

B. For candidal vaginitis
   1. Place one drop of vaginal specimen on a slide
   2. Add one drop of 10% KOH solution and mix specimen with wooden stick
   3. Apply coverslip and briefly heat preparation over a flame or lightbulb
   4. Scan via microscope under low power, then high power
   5. Results indicative of infection
      a. *Candida* appear as oval cells that may produce germ tubes (pseudohyphae) or small oval projections (budding)
      b. Presence of large numbers of cells, budding and pseudohyphae are indicative of a candidal infection

C. For corynebacterial vaginitis
1. Obtain vaginal specimen from the *vagina, not* from the endocervix
2. Prepare wet mount as stated for *Trichomonas* (see A)
3. Examine under the microscope
4. Microscopic clues to corynebacterial vaginitis include:
   a. A predominant flora of small, pleomorphic, gram-negative rods often seen in sheets
   b. The presence of "clue cells," or vaginal epithelial cells studded with coccobacilli
   c. Observation of few polymorphonuclear leukocytes in relation to the number of epithelial cells present

Note: Diagnosis of candidal vaginitis, and corynebacterial vaginitis also can be made via Gram stain and culture

Reference

Rein MF: *Vaginal Discharge* (Fact Sheet, Health and Human Services, Public Health Services, Center for Disease Control, Venereal Disease Control Division). Washington, DC, U.S. Government Printing Office, 1980, reproduced, with permission of U.S. Department of Health, Education, and Welfare Public Health Service, Communicable Disease Center, Atlanta.

STOOL FOR OCCULT BLOOD: GUAIAC METHOD

Examination of stool for occult blood, or blood not readily observed by direct visualization, can be done in several ways. This procedure will discuss only the guaiac method.

Equipment Needed:

Developing solution, filter paper, glove or wooden applicator

Procedure

A. Collect small stool specimen on one end of wooden applicator directly from stool or on gloved finger during rectal exam

B. Apply thin film of specimen to filter paper
C. Collect a second specimen from a different part of stool or different area of rectum and apply to a second piece of filter paper
D. Apply two drops of developing solution to specimen on filter paper, and read results between 30-60 seconds later

Results:

A. Test is positive for occult blood if any trace of blue appears on filter paper
B. For accurate screening, a series of at least three specimens should be collected and tested

Cautions

A. Certain foods, medications, and vitamin C alter results of guaiac tests
   1. Red meats, medications causing GI irritations (e.g., aspirin, indomethacin, corticosteroids, phenylbutazone, reserpine, etc.), certain perosidase containing vegetables and fruits (e.g., fresh tomatoes and cherries, and fresh or cooked turnips)
   2. Ascorbic acid (vitamin C) can produce false-negative results if as little as 1-2 g is ingested per day
B. If one of the three specimens tested is positive, instruct the patient to alter dietary intake for 3-5 days before beginning a second series of specimen collections
C. Patients collecting specimens at home should be instructed to return specimens for testing within 2 days of stool collection to minimize changes in test reliability

References:

Fleming RA: *Primary Care Techniques.* St Louis, CV Mosby Co, 1980.

Hill SC: Fecal occult blood: Efficacy of testing measures. *Nurse Pract,* Sept/Oct 1980, p 15-21.

KOH EXAMINATION OF SKIN SCRAPING

To aid in diagnosing fungal infections of the skin the following procedure is done.

Equipment Needed:

Glass slide and coverslip, no. 11 or no. 15 knife blade, 10% potassium hydroxide (KOH), heat source

Procedure:

A. Scrape a small amount of stratum corneum with a no. 11 or no. 15 knife blade from the active border of a suspected lesion
B. Transfer specimen to glass slide and apply coverslip
C. One or two drops of KOH solution is added to edge of coverslip and allowed to flow under it and mix with specimen
D. Gently heat slide over light bulb or flame until specimen clears or becomes translucent. (Heat dissolves the keratin material)
E. Observe slide under low power (10x) and high power (40x) for the hyphae of fungus growth

References:

Sonnenivirth AC, Jarett L (eds): *Gradwohl's Clinical Laboratory Methods and Diagnosis,* ed 8. St. Louis, CV Mosby Co, 1980.

Bibliography

CHAPTER 1: THE NURSING PROCESS

Campbell C: *Nursing Diagnosis and Intervention in Nursing Practice.* New York, John Wiley, 1984.

Carpenito L: *Nursing Diagnosis: Application to Clinical Practice.* Philadelphia, J.B. Lippincott, 1983.

Doenges et al: *Nursing Care Plans.* Philadelphia, FA Davis Co, 1984.

Gordon M: *Nursing Diagnosis: Process and Application,* ed 2. New York, McGraw-Hill, 1987.

Griffith JW, Christensen P: *Nursing Process.* St. Louis, CV Mosby, 1982.

Iyer PW et al: *Nursing Process and Nursing Diagnosis.* Philadelphia, WB Saunders, 1986.

Lederer JR et al: *Care Planning: A Nursing Diagnosis Approach.* Menlo Park, CA, Addison-Wesley, 1986.

Yura H, Walsh MB: *The Nursing Process,* ed 4. Norwalk, Conn, Appleton-Century-Crofts, 1983.

CHAPTER 2: PROBLEM ORIENTATION

Vaughan-Wrobel BC, Henderson B: *The Problem Oriented System in Nursing,* ed 2. St. Louis, CV Mosby Co, 1981.

Weed LL: *Medical Records, Medical Education and Patient Care: The Problem Oriented Record as a Basic Tool.* Cleveland, Case Western University Press, 1970.

CHAPTER 3: THE PROCESS OF INTERVIEWING

Coulehan JL, Block MR: *The Medical Interview: A Primer for Students of the Art.* Philadelphia, FA Davis Co, 1986.

Enelow AJ, Swisher SN: *Interviewing and Patient Care,* ed 3. New York, Oxford University Press, 1986.

623

Reiser DE, Schroeder AK: *Patient Interviewing: The Human Dimension.* Baltimore, Williams & Wilkins, 1980.

CHAPTERS 4 AND 5: THE HEALTH HISTORY

Barnard M et al: *Human Sexuality for Health Professionals.* Philadelphia, WB Saunders Co, 1978.

Blacklow RS: *MacBryde's Signs and Symptoms,* ed 6. Philadelphia, JB Lippincott Co, 1983.

Jacobs MM, Geels W: *Signs and Symptoms in Nursing.* Philadelphia, JB Lippincott Co, 1985.

CHAPTERS 6 AND 7: THE PHYSICAL EXAMINAITON AND GENERAL SURVEY

Bates B: *A Guide to Physical Examination,* ed 4. Philadelphia, JB Lippincott Co, 1987.

Clain A: *Hamilton Bailey's Demonstrations of Physical Signs in Clinical Surgery,* ed 17. London, Wright, 1986.

Delp MH, Manning RT: *Major's Physical Diagnosis,* ed 9. Philadelphia, WB Saunders Co, 1981.

CHAPTER 8: THE INTEGUMENT, MASSES, AND LYMPHATICS

Fitzpatrick T et al.: *Color Atlas and Synopsis of Clinical Dermatology.* New York, McGraw-Hill, 1983.

Lamberg S: *Dermatology in Primary Care.* Philadelphia, WB Saunders Co, 1986.

Lookingbill D, Marks JG: *Principles of Dermatology.* Philadelphia, WB Saunders Co, 1986.

Rosen T, Lanning M, Hill M: *Nurse's Atlas of Dermatology.* Boston, Little, Brown & Co, 1983.

Sauer GC: *Manual of Skin Diseases,* ed 5. Philadelphia, JB Lippincott Co, 1986.

CHAPTERS 9, 10 AND 11:
THE HEAD, FACE, AND NECK; THE EYES;
AND THE EAR, NOSE, MOUTH, AND PHARYX

Ballender JJ: *Diseases of the Nose, Throat, Ear, Head and Neck,* ed 13. Philadelphia, Lea & Febiger, 1985.

Brown MS, Alexander MM: Physical examination, Part 7: Examining the ear. *Nursing '74* (Feb) 1974, 4:48.

Brown MS, Alexander MM: Physical examination, Part 9: Examining the nose. *Nursing '74* (July) 1974, 4:35.

Deweese DD, Saunders W: *Textbook of Otolaryngology,* ed 6. St. Louis, CV Mosby, 1982.

Nover A: *The Ocular Fundus: Methods of Examination and Typical Findings,* ed 4. Philadelphia, Lea & Febiger, 1981.

Wilensky JT, Read JM (eds): *Primary Ophthalmology.* Orlando, Florida, Grune & Straton, 1984.

CHAPTER 12: THE THORAX AND LUNGS

Holt T: *Assessment-Based Respiratory Care.* New York, John Wiley, 1986.

Wilkins R et al: *Clinical Assessment in Respiratory Care.* St. Louis, CV Mosby, 1985.

CHAPTER 13: THE BREAST

American Cancer Society: *How to Examine Your Breasts.* New York, American Cancer Society, 1984.

American Cancer Society: *Cancer Facts and Figures 1987.* New York, American Cancer Society, 1987.

Annovier C: *Female Breast Examination: A Theoretical Guide to Breast Diagnosis.* New York, Springer-Verlag, 1986.

Huguley CM Jr, Brown RL: The value of breast self-examination. *Cancer* 1981, 47:989.

Winchester DP, Sener S, Immerman S, et al: A systematic approach to the evaluation and management of breast masses. *Cancer* 1983;51:2535.

CHAPTER 14: THE HEART

Braunwald E: *Heart Disease,* ed 2. Philadelphia, WB Saunders Co, 1984.

Hurst JW et al: *The Heart, Arteries, and Veins,* ed 6. McGraw-Hill, New York, 1986.

Perloff J: *Physical Examination of the Heart and Circulation.* Philadelphia, WB Saunders Co, 1982.

CHAPTER 15: THE ABDOMEN

GI Series: *Physical Examination of the Abdomen.* Richmond, Va, AH Robins Co.

Berk JE (ed): *Bockus Gastroenterology,* ed 4. Vol I. Philadelphia, WB Saunders Co, 1985.

Silen W: *Cope's Early Diagnosis of the Acute Abdomen,* ed 17. New York, Oxford University Press, 1987.

Spiro HM: *Clinical Gastroenterology,* ed 3. New York, Macmillan Publishing Co, 1983.

Strange J: *Gastrointestinal Problems,* Nursing Assessment Series 4. Oradell, NJ, Medical Economics, 1985.

CHAPTER 16: THE EXTREMITIES AND BACK

American Academy of Orthopedic Surgeons: *Joint Motion: Method of Measuring and Recording.* Chicago, Churchill, 1972.

Esch D, Lepley M: *Evaluation of Joint Motion: Methods of Measurement and Recording.* Minneapolis, University of Minnesota Press, 1974.

Hoppenfeld S: *Physical Examination of the Spine and Extremities.* New York, Appleton-Century-Crofts, 1976.

Polley HF, Hunder GG: *Rheumatologic Interviewing and Physical Examination of the Joints,* ed 2. Philadelphia, WB Saunders Co, 1978.

CHAPTER 17: THE MALE GENITALIA AND RECTAL SYSTEMS

Harrison JH et al (eds): *Campbell's Urology,* Vol I, ed 4. Philadelphia, WB Saunders Co, 1978.

Smith DR: *General Urology,* ed 11. Los Altos, Calif, Lange Medical Publications, 1984.

CHAPTER 18: THE FEMALE GENITAL ORGANS

Danforth DN (ed): *Obstetrics and Gynecology,* ed 4. Hagerstown, Penn, Harper and Row, 1982.

Hacker N, Moore JG: *Essentials of Obstetrics and Gynecology.* Philadelphia, WB Saunders Co, 1986.

Jones HW Jr, Jones GS: *Novak's Textbook of Gynecology,* ed 10. Baltimore, Williams & Wilkins Co, 1981.

Magee J: The pelvic examination: A view from the other end of the table. *Annals of Internal Medicine,* 1975, 83: 563.

Romney SL, Gray MJ, Little AB, et al: *Gynecology and Obstetrics: The Health Care of Women,* ed 2. McGraw-Hill Book Co., New York, 1980.

CHAPTER 19: THE NEUROLOGIC AND MENTAL EXAMINATION

DeJong RN: *The Neurologic Examination,* ed 4. Hagerstown, Penn, Harper and Row, 1979.

Harrison: *Neurologic Skills.* Stoneham, Mass, Butterworth.

Mancall EL: *Essentials of the Neurological Examination,* ed 2. Philadelphia, FA Davis Co, 1981.

Rowland LP: *Merritt's Textbook of Neurology,* ed 7. Philadelphia, Lea & Febiger, 1984.

Strub RL, Black FW: *The Mental Status Examination in Neurology,* ed 2. Philadelphia, FA Davis Co, 1985.

Van Allen MW: *Pictorial Manual of Neurological Tests,* ed 2. Chicago, Year Book Medical Publishers, 1981.

CHAPTER 21: NUTRITIONAL ASSESSMENT

Bray GA (ed): *Obesity in America.* Washington, DC, Dept. of Health, Education, and Welfare, Pub No 79-359 (NIH), 1979.

Christakis G (ed): Nutritional assessment in health programs. *Am J Public Health,* 1973;63(Nov Suppl).

Goodhart RS, Shils M: *Modern Nutrition in Health and Disease,* ed 6. Philadelphia, Lea & Febiger, 1980.

Krause M, Mahan LK: *Food, Nutrition and Diet Therapy,* ed 7. Philadelphia, WB Saunders Co, 1984 (Unit 2, Nutritional Status of the Individual).

CHAPTER 22:
THE LABORATORY EXAMINATION

American Cancer Society: *Cancer Facts and Figures 1987.* New York, American Cancer Society, 1987.

Koepke JA: *Guide to Clinical Laboratory Diagnosis,* ed 2. New York, Appleton-Century-Crofts, 1979.

Ravel R: *Clinical Laboratory Medicine,* ed 4. Chicago, Year Book Medical Publishers, 1984.

Tilkian S, et al: *Clinical Implications of Laboratory Tests,* ed 3. St. Louis, CV Mosby Co, 1983.

Widmann FK: *Clinical Interpretation of Laboratory Tests,* ed 9. Philadelphia, FA Davis Co, 1983.

CHAPTER 23: PRENATAL ASSESSMENT

Benson RC: *Current Obstetric and Gynecologic Diagnosis and Treatment,* ed 5. Los Altos, Calif, Lange Medical Publications, 1984.

Hacker NF, and Moore JG: *Essentials of Obstetrics and Gynecology.* Philadelphia, WB Saunders Co, 1986.

Pritchard JA, MacDonald PC, Gant N: *Williams' Obstetrics,* ed 17. New York, Appleton-Century-Crofts, 1985.

Romney SL, Gray MJ, Little AB, et al: *Gynecology and Obstetrics: The Health Care of Women,* ed 2. New York, McGraw-Hill Book Co, 1980.

CHAPTERS 24 AND 25:
ASSESSMENT OF THE NEWBORN AND
ASSESSMENT OF THE INFANT AND CHILD

Alexander MM, Brown MD: *Pediatric History Taking and Physical Diagnosis for Nurses,* ed 2. New York, McGraw-Hill Book Co, 1979.

Avery ME, Taeusch HW Jr: *Schaffer's Diseases of the Newborn,* ed 5. Philadelphia, WB Saunders Co, 1984.

Barness LA: *Manual of Pediatric Physical Diagnosis,* ed 4. Chicago, Year Book Medical Publishers, 1972.

Behrman RE, Vaughan VC (eds): *Nelson Textbook of Pediatrics,* ed 12. Philadelphia, WB Saunders Co, 1983.

Brodish MS: Perinatal assessment. *J Obstet Gynecol Neonatal Nurs* Jan/Feb 1981, 10:42-46.

Chinn PL, Leitch C: *Child Health Maintenance: A Guide to Clinical Assessment,* ed 2. St. Louis, CV Mosby Co, 1979.

Dubowitz L, Dubowitz V: *Neurological Assessment of the Pre-Term and Full-Term Infant.* Clinics in Developmental Medicine Series, Vol 79. Philadelphia, JB Lippincott Co, 1981.

Frankenburg WK, Camp B (eds): *Pediatric Screening Tests Manual.* Springfield, Ill, CC Thomas, 1975.

Green, Morris, Green, Richmond: *Pediatric Diagnosis* (Chapter 1). Philadelphia, WB Saunders Co, 1986.

Kempe CH et al (eds): *Current Pediatric Diagnosis and Treatment*, ed 8. Los Altos, Calif, Lange Medical Publications, 1984.

O'Doherty N: *Atlas of the Newborn,* ed 2. Boston, Kluwer Academic Publishers, 1985.

Powell ML: *Assessment and Management of Developmental Changes in Children,* ed 2. St. Louis, CV Mosby Co, 1981.

CHAPTER 26:
ASSESSMENT OF THE ADOLESCENT

Hoffman A: *Adolescent Medicine.* Menlo Park, Calif, Addison-Wesley Publishing Co, 1983.

Julian DG, Wenger NK (eds): *Cardiac Problems of the Adolescent & Young Adult.* Stoneham, Mass, Butterworth, 1985.

Kagan J et al (eds): *Twelve to Sixteen: Early Adolescence.* New York, WW Norton & Co, 1972.

Kalafatich A: *Approaches to the Care of Adolescents.* New York, Appleton-Century-Crofts, 1975.

Miller WE: Lower class culture as a generating milieu of gang delinquency, in Wender AE, Angus DL (eds): *Adolescence Contemporary Studies.* New York, Van Nostrand, Reinhold Co, 1968, pp 189-204.

Tanner JM: *Growth at Adolescence,* ed 2. Oxford, England, Blackwell Scientific Publications, 1973.

CHAPTER 27:
ASSESSMENT OF THE AGED

Burnside IM: *Nursing and the Aged,* ed 2. New York, McGraw-Hill Book Co, 1980.

Burnside IM: *Psychosocial Nursing Care of the Aged,* ed 2. New York, McGraw-Hill Book Co, 1980.

Busse E, Pfeiffer E: *Behavior & Adaptation in Late Life,* ed 2. Boston, Little, Brown and Co, 1977.

Eliopoulos C: *Health Assessment of the Older Adult.* Menlo Park, Calif, Addison-Wesley Publishing Co, 1984.

Steinberg FU (ed): *Cowdry's Care of the Geriatric Patient,* ed 5. St. Louis, CV Mosby Co, 1976.

Yurick AG et al: *The Aged Person and the Nursing Process,* ed 2. Norwalk, Conn, Appleton-Century-Crofts, 1984.

CHAPTER 28:
PSYCHIATRIC MENTAL HEALTH ASSESSMENT

Hamilton M: Assessment of anxiety. *British Journal of Medical Psychology* 1959;32:54-55.

Kaplan H, Sadock B: in Chapter 12, Diagnosis and Psychiatric Examination of the Psychiatric Patient, in *Comprehensive Textbook of Psychiatry,* ed 4. Baltimore, Williams & Wilkins Co, 1985.

Kolb LC, Brodie HK: *Modern Clinical Psychiatry,* ed 10. (Chapter 8). Philadelphia, WB Saunders Co, 1982.

McFarland G, Wasli E: *Nursing Diagnosis and Process in Psychiatric Mental Health Nursing.* Philadelphia, JB Lippincott Co, 1986.

CHAPTER 29:
EXAMINATION OF THE COMATOSE PATIENT

Plum F, Posner JA: *Diagnosis of Stupor and Coma,* ed 3, rev'd. Philadelphia, FA Davis Co, 1982.

Index